Lecture Notes in Computer Science 11924

More information about this series at http://www.springer.com/series/7409

Hsinchun Chen · Daniel Zeng ·
Xiangbin Yan · Chunxiao Xing (Eds.)

Smart Health

International Conference, ICSH 2019
Shenzhen, China, July 1–2, 2019
Proceedings

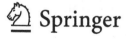 Springer

Editors
Hsinchun Chen
The University of Arizona
Tucson, AZ, USA

Xiangbin Yan
University of Science
and Technology Beijing
Beijing, China

Daniel Zeng
College of Management
The University of Arizona
Tucson, AZ, USA

Chunxiao Xing
Tsinghua University
Beijing, China

ISSN 0302-9743   ISSN 1611-3349   (electronic)
Lecture Notes in Computer Science
ISBN 978-3-030-34481-8   ISBN 978-3-030-34482-5   (eBook)
https://doi.org/10.1007/978-3-030-34482-5

LNCS Sublibrary: SL3 – Information Systems and Applications, incl. Internet/Web, and HCI

This Springer imprint is published by the registered company Springer Nature Switzerland AG
The registered company address is: Gewerbestrasse 11, 6330 Cham, Switzerland

Preface

ICSH 2019, held July 1–2, 2019, in Shenzhen, China, is the 7th International Conference for Smart Health. In this edition, we created a bridge to promote lively exchange and collaborations between the growing international smart health research scholars and communities, and to advance our understanding about the technical, practical, economic, behavioral, and social issues centered on smart health. ICSH 2019 was a unique forum for researchers with cross-disciplinary interests to meet and interact.

This volume contains the 34 papers, out of a total of 43 submissions, accepted to be presented in ICSH 2019. Each submission, received at least three reviews. We thank all authors who submitted their work for consideration to ICSH 2019 and we specially thank the Program Committee, whose many thorough reviews helped us select the papers presented. The success of the scientific program is due to their hard work.

Apart from the 34 accepted papers, the scientific program included four invited keynote speeches, given by:

- Hsinchun Chen on "AI for Health Analysts: SilverLink for Proactive Mobile Health"
- Kwok Leung Tsui on "Big Data Opportunities: Systems Monitoring and Personalized Health Management"
- Guodong (Gordon) Gao on "Research Ideas in the 5G Era"
- Gang Chen on "Analysis of 300,000 genomes from DTC Testing and Cohort Studies for Population Genomics"

We thank the invited speakers for accepting our invitation and for their excellent presentations at the conference.

July 2019

Hsinchun Chen
Daniel Zeng
Xiangbin Yan
Chunxiao Xing

Organization

Conference Co-chairs

Hsinchun Chen	University of Arizona, USA
Daniel Zeng	University of Arizona, USA, and Chinese Academy of Sciences, China
Xiangbin Yan	University of Science and Technology Beijing, China
Chunxiao Xing	Tsinghua University, China

Honorary Co-chairs

Yijun Li	Harbin Institute of Technology, China
Weicai Wang	University of Science and Technology Beijing, China
Yong Tan	University of Washington, USA
Ting-Peng Liang	National Sun Yat-Sen University, Taiwan, China

Program Co-chairs

Ahmed Abbasi	University of Virginia, China
Mingxin Gan	University of Science and Technology Beijing, China
Jiang Wu	Wuhan University, China
Eric Zheng	University of Texas at Dallas, USA

Publication Co-chairs

Xin Li	City University of Hong Kong, Hong Kong, China
Jiahua Jin	University of Science and Technology Beijing, China

Publicity Co-chairs

Xiaoxia Huang	University of Science and Technology Beijing, China
Xitong Guo	Harbin Institute of Technology, China
Harry Wang	University of Delaware, USA

Local Arrangement Co-chairs

Wei Gu	University of Science and Technology Beijing, China
Xiaolong Zheng	Chinese Academy of Sciences, China
Bo Fan	Shanghai Jiaotong University, China

Program Committee

Muhammad Amith	Texas Medical Center, USA
Lu An	Wuhan University, China
Mohd Anwar	North Carolina A&T State University, USA
Ian Brooks	University of Illinois at Urbana-Champaign, USA
Lemen Chao	Renmin University of China, China
Michael Chau	University of Hong Kong, Hong Kong, China
Ting Chen	Tsinghua University, China
Qin Chen	University of Science and Technology Beijing, China
Chien-Chin Chen	National Taiwan University, Taiwan, China
Chih-Lin Chi	University of Minnesota, USA
Hongfei Cui	University of Science and Technology Beijing, China
Shufen Dai	University of Science and Technology Beijing, China
Yimeng Deng	National University of Singapore, Singapore
Prasanna Desikan	Blueshield of California, USA
Shaokun Fan	Oregon State University, USA
Haiqi Feng	Central University of Finance and Economics, China
Qianjing Feng	Southern Medical University, China
Mingxin Gan	University of Science and Technology Beijing, China
Chunmei Gan	Sun Yat-sen University, China
Gordon Gao	University of Maryland, USA
Huiying Gao	Beijing Institute of Technology, China
Kaiye Gao	Beijing Information Science and Technology University, China
Hung-Yu Kao	National Cheng Kung University, Taiwan, China
Yan Li	City University of Hong Kong, Hong Kong, China
Tianxing Li	Fu Jen Catholic University, Taiwan, China
Chunxiao Li	Arizona State University, USA
Jiexun Li	Western Washington University, USA
Mingyang Li	University of South Florida, USA
Jiao Li	Chinese Academy of Medical Sciences, China
Ye Liang	Beijing Foreign Studies University, China
Furen Lin	National Tsing Hua University, Taiwan, China
Yu-Kai Lin	Florida State University, USA
Hongyan Liu	Tsinghua University, China
Xuejuan Liu	University of Science and Technology Beijing, China
Yidi Liu	City University of Hong Kong, Hong Kong, China
Shuzhu Liu	National Pingtung University of Science and Technology, Taiwan, China
Xiao Liu	University of Utah, USA
Luning Liu	Harbin Institute of Technology, China
Long Lu	Wuhan University, China
Quan Lu	Wuhan University, China
Yingxue Ma	University of Science and Technology Beijing, China
James Ma	University of Colorado, USA

Abhay Mishra	Georgia State University, USA
Robert Moskovitch	Ben Gurion University, Israel
Cath Oh	Georgia State University, USA
V. Panduranga Rao	Indian Institute of Technology Hyderabad, India
Raj Sharman	State University of New York, University at Buffalo, USA
Xiaolong Song	Dongbei University of Finance and Economics, China
Weiquan Wang	City University of Hong Kong, Hong Kong, China
Alan Wang	Virginia Polytechnic Institute and State University, USA
Yu Wang	Virginia Polytechnic Institute and State University, USA
Xi Wang	Central University of Finance and Economics, China
Qiang Wei	Tsinghua University, China
Zoie Wong	St. Luke's International University, Japan
Jiang Wu	Wuhan University, China
Mengmeng Wu	Alibaba Group, China
Yi Wu	Tianjin University, China
Dong Xu	University of Arizona, USA
Jennifer Xu	Bentley College, USA
Kaiquan Xu	Nanjing University, China
Xiangbin Yan	University of Science and Technology Beijing, China
Lucy Yan	Indiana University at Bloomington, USA
Zhijun Yan	Beijing Institute of Technology, China
Jonathan Ye	University of Auckland, New Zealand
Shuo Yu	University of Arizona, USA
Anna Zaitsev	University of Sydney, Australia
Bin Zhang	University of Arizona, USA
Tingting Zhang	University of Science and Technology Beijing, China
Qingpeng Zhang	City University of Hong Kong, Hong Kong, China
Kang Zhao	University of Iowa, USA
Lina Zhou	University of Maryland, Baltimore, USA
Hongyi Zhu	University of Arizona, USA
Bin Zhu	Oregon State University, USA
Hou Zhu	Sun Yat-sen University, China
Zhiya Zuo	University of Iowa, USA

Contents

Social, Psychosocial and Behavioral Determinants of Health

Data science/Analytics/Clinical and Business Intelligence

Clinical Informatics and Clinician Engagement

Precision Medicine and Telehealth

Estimation of Potential Richness of Dark Matters in "Pan Metagenome" Using Species Appearance Model

Hongfei Cui[✉]

DonLinks School of Economics and Management,
University of Science and Technology Beijing, Beijing, China
Cuihf06@hotmail.com

Abstract. The study of complexity of metagenome populations is crucial in understanding different microbial communities. The potential number of microbes in the environment is much higher than our knowledge. However, most metagenomic projects only contain tens to hundreds of samples. Most of the microbes can hardly be sampled under such small sample size. Thus, there are many "dark matters" that never been observed. Here in this study, we proposed a statistical model, named SAM (Species Appearance Model), which uses only one to two hundred samples to optimize the parameters, and estimate the potential richness of dark matters when the data size is much higher. An index named ESS (Estimated saturated sample size) were also proposed as an indicator of the complexity of the metagenome population. In the dataset of the American Gut Project (AGP), SAM can precisely predict the OTU richness of pan metagenome with more than 1000 samples using only 200 samples. The ESS of AGP is $\sim 25{,}000$, which means the AGP population is very complex. Using our SAM model, researchers can estimate and decide how many samples they need to collect when initiating a new metagenomic project. Different ESS values of different metagenomic populations can also serve as a guidance of understanding their different complexities.

Keywords: Metagenome · Dark matter · Prevalence distribution · Microbiota complexity

1 Introduction

Microbes are important for human health. Up to 90% cells inside or on the surface of our human body are microbes, including bacteria, archaea, viruses or other forms of microbes [1]. They appear in any body site and can deeply influence our live. Some of them are pathogens that may cause serious diseases [2, 3]. However, most of them are harmless, or even beneficial to our health, by producing nutriment that we cannot synthesize by ourselves or competing against foreign pathogens [4, 5]. For these reasons, there are researchers agree that a human is actually a "superorganism" that consist of his/her symbiotic microorganisms and himself/herself [6].

Human microbes often exist in the form of "community", which is called "microbiota". They exchange substances, benefit from or compete with each other [7, 8],

© Springer Nature Switzerland AG 2019
H. Chen et al. (Eds.): ICSH 2019, LNCS 11924, pp. 3–15, 2019.
https://doi.org/10.1007/978-3-030-34482-5_1

and interact with human beings [9–12]. As the development of the next generation sequencing technique, "metagenome" sequencing, which sequences marker genes or full genomes of all microbial genomes from a specific environment (from a human niche or from nature), becomes a mainstream manner in microbiota study. Using metagenome sequencing, researchers have found that the composition of human microbiota have close associations with our habits such as diet [13] and smoking [14], and with some diseases such as obesity [15–17], diabetes [18], cirrhosis [19], inflammatory bowel disease (IBD) [20] and so on.

Richness is a basic statistic to shape the composition of a microbiota, which means how many species (or other taxonomic units, e.g., OTUs) are existing in the microbiota. Different kinds of human niches often have different microbial richness, which reflect their different biological characters. Moreover, for each specific body niche, the microbe composition of an individual can be regarded as a result of random sampling from his/her living environment and selecting by human niche environment. Thus, studying the microbial richness of all metagenome samples from a specific body site (we call this "pan metagenome") can help us understand the specific characteristics of the niche, and the homogeneity/heterogeneity of different individuals about the niche.

There are many metagenomic projects that collecting and sampling hundreds or thousands of samples. For example, HMP (Human Microbiome Project [21]), MetaHIT (Metagenomics of the Human Intestinal Tract [22]), Lifeline-Deep [23], GEM (The Genetic, Environmental and Microbial Project [24]) and FGFP (Belgian Flemish Gut Flora Project [25]). Now the metagenomic study even enters an age of "ten thousand samples". Till now, the American Gut Project (AGP [26]) has collected and sequenced more than 15,000 samples. One of their main targets is to shape the global microbial diversity in their specific body site. However, most of these projects focus on gut microbiome, and only several human populations were studied.

In fact, when launch a new metagenomic study on other body sites or other populations, most research teams can only sequence tens of samples restricted by time, human, physical and financial resources. As the pool of microbes in the living environment is far beyond our understanding [27], and each individual only carries a very small part, there is a huge amount of "dark matters" that cannot be sampled and sequenced, especially under small sample size. Hence, using data with a small sample size to predict the richness of pan metagenome is meaningful for researchers to estimate the number of potential dark matters, and to understand the global feature of the body niche and the human population.

Now there lacks the research on estimating richness of metagenome. However, in the area of bacteria genome study, there is a similar question: to estimate the total number of possible genes of different strains from a same taxonomic unit. There are some works trying to solve the problem by modeling the number of genes in each strain [28, 29]. Here we propose a model specialized for metagenome, named SAM (Species Appearance Model), to help estimating the species/OTU richness of pan metagenome in a specific body site of specific human population. To evaluate the performance of our SAM model, we downloaded the gut OTU table from the American Gut Project which a dataset with extremely large size ($\sim 15{,}000$ fecal samples), trained the model using 50, 100, 200, 300, 400, or 500 of samples and estimate the richness of when sample size goes larger. Results show that our SAM model can precisely predict the species/OTU richness of pan metagenome, especially when the dataset contains less than 2000 samples. Predicting using 200 samples gives the best results. Besides, we defined an index, ESS (Estimated Saturated Sample size), which represents the predicted minimum sample size that adding a new sample only brings less than 0.1 expected new observed species/OTUs. We hope the index can serve as a new measurement to understanding a specific metagenome population, and we also hope our work can provide users a guidance when deciding the final sample size of their metagenome projects.

2 Materials and Methods

2.1 Data

To full investigate how the "dark matters" were observed when the number of samples increased to a large number, we chose the American Gut Project [26], which is the largest human metagenome dataset in present. We downloaded the gut OTU table (11-packaged/fecal/100nt/ag_fecal.biom) from the latest version of AGP (updated in 2018/01/08, ftp://ftp.microbio.me/AmericanGut/latest/). The original file was saved in binary and we manually converted it into plain text.

The original gut OTU table contains 15,158 samples and 24,114 OTUs. The OTUs were picked using 97% similarity using SortMeRNA by the AGP consortium. Each cell in the table presents the abundance of its corresponding OTU in a specific sample.

We did a simple quality control for samples. Only samples that contain no less than 50 OTUs were kept. After the quality control step, 462 samples were filtered out (3.05%), and 14,696 samples were left. Finally, there are 24,098 OTUs occur in at least one sample.

2.2 Definitions and Symbols in this Paper

Concepts Used in this Paper

Pan metagenome: the summation of all the metagenome samples collected in a project, which targets to a specific human niche environment and a specific human population.

Richness: number of species/OTUs in a given metagenome sample, or a pan metagenome.

Estimated saturated sample size (ESS): the expected minimum sample size that adding one newly sampled individual will expectedly bring less than 0.1 (this number can also be customized by users, for example, 0.5 or 1) new observed species/OTUs. When sample size reaches the ESS number, effect of sequencing new samples is limited in discovering new species/OTUs. Therefore, we call this condition as "saturated".

Symbols Used in this Paper

M: number of species/OTUs in the entire species/OTU pool.

Φ: prevalence distribution, in which $\Phi(x)$ stands for the probability that a species or an OTU appear in and only in x proportion of samples. $x \in [0, 1]$.

n: number of samples in a metagenome dataset.

$T(k|n)$: the expected number of taxonomic units (species/OTUs) that appear in k out of n samples.

T pan (n): the expected richness of pan metagenome with n samples.

2.3   Assumptions in Species Appearance Model (SAM)

First, we assumed that the prevalence distribution of species/OTUs follows a "U"-like or "L"-like shape. Figure 1 shows the observed prevalence distributions under 100, 1,000 and 10,000 AGP sample size, respectively. The larger sample size is, the more observed prevalence be closed with real prevalence. Figure 2 shows a "U"-like prevalence distribution in the HMP tongue dorsum (TD) dataset. When the taxonomy units were annotated using known reference (for example, in the HMP TD dataset, the species abundance table were calculated by a reference-based method, MetaPhlan2) in higher taxonomy level (for example, species or genus, compared with 97% OTUs), the observed prevalence distribution is more likely to be "U"-like.

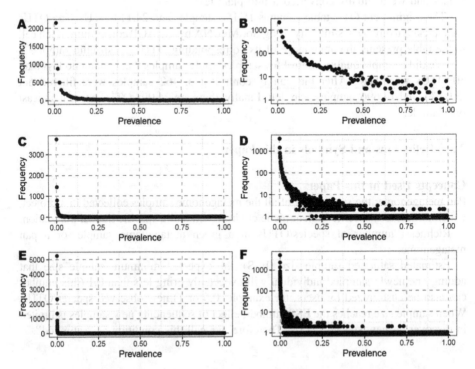

Fig. 1. "L"-like prevalence distributions of (A, B) 100, (C, D) 1,000 and (E, F) 10,000 AGP samples. B, D, and F are in log10 scale.

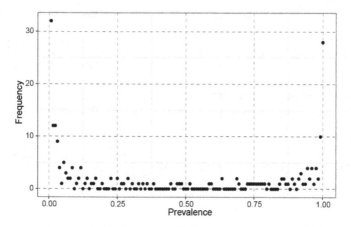

Fig. 2. "U"-like prevalence distributions of species in HMP tongue dorsum samples

We can see that no matter how many samples were chosen to construct the prevalence distribution, the shapes are similar. Most OTUs were rare that only appear in less than 5% samples. In the case of "U"-like distribution, many OTUs are also widespread that appear in more than 95% samples. No matter "L"-like or "U"-like prevalence distribution, we can model them by beta distribution, which is a very useful family to fit distributions on the interval of $[0, 1]$. Hence, we propose our first assumption in SAM model: the prevalence distribution of taxonomic units (species/OTUs) in metagenomic samples can be fit by a beta distribution (Assumption 1):

$$\Phi(x) = \frac{\Gamma(\alpha + \beta)}{\Gamma(\alpha)\Gamma(\beta)} x^{\alpha - 1}(1 - x)^{\beta - 1} \tag{1}$$

where $\Phi(x)$ has been described in Sect. 2.2, and α and β are parameters.

We also have two assumptions about the size of microbial pool: (1) the whole microbial pool contains infinite many taxonomies (Assumption 2), and (2) when sample size goes large, the number of new-observed taxonomies brought by a new sample is finite (Assumption 3).

2.4   Excepted Observing Prevalence Distribution and Pan Metagenome Richness Inferred from SAM Model

The collection and sequencing of metagenome samples can be regarded as a random sampling procedure from environment. For a taxonomy that occurs in x fraction of samples, the probability that k out of n samples contain microbes of this taxonomy is:

$$g(k|x, n) = \binom{n}{k} x^k (1 - x)^{n-k} \tag{2}$$

Then the fraction of microbes that occur in k out of n samples can be calculated by:

$$f(k|n) = \int_0^1 \Phi(x)g(k|x,n)dx = \binom{n}{k} \frac{\Gamma(k+\alpha)\Gamma(n-k+\beta)}{\Gamma(n+\alpha+\beta)} \frac{\Gamma(\alpha+\beta)}{\Gamma(\alpha)\Gamma(\beta)} \quad (3)$$

which follows a beta-binomial distribution.

Then the expression of expected taxonomy number that appear in k out of n samples is:

$$T(k|n) = Mf(k|n) = M\int_0^1 \Phi(x)g(k|x,n)dx = M\binom{n}{k} \frac{\Gamma(k+\alpha)\Gamma(n-k+\beta)}{\Gamma(n+\alpha+\beta)} \frac{\Gamma(\alpha+\beta)}{\Gamma(\alpha)\Gamma(\beta)} \quad (4)$$

From the definition of richness of pan metagenome, when collecting n samples, the richness can be calculated as:

$$T_{pan}(n) = M - T(0|n) = M - M\frac{\Gamma(n+\beta)}{\Gamma(n+\alpha+\beta)} \frac{\Gamma(\alpha+\beta)}{\Gamma(\beta)} = M\left(1 - \frac{\frac{\Gamma(n+\beta)}{\Gamma(\beta)}}{\frac{\Gamma(n+\alpha+\beta)}{\Gamma(\alpha+\beta)}}\right) \quad (5)$$

Note that there is an alternative expression for $\frac{\Gamma(k+\alpha)}{\Gamma(\alpha)}$:

$$\frac{\Gamma(k+\alpha)}{\Gamma(\alpha)} = (k-1+\alpha)...(\alpha+1)\alpha = \alpha\prod_{i=1}^{k-1}(\alpha+i) \quad (6)$$

After simplifying, $T_{pan}(n)$ becomes:

$$T_{pan}(n) = M\left[1 - \prod_{i=0}^{n-1}\frac{\beta+i}{\alpha+\beta+i}\right] \quad (7)$$

When the $(n+1)th$ sample was added, the pan species number becomes:

$$T_{pan}(n+1) = M\left[1 - \prod_{i=0}^{n}\frac{\beta+i}{\alpha+\beta+i}\right] = M\left[1 - \frac{\beta+n}{\alpha+\beta+n}\prod_{i=0}^{n-1}\frac{\beta+i}{\alpha+\beta+i}\right] \quad (8)$$

So the expected number of species that the $(n+1)$th sample brings is:

$$T_{new}(n) = T_{pan}(n+1) - T_{pan}(n) = \frac{M\alpha}{\alpha+\beta+n}\prod_{i=0}^{n-1}\frac{\alpha+i}{\alpha+\beta+i} \quad (9)$$

From Assumption 3, $T_{new}(n)$ should be finite, so $M\alpha$ should be a finite constant. Let $\theta = M\alpha$, from Assumption 2, $M \to \infty$, so α is very small number that goes to zero ($\alpha \to 0$). Then under the limit $M \to \infty$ and $\alpha \to 0$ and substitution $\theta = M\alpha$, after simplifying, we can get the expected observing prevalence distribution:

$$T(k|n) = \frac{\theta}{k} \frac{n(n-1)\ldots(n-k+1)}{(\beta+n-k)\ldots(\beta+n-1)} (1 \le k \le n) \tag{10}$$

And the expected richness of pan metagenome is:

$$T_{pan}(n) = M\left[1 - \prod_{i=0}^{n-1} \frac{\beta+i}{\alpha+\beta+i}\right] = M\alpha \sum_{i=0}^{n-1} \frac{1}{i+\beta} = \theta \sum_{i=0}^{n-1} \frac{1}{i+\beta} \tag{11}$$

Then the number of taxonomy that the (n + 1)th sample brings is:

$$T_{new}(n) = T_{pan}(n+1) - T_{pan}(n) = \frac{\theta}{n+\beta} \tag{12}$$

From the definition of the Estimated saturated sample size (ESS):

$$T_{new}(ESS) = \frac{\theta}{ESS+\beta} = 0.1 \tag{13}$$

Then:

$$ESS = 10\theta - \beta \tag{14}$$

2.5   Fit SAM Model

The SAM model has two unknown parameters: θ and β. From the expression of $T(k|n)$, we can see that the shape of observing prevalence distribution is only decided by β. Therefore, we designed a loss function that reflect the difference between the shape of expected observing prevalence distribution inferred from SAM model compared with the shape of real observed prevalence distribution. The real observed prevalence distribution can be calculated from real sample-taxonomy table:

$$\widehat{T}(k|n) = \sum_{i=1}^{M} I_k(i) \tag{15}$$

in which M is the total number of taxonomic units in the environment pool, and $I_k(i)$ is an indicator that the i-th taxonomy appears in and only in k out of n samples.

The observed richness of pan metagenome is:

$$\widehat{T}_{pan}(n) = \sum_{k=1}^{n} \widehat{T}(k|n) \tag{16}$$

The loss function is designed as:

$$\text{Loss} = \sum_{k=1}^{n} \left(\frac{T(k|n)}{T_{\text{pan}}(n)} - \frac{\widehat{T}(k|n)}{\widehat{T}_{\text{pan}}(n)} \right)^2 \left(\frac{T(k|n)}{T_{\text{pan}}(n)} \right)^2 \tag{17}$$

By fitting the SAM model by minimizing the loss function, we can get an optimized value of $\beta = \beta^*$. We then estimate the richness of pan metagenome as observed, in other word, we set $T^*_{pan}(n) = \widehat{T}_{pan}(n)$. Then from the expression of $T_{pan}(n)$, θ can be calculated as:

$$\theta^* = \frac{\widehat{T}_{\text{pan}}(n)}{\sum_{i=0}^{n-1} \frac{1}{i+\beta^*}} \tag{18}$$

2.6   Experiments and Evaluation

We designed a series of experiments to evaluate the performance of our estimation. In each experiment (Fig. 3), we only used n ($n = 50, 100, 200, 300, 400$, or 500) samples to fit the SAM model, and got the optimized β and θ. Then we predict the richness of pan metagenome when sample size grows (from n to 14000, listed in Table 1). We replied each experiment for 10 times, and recorded the minimum, maximum and average predicted richness in each sample size. At the same time, we down-sampled the original dataset, 10 times in each sample size, as the groundtruth of pan metagenome richness. We finally compared the predicted richness against groundtruth, to show the performance of the results.

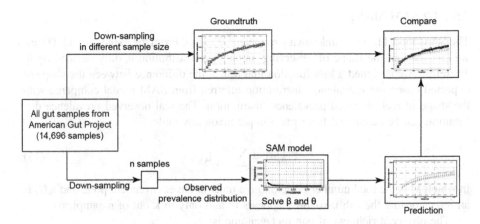

Fig. 3. Pipeline of each experiment

Table 1. Experiments in this study

# Samples	Predicted sample size	# Replications
50	(100, 200, ..., 5000), (6000, 7000, ..., 14000)	10
100	(200, 300, ..., 5000), (6000, 7000, ..., 14000)	10
200	(300, 400, ..., 5000), (6000, 7000, ..., 14000)	10
300	(400, 500, ..., 5000), (6000, 7000, ..., 14000)	10
400	(500, 600, ..., 5000), (6000, 7000, ..., 14000)	10
500	(600, 700, ..., 5000), (6000, 7000, ..., 14000)	10

3 Results

3.1 Data Review of American Gut Project

The original AGP dataset contains 15,158 samples and 24,114 OTUs. About 90% of samples (13,489 out of 15,158, 88.99%) contain 200 to 1,000 OTUs. The OTU richness in the AGP database approximately follows a log-normal-like distribution (Fig. 4). We did a quality control by filtering out samples with less than 50 OTUs (red dashed line in Fig. 4). Only 3.05% (462) of OTUs were discarded.

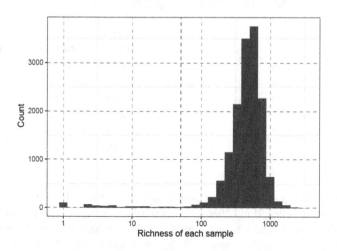

Fig. 4. Distribution of OTU Richness in AGP sample (Colour figure online)

After the quality control step, 14,696 samples were kept, and 24,098 OTUs occurred in at least one samples. Among the 24,098 OTUs, 22.85% (5,507) occur in only one samples. There are 91.43% (22,033) OTUs appear in less than 5% of samples. Only 0.03% (8) OTUs can appear in more than 95% (13,961) of samples. From this angle of view, the discrepancy among gut samples are fairly high. Using down sampling method, we also studied the observed OTU prevalence distribution with smaller sample size (Sect. 2.3 in Materials and methods). Results show that the observed prevalence distribution curve seems "softer" when sample size goes down (Fig. 1). For example, in an experiment that sampling 100 samples, about 66.78% (4,041 out of 6,051) of OTUs appear in less than 5% of samples, and 0.18% (11) OTUs appear in more than 95% of samples.

3.2 Performance in Predicting Richness of Pan Metagenome Using SAM

We designed a series of experiments to study the performance of our SAM model, and the relationship between the sample size that were used to fit the model and the final effect. We tried to use 50, 100, 200, 300, 400 or 500 samples to get the optimized β and θ in the SAM model, and predicted the richness of pan metagenome with sample size 100 to 14,000 (Table 1). When using 200 samples, our model can give the best results (Table 2, Figs. 5 and 6). Besides, the variation of predicted richness when using 200 sub-samples is small (Table 2, Figs. 5 and 6), especially when predicted sample size goes bigger (Fig. 6).

Table 2. Performance when using different sample sizes

Sample size	Beta (average)	Theta (average)	Performance when predict richness of 1000 metagenome samples	
			Error (%)	Variation (max-min)
50	5.66	1905.12	20.42%	2450.72
100	7.99	2169.90	11.84%	3029.91
200	11.62	2483.87	4.90%	1598.09
300	11.71	2410.89	10.89%	2429.84
400	2.33	1395.51	13.15%	1626.48
500	2.45	1422.87	11.29%	1178.82

From the results, we can see that only increasing the sample size does not necessarily make results better. It may because when using too many samples, the observed prevalence distribution tends to concentrate in the left side too much (Fig. 1), and number of OTUs with higher prevalence becomes too small, which is not good for accurate fitting of SAM model.

As we only use as few as 200 samples, our model is satisfactory when predicting richness of pan metagenome with sample size that not too big, especially under 2000 samples. When predict in more than 5000 samples, our model tends to underestimate the richness, which may because the natural complexity increasing when the population size is very large. However, our model can still give instructive understanding of metagenome population complexity.

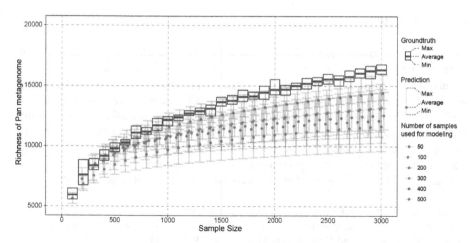

Fig. 5. Predicted richness of pan metagenome vs. groundtruth (zoomed in to the region of less than 3,000 samples)

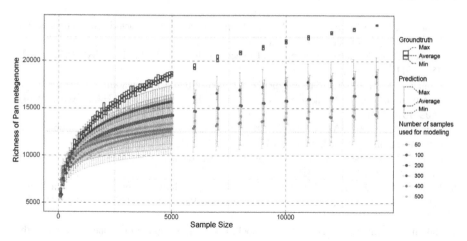

Fig. 6. Predicted richness of pan metagenome vs. groundtruth

Using the average parameters ($\beta = 11.62$, $\theta = 2483.87$) obtained by 200 samples, we can estimate the ESS of the gut metagenome population of American Gut Project: ESS $= 10\theta - \beta = 24,827$. As the real complexity of the AGP population may be much higher than expected, the observed OTU may need even more than 25,000 samples to be saturated. This means that the AGP population is very complex, in the angle of OTUs.

4 Conclusion

In this paper, a model named SAM (Species Appearance Model) were proposed to estimate the taxonomic richness of pan metagenome with any sample size. When testing in the American Gut Project (AGP) dataset, our model needs only 200 samples, and can precisely predict richness of more than 2000 samples. We also proposed an ESS index (Estimated Saturated Sample size) to describe the overall complexity of the metagenome population. The ESS of the AGP dataset is about 25,000, which implies the population is complex. We hope our study can provide a new angle of understanding different metagenome population, and help researchers in this area in deciding the sample size when initiating their projects on a new metagenomic population.

Acknowledgements. This work is a continuation of the author's doctoral research. The author thanks Prof. Xuegong Zhang for his inspirations about this work. This work was supported by the National Key Research and Development Project 2018YFC0910400.

References

1. Lundberg, J.O., Weitzberg, E., Cole, J.A., Benjamin, N.: Nitrate, bacteria and human health. Nat. Rev. Microbiol. **2**(7), 593–602 (2004)
2. Relman, D.A.: Microbial genomics and infectious diseases. N. Engl. J. Med. **365**(4), 347–357 (2011)
3. Loman, N.J., et al.: A culture-independent sequence-based metagenomics approach to the investigation of an outbreak of Shiga-toxigenic Escherichia coli O104:H4. JAMA **309**(14), 1502–1510 (2013)
4. Kamada, N., Chen, G.Y., Inohara, N., Nunez, G.: Control of pathogens and pathobionts by the gut microbiota. Nat. Immunol. **14**(7), 685–690 (2013)
5. Gallo, R.L., Hooper, L.V.: Epithelial antimicrobial defence of the skin and intestine. Nat. Rev. Immunol. **12**(7), 503–516 (2012)
6. Kramer, P., Bressan, P.: Humans as superorganisms: how microbes, viruses, imprinted genes, and other selfish entities shape our behavior. Perspect. Psychol. Sci. **10**(4), 464–481 (2015)
7. Rakoff-Nahoum, S., Foster, K.R., Comstock, L.E.: The evolution of cooperation within the gut microbiota. Nature **533**(7602), 255–259 (2016)
8. Coyte, K.Z., Schluter, J., Foster, K.R.: The ecology of the microbiome: networks, competition, and stability. Science **350**(6261), 663–666 (2015)
9. Cho, I., Blaser, M.J.: The human microbiome: at the interface of health and disease. Nat. Rev. Genet. **13**(4), 260–270 (2012)
10. Clemente, J.C., Ursell, L.K., Parfrey, L.W., Knight, R.: The impact of the gut microbiota on human health: an integrative view. Cell **148**(6), 1258–1270 (2012)
11. Dinan, T.G., Stilling, R.M., Stanton, C., Cryan, J.F.: Collective unconscious: how gut microbes shape human behavior. J. Psychiatr. Res. **63**, 1–9 (2015)
12. Bravo-Blas, A., Wessel, H., Milling, S.: Microbiota and arthritis: correlations or cause? Curr. Opin. Rheumatol. **28**(2), 161–167 (2016)
13. David, L.A., et al.: Diet rapidly and reproducibly alters the human gut microbiome. Nature **505**(7484), 559–563 (2014)

14. Morris, A., et al.: Comparison of the respiratory microbiome in healthy nonsmokers and smokers. Am. J. Respir. Crit. Care Med. **187**(10), 1067–1075 (2013)
15. Devaraj, S., Hemarajata, P., Versalovic, J.: The human gut microbiome and body metabolism: implications for obesity and diabetes. Clin. Chem. **59**(4), 617–628 (2013)
16. Bouter, K.E., van Raalte, D.H., Groen, A.K., Nieuwdorp, M.: Role of the gut microbiome in the pathogenesis of obesity and obesity-related metabolic dysfunction. Gastroenterology **152** (7), 1671–1678 (2017)
17. Tilg, H., Kaser, A.: Gut microbiome, obesity, and metabolic dysfunction. J. Clin. Invest. **121** (6), 2126–2132 (2011)
18. Qin, J., et al.: A metagenome-wide association study of gut microbiota in type 2 diabetes. Nature **490**(7418), 55–60 (2012)
19. Qin, N., et al.: Alterations of the human gut microbiome in liver cirrhosis. Nature **513**(7516), 59–64 (2014)
20. Saulnier, D.M., et al.: Gastrointestinal microbiome signatures of pediatric patients with irritable bowel syndrome. Gastroenterology **141**(5), 1782–1791 (2011)
21. Human Microbiome Project C: Structure, function and diversity of the healthy human microbiome. Nature **486**(7402), 207–214 (2012)
22. Qin, J., et al.: A human gut microbial gene catalogue established by metagenomic sequencing. Nature **464**(7285), 59–65 (2010)
23. Bonder, M.J., et al.: The effect of host genetics on the gut microbiome. Nat. Genet. **48**(11), 1407–1412 (2016)
24. Turpin, W., et al.: Association of host genome with intestinal microbial composition in a large healthy cohort. Nat. Genet. **48**(11), 1413–1417 (2016)
25. Falony, G., et al.: Population-level analysis of gut microbiome variation. Science **352**(6285), 560–564 (2016)
26. McDonald, D., Birmingham, A., Knight, R.: Context and the human microbiome. Microbiome **3**, 52 (2015)
27. Lloyd, K.G., Steen, A.D., Ladau, J., Yin, J., Crosby, L.: Phylogenetically novel uncultured microbial cells dominate earth microbiomes. mSystems **3**(5) (2018)
28. Lapierre, P., Gogarten, J.P.: Estimating the size of the bacterial pan-genome. Trends Genet. **25**(3), 107–110 (2009)
29. Collins, R.E., Higgs, P.G.: Testing the infinitely many genes model for the evolution of the bacterial core genome and pangenome. Mol. Biol. Evol. **29**(11), 3413–3425 (2012)

Prediction of Hospital Readmission for Heart Disease: A Deep Learning Approach

Jingwei Da[1], Danni Yan[1], Sijia Zhou[2], Yidi Liu[2], Xin Li[2], Yani Shi[3], Jiaqi Yan[1(✉)], and Zhongmin Wang[4]

[1] School of Information Management, Nanjing University, Nanjing 210023, China
jiaqiyan@nju.edu.cn
[2] Department of Information Systems, City University of Hong Kong, Kowloon, Hong Kong, China
[3] School of Economics and Management, Southeast University, Nanjing 211189, China
[4] Jiangsu Province Hospital, The First Affiliated Hospital of Nanjing Medical University, Nanjing 210029, China

Abstract. Hospital readmissions consume large amounts of medical resources and negatively impact the healthcare system. Predicting the readmission rate early one can alleviate the financial and medical consequences. Most related studies only select the patient's structural features or text features for modeling analysis, which offer an incomplete picture of the patient. Based on structured data (including demographic data, clinical data, administrative data) and medical record text, this paper uses deep learning methods to construct an optimal model for hospital readmission prediction, tested on a dataset of heart disease patients' 30-day readmission. The results show that when only structured data is used, the deep learning model is much better than the Naive Bayes model and slightly better than the Support Vector Machine model. Adding a text model to the deep learning model improves performance, increasing accuracy and F1-score by 2% and 6%, respectively. This indicates that textual information contributes greatly to hospital readmission predictions.

Keywords: Hospital readmission · Predictive analytics · Deep learning

1 Introduction

Hospital readmission is a vital problem in disease management. It is defined as admission within a short period of time after discharge; within 30 days is considered to have clinical significance [1]. Hospital readmission rate is one of the main indicators for evaluating hospitals' medical quality and management level. Hospital readmission disrupts patients' lives and consumes medical resources, which has a negative impact on the medical system [2]; 30-day readmissions lead to an annual cost of $26 billion dollars [3]. However, studies have found that 9% to 48% of hospital readmission can be avoided [4]. Predicting the readmission rate early on can identify patients with high risk of readmission and lead to taking timely measures to avoid such occurrence.

© Springer Nature Switzerland AG 2019
H. Chen et al. (Eds.): ICSH 2019, LNCS 11924, pp. 16–26, 2019.
https://doi.org/10.1007/978-3-030-34482-5_2

Related studies often use traditional statistical methods and machine learning methods to build hospital readmission prediction models. However, the traditional prediction methods (such as logistic regression model and Cox proportional risk model) have insufficient prediction accuracy, so they cannot provide effective decision support for hospital readmission management. As for machine learning methods, most prediction models are based on structured data. Although structured data contains features that are well-established predictors of readmission, they offer an incomplete picture of the patient. The medical record text contains information related to readmission, including the patient history, ongoing conditions, and the treatments and procedures attempted during the hospitalization. Nevertheless, few studies combine structured data with text for prediction. One reason could be that it is difficult to process and extract features from text data, although it contains rich information. Deep learning methods have significant advantages in text processing, which implement end-to-end learning and make better use of word order features. With deep learning methods, a hospital readmission prediction model can be constructed based on structured data and unstructured medical records, thereby more accurately predicting readmission.

Since heart disease is a common chronic disease leading to frequent hospital readmission, this paper takes heart disease as an example to study hospital readmission prediction. Based on structured data (including demographic data, clinical data, administrative data) and medical record text data, this paper uses deep learning methods to construct an optimal model for hospital readmission prediction of heart disease patients within 30 days.

The organization of the paper is as follows. Section 2 reviews the literature on hospital readmissions. Section 3 briefly introduces our method, namely Deep Learning Model with All Data (DL-ALL). The experiment and results are presented in Sect. 4. In Sect. 5, conclusions are drawn.

2   Literature Review

The existing research on hospital readmission is mainly divided into two aspects. The first aspect focuses on factors affecting hospital readmission, including econometric issues. Such research uses regression analysis and other methods to find out whether different factors have an impact on hospital readmission and the extent of their impact [5, 6]. The second approach is to build a prediction model using relevant factors to predict the probability of hospital readmission [7, 8].

From a prediction methods perspective, previous studies mainly used traditional machine learning methods, such as linear regression, logical regression, Support Vector Machine (SVM), Naive Bayes and Decision Tree. For example, in 2011, Omar and David et al. [9] analyzed the influencing factors of 10,946 patients' readmission by establishing a multivariable logistic regression model. In 2014, Braga and Portela [10] used SVM and Decision Tree to predict the risk index of patients who had been discharged from the intensive care unit (ICU) and readmitted. Eigner et al. [11] used state-of-the-art sampling and ensemble methods to build a prediction model to predict the unplanned hospital readmission of patients after hysterectomies in Australia. Recently, as a special type of machine learning method, deep learning has shown excellent performance in visual recognition, speech recognition, text processing and other aspects. Therefore, some researchers applied deep learning methods to hospital readmission prediction. For example, Wang et al. [12] developed a cost-sensitive deep learning approach combining Convolutional Neural Network (CNN) and Multi-Layer Perceptron (MLP) for readmission prediction. Rajkomar et al. [13] also developed an approach that ensembles three deep learning models (LSTM, an attention-based TANN, neural network with boosted time-based decision stumps) to predict the risk of 30-day unplanned readmission.

From a feature selection perspective, most studies used structured data to build prediction models. For instance, McManus's [7] hospital readmission prediction model for patients with acute coronary syndrome in the United States was built based on medical insurance claim data and other clinical, social psychology and socio-demographic data. However, structured data only contains a part of feature information extracted from patients' medical record information, not their complete information. With the development of natural language processing technology and deep learning, some scholars used deep learning methods to study text data of electronic medical records. In 2018, Xiao et al. [14] built a model based on clinical events (including disease, lab test and medication codes) from an EHR repository of a Congestive Heart Failure (CHF) cohort to predict the readmission risk of patients with heart failure. Craig et al. [15] developed a model based on physicians' discharge notes on 141,226 inpatients to predict an unplanned readmission to the hospital within 30 days. The above studies only select the patients' structural features or text features, respectively, for modeling analysis. Golas et al. [16] were the first to combine structured data (demographic, admissions, diagnosis, lab, medications and procedures data) with unstructured data (physician notes, discharge summaries) to build a model for predicting 30-day readmission risk in patients with heart failure. The study proved that the performance of deep learning methods is better than other traditional methods. However, the study used the bag of words model to process text, which may ignore the word order information of text that could influence the model results.

In summary, traditional machine learning methods are generally based on structured data to build models. The patient information in structured data is incomplete, and prediction accuracy will be affected by feature selection. In contrast, deep learning and natural language processing methods can predict hospital readmission based on complete patient information (including structured data and text data), and the effect of the prediction model is superior to traditional models. Although previous studies have combined structured data with text data for readmission prediction, they ignore the text word order information in text processing, which may influence the model results. Character-level convolutional neural network (Char-CNN) [17] extracts high-level abstract concepts from text processing at the character level. It does not need to understand the word order of the text and other information. And it will not be restricted by medical terms when processing medical records. So, this paper uses Char-CNN to process medical record text and build a hospital readmission prediction model with a combination of structured data and text data.

3 Method

Deep learning is simply a neural network (NN) of multiple layers and structures that learns representations of data with multiple levels of abstraction. Different from conventional machine learning techniques that have limited ability to enhance by getting exposed to more data, deep learning has the capacity to scale effectively even with raw data [18]. Convolutional Neural Networks (CNN) is one of the classic deep learning models. CNN is a neural network that can make use of the internal structure of data and utilize multiple layers with convolution filters applied to local features, wherein each computation unit responds to a small region of input data [19]. CNN models have shown impressive results in the areas of computer vision and natural language processing.

Character-level Convolutional Neural Network (Char-CNN) regards text as a kind of original signal at the character level. It processes text at character level and extracts high-level abstract concepts without using pre-trained word vectors, grammar and syntactic structures [20]. Medical record text processing will be not restricted by medical terms. Before applying the Char-CNN model, we first create a character table. Each character can be transformed into a one-hot vector correspondingly based on the character table. Then a sentence composed of multiple characters is transformed into a vector matrix composed of character one-hot vectors. Taking the vector matrix as an input, the model makes a classification prediction through an embedding layer, several convolution layers, pooling layers and connection layers.

Based on structured data, we use the deep learning method to build a Deep Learning Model with Structured Data (DL-Structured). DL-Structured consists of five dense layers with 128, 64, 16, 16 and 2 hidden neurons respectively. We add a dropout layer with a dropout probability of 0.5 between the first and second layer to reduce over-fitting. Since the classifier distinguishes between two classes (0 means no readmission, 1 means readmission), the Softmax activation function was chosen for the output layer. ReLU was chosen for all other layers because it leads to efficient computation and fewer vanishing gradient problems. Training is done through Adam at learning rate 0.001. Figure 1 shows the architecture of DL-Structured.

A Deep Learning Model with All Data (DL-ALL) adds a text model based on DL-Structured. The text model includes three inputs based on the three parts of the text, namely, Medical history, Family disease history and Personal lifestyle history. The text model includes a word embedding layer, a convolutional layer, a max pooling layer and a dense layer. Then text data vectors and structured data vectors are concatenated as an input to connect with a fully connected layer for final classification. The Softmax activation function was chosen for the output layer, and ReLU was chosen for all layers other than the output layer. Training is done through Adam at learning rate 0.001. Figure 2 shows the architecture of DL-ALL.

The text model accepts a sequence of encoded characters as input. We leverage character embedding to map individual characters into distributed representation (character embedding). With an embedding table of 200 * 3000 (200 characters and a vector with size 3000 for each character), we feed the textual data into the convolutional layer with a matrix of 200 (number of characters in each input) * 64.

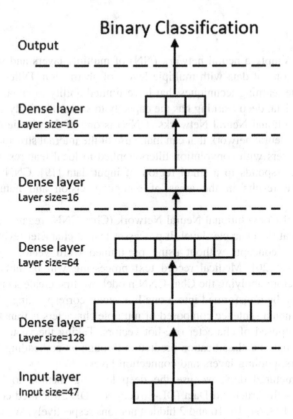

Fig. 1. Architecture of DL-Structured

4   Experiment

4.1   Data

The study uses a dataset of hospitalization records for heart disease patients from 2017 to 2018 provided by a large public hospital in China. The dataset only includes records with the "heart disease" keyword in the disease name, and each record includes structured data and text data. The dataset contains 4020 patient records, each of which represents a patient's single hospitalization record.

The data contains structured data and text data. Table 1 shows the description of structured data. The structured data contains 9 variables: Demographic Data (gender, marital status), Clinical Data (systolic blood pressure, diastolic blood pressure) and Administrative Data (hospitalization days, ICD_10 codes, metoprolol use, Irbesartan use, surgery). Text data is divided into three parts by content, including patient's Medical history, Family disease history and Personal lifestyle history. The Medical history contains the patient's past medical history, treatment and allergy history. The Family disease history includes the patient's family hereditary diseases and infectious

Binary Classification

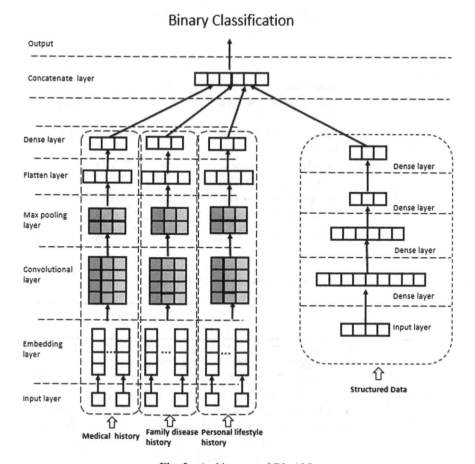

Fig. 2. Architecture of DL-ALL

diseases, and the Personal lifestyle history includes the patient's living conditions and habits. Table 2 shows example of text data.

There are some problems in the original data that need to be cleaned, such as missing values, redundancy and duplication. For missing values, average values are used to fill in numerical variables, and records with missing values in other variables are deleted. For text data, we remove stop words and special characters based on the common stop words list. In our study, only the second admission after discharge was counted when judging whether hospital readmission occurred. If one patient has several hospital admissions, then each admission can be counted respectively. For example, the third admission is recorded as the second hospital readmission.

After data processing, the final data contains 3740 records, each of which includes the basic information field, single hospitalization information field of a patient and whether the patient was readmitted within 30 days after discharge. Of all records, 1774 records are marked as readmission within 30 days, with a readmission rate of 47.4%.

Table 1. Description of structured data

Feature classification	Feature name	Type	Description (dc = distinct count)
Demographic data	Gender	Categorical	Male (64.9%); Female (35.1%)
	Marital status	Categorical	dc = 4
Clinical data	Systolic blood pressure	Numeric	Mean = 129.582; Std = 18.512
	Diastolic blood pressure	Numeric	Mean = 72.314; Std = 12.130
Administrative data	Length of stay	Numeric	Mean = 14.879; Std = 10.311
	ICD_10	Categorical	dc = 36
	Metoprolol use	Boolean	Yes (32.9%); No (67.1%)
	Irbesartan use	Boolean	Yes (5.8%); No (94.2%)
	Surgery	Boolean	Yes (5.6%); No (94.4%)

Table 2. Example of text data

Feature Name	Example
Medical History	既往否认XXXX病史；有XXXX病史，现予XXXX药物预防治疗；否认XXXX等传染性疾病史；有XXXXX过敏史；2009年12月因XXX病行XXX手术，手术过程顺利，术后患者恢复良好，未遗留后遗症；否认其他手术及重大外伤史，预防接种随社会。 (Including the patient's past medical history, current medical history, treatment measures, history of infectious diseases, history of allergies, history of surgery, detailed information on surgery, and vaccination.)
Family Disease History	否认"高血压、糖尿病、血友病"等家族遗传性疾病史。 (Including the history of family genetic diseases including hypertension, diabetes, and hemophilia.)
Personal Lifestyle History	出生并生长于原籍，退休后定居XX，否认其他异地久居史，否认有毒有害物质接触史。有吸烟史X年，20支/天，已戒烟X年。少量饮酒史。适龄婚配，配偶及子女体健。(Including the patient's birth information, residency information, history of exposure to toxic and hazardous substances, smoking history, drinking history, marriage, and family members' health status.)

4.2 Experimental Procedure

To evaluate the model, we split data into training and testing sets with a proportion of 4:1. Then, we perform 10-fold cross-validation with the training set to tune the parameters. The training set is divided into 10 equal folds, and each fold is considered as validation data to validate the model built on the remaining 9 folds. As each fold is considered once as validation data, we will get a validation result of the model accordingly. In order to reduce variability, we use averaged validation results to represent the model performance. We tune the parameters based on the model performance each time. An optimal model performance corresponds to the optimal parameters. After parameter tuning, we will train the model based on the original training set with the optimal parameters and evaluate the model based on the test set.

4.3 Evaluation Metrics

We use accuracy, precision, recall and the F1-score to assess the performance of the different models. Accuracy measures the proportion of correctly predicted samples to the total number of samples. Precision measures the proportion of truly readmitted samples in identified readmission samples. Recall measures the proportion of correctly identified samples in real readmission samples. The F1-score combines precision and recall as an overall assessment of the performance.

4.4 Model Based on Structured Data

To assess the performance of the deep learning model, we use Support Vector Machine (SVM) and Naive Bayes (NB) as our baseline [21,22]. They are widely used methods in hospital readmission prediction.

The results of our experiments are shown in Table 3.

Table 3. Performance of models based on structured data

	NB	SVM	DL-Structured
Accuracy	0.733	0.756	**0.759**
Precision	0.724	0.789	**0.790**
Recall	0.673	0.641	**0.647**
F1-score	0.698	0.707	**0.712**

As we can see from Table 3, DL-Structured is much better than the NB model and slightly better than the SVM model. Both the SVM model and the deep learning model have an accuracy of more than 0.75, indicating that the prediction accuracy of both is better. And they can make a more accurate prediction of readmission based on the existing structured data.

4.5 Model Based on Structured Data and Text

The results of our experiments are shown in Table 4.

Table 4. Performance of DL-ALL

	DL-Structured	DL-ALL
Accuracy	0.759	**0.781**
Precision	0.790	**0.774**
Recall	0.647	**0.734**
F1-score	0.712	**0.755**

We can see from Table 4 that DL-ALL performs better than DL-Structured. The accuracy and F1-score of DL-ALL are increased by 2% and 6% respectively, which indicates that the deep learning model has a better performance after adding text to it. This indicates that the feature information included in the medical record text contributes greatly to hospital readmission predictions.

5 Conclusion

In this research, we build a novel hospital readmission prediction model to help monitor hospital readmission probability. Using heart disease as an example, we build a 30-day readmission prediction model based on patients' structured data and text data using a deep learning method. We found that the deep learning model with textual and structural data outperforms all other models. The deep learning model with only structural data as input also outperforms other machine learning models.

We contribute to both academic research and medical practice. We demonstrate that the use of textual data can dramatically improve readmission prediction performance. We build a novel deep learning model with both textual and structural data as input and gain excellent performance in heart disease readmission prediction. In practice, hospitals should consider including textual input to aid their readmission prediction. Medical record text contains abundant feature information. Adding it to the prediction model can improve the prediction accuracy of the model, which can help doctors more effectively identify and pay attention to high-risk patients in advance, so as to take effective intervention measures in time and reduce the readmission rate. They should also consider leveraging deep learning methods when conducting readmission prediction even if there is no available textual data, as deep neural net also outperforms other baselines without text.

There are some limitations in our study. First, our data comes from one hospital, so there may exist some errors when judging whether a patient has readmitted within 30 days. A patient may have been readmitted to other hospitals within 30 days after discharge. Second, we only use part of the data of the medical record text, excluding some professional data such as examination report. In future research, we plan to use more comprehensive data to predict. Third, we only use the Char-CNN model to process medical record text. In the future, we can study more models to get a more accurate prediction model.

Acknowledgements. This work was supported in part by the National Natural Science Foundation of China under Grant 71701091 and Grant 71701043, in part by the CityU SRG under Grant 7005195, in part by the Fundamental Research Funds for the Central Universities under Grant 2242019K40157, and in part by the Chinese Ministry of Education Project of Humanities and Social Science under Grant 17YJC870020.

References

1. Basu Roy, S., et al.: Dynamic hierarchical classification for patient risk-of-readmission. In: Proceedings of the 21st ACM SIGKDD International Conference on Knowledge Discovery and Data Mining, pp. 1691–1700. ACM (2015)
2. Mcilvennan, C.K., Eapen, Z.J., Allen, L.A.: Hospital readmissions reduction program. Circulationl **31**(20), 1796–1803 (2015)
3. Center for Health Information and Analysis: Performance of the Massachusetts Health Care System Series: A Focus on Provider Quality (2015)
4. Benbassat, J., Taragin, M.: Hospital readmissions as a measure of quality of health care: advantages and limitations. Arch. Intern. Med. **160**(8), 1074–1081 (2000)
5. Kamalesh, M., Subramanian, U., Ariana, A., Sawada, S., Peterson, E.: Diabetes status and racial differences in post–myocardial infarction mortality. Am. Heart J. **150**(5), 912–919 (2005)
6. Mahmoud, A.N., et al.: Prevalence, causes, and predictors of 30 day readmissions following hospitalization with acute myocardial infarction complicated by cardiogenic shock: findings from the 2013–2014 National readmissions database. J. Am. Heart Assoc. **7**(6), e008235 (2018)
7. McManus, D.D., Saczynski, J.S., Lessard, D., Waring, M.E., Allison, J., Parish, D.C., TRACE-CORE Investigators.: Reliability of predicting early hospital readmission after discharge for an acute coronary syndrome using claims-based data. Am. J. Cardiol. **117**(4), 501–507 (2016)
8. Yu, S., Farooq, F., Van Esbroeck, A., Fung, G., Anand, V., Krishnapuram, B.: Predicting readmission risk with institution-specific prediction models. Artif. Intell. Med. **65**(2), 89–96 (2015)
9. Hasan, O., et al.: Hospital readmission in general medicine patients: a prediction model. J. Gen. Intern. Med. **25**(3), 211–219 (2010)
10. Braga, P., Portela, F., Santos, M.F., Rua, F.: Data mining models to predict patient's readmission in intensive care units. In: Proceedings of the 6th International Conference on Agents and Artificial Intelligence, ICAART 2014, vol. 1, pp. 604–610. SCITEPRESS (2014)
11. Eigner, I., Reischl, D., Bodendorf, F.: Development and evaluation of ensemble-based classification models for predicting unplanned hospital readmissions after hysterectomy (2018)
12. Wang, H., Cui, Z., Chen, Y., Avidan, M., Abdallah, A.B., Kronzer, A.: Predicting hospital readmission via cost-sensitive deep learning. IEEE/ACM Trans. Comput. Biol. Bioinform. (TCBB) **15**(6), 1968–1978 (2018)
13. Rajkomar, A., et al.: Scalable and accurate deep learning with electronic health records. NPJ Digit. Med. **1**(1), 18 (2018)
14. Xiao, C., Ma, T., Dieng, A.B., Blei, D.M., Wang, F.: Readmission prediction via deep contextual embedding of clinical concepts. PLoS ONE **13**(4), e0195024 (2018)
15. Craig, E., Arias, C., Gillman, D.: Predicting readmission risk from doctors' notes. arXiv preprint arXiv:1711.10663 (2017)
16. Golas, S.B., et al.: A machine learning model to predict the risk of 30-day readmissions in patients with heart failure: a retrospective analysis of electronic medical records data. BMC Med. Inf. Decis. Making **18**(1), 44 (2018)
17. Zhang, X., Zhao, J., LeCun, Y.: Character-level convolutional networks for text classification. In: Advances in Neural Information Processing Systems, pp. 649–657 (2015)
18. LeCun, Y., Bengio, Y., Hinton, G.: Deep learning. Nature **521**(7553), 436–444 (2015)

19. Cheng, Y., Wang, F., Zhang, P., Hu, J.: Risk prediction with electronic health records: a deep learning approach. In: Proceedings of the 2016 SIAM International Conference on Data Mining, pp. 432–440. Society for Industrial and Applied Mathematics (2016)
20. Saxe, J., Berlin, K.: eXpose: a character-level convolutional neural network with embeddings for detecting malicious URLs, file paths and registry keys. arXiv preprint arXiv:1702.08568 (2017)
21. Hearst, M.A., Dumais, S.T., Osuna, E., et al.: Support vector machines. IEEE Intell. Syst. Appl. **13**(4), 18–28 (1998)
22. Rish, I.: An empirical study of the naive Bayes classifier. In: Workshop on Empirical Methods in Artificial Intelligence, IJCAI 2001, vol. 3, no. 22, pp. 41–46 (2001)

DEKGB: An Extensible Framework for Health Knowledge Graph

Ming Sheng[1], Yuyao Shao[2], Yong Zhang[1(✉)], Chao Li[1],
Chunxiao Xing[1], Han Zhang[3], Jingwen Wang[2], and Fei Gao[4]

[1] RIIT&BNRCIST&DCST, Tsinghua University, Beijing 100084, China
{shengming, zhangyong05, lichao, xingcx}@tsinghua.edu.cn
[2] Beijing Foreign Studies University, Beijing 100089, China
{shaoyuyao, wjw}@bfsu.edu.cn
[3] Beijing University of Posts and Telecommunications, Beijing 100876, China
zhanghan3281@bupt.edu.cn
[4] Henan Justice Police Vocational College, Zhengzhou 450046, China
68521617@qq.com

Abstract. With the progress of medical informatization and the substantial growth of clinical data, knowledge graph is playing an increasingly important role in medical domain. Medical domain is highly specialized with abundant high-quality ontologies, and has many professional sub-fields such as cardiovascular diseases, diabetes mellitus and so on. It is very difficult to build a health knowledge graph for all of the diseases because of data availability and deep involvement of doctors. In this paper, we propose an efficient and extensible framework, DEKGB, to construct knowledge graphs for specific diseases based on prior medical knowledge and EMRs with doctor-involved. After that, we present the detailed process how DEKGB is applied to extend an existing health knowledge graph to include a new disease. It is confirmed that using this framework, doctors can get highly specialized health knowledge graphs conveniently and efficiently.

Keywords: Health knowledge graph · Extensibility · Conceptual graph · Instance graph

1 Introduction

Knowledge graphs have been in the focus of research since 2012 when the term was firstly proposed by Google, as an enhancement of their search engine with semantics [1]. A popular definition of knowledge graph is a graph-based data structure composed of nodes (entities) and labeled edges (relationships between entities) [2]. In general, we define knowledge graphs with only concept nodes as Concept Knowledge Graph (CKG), knowledge graphs with both instance nodes and event nodes as Instance Knowledge Graph (IKG), and knowledge graphs covering CKG and IKG as Factual Knowledge Graph (FKG).

Current health knowledge graphs usually cover wide areas of medical knowledge: all proteins (UniProt), as many drugs as possible (Drugbank), as many drug-drug

© Springer Nature Switzerland AG 2019
H. Chen et al. (Eds.): ICSH 2019, LNCS 11924, pp. 27–38, 2019.
https://doi.org/10.1007/978-3-030-34482-5_3

interactions as are known (Sider), and massively integrated knowledge graphs such as Bio2RDF and LinkedLifeData [3]. However, the knowledge graphs covering wide areas may contain inaccurate and irrelevant knowledge so as to be difficult in actual use. For user-friendly and accurate purpose, health knowledge graphs should be tailored for doctors in specific diseases. Meanwhile another problem may occur. Building a new knowledge graph for a new disease from scratch in medical domain is time consuming because there are many repetitive procedures such as data alignment. So a construction framework for knowledge graph in a specific disease is necessary. Currently, the construction framework for general knowledge graphs mainly includes knowledge representation, knowledge graph building tools such as extraction tools, and knowledge storage and application. However, general strategies cannot be directly applied to domain-specific knowledge graphs, let alone to more sophisticated disease-specific knowledge graphs. The reason is that specific entities and relations from specific data sources need to be extracted, and specialized semantic networks for different diseases need to be constructed. In medical domain, there are many complex concepts and relations, diverse diseases, which require large amount of prior knowledge from doctors to clarify them. What's more, the doctors' actual demands may be various. So the help from doctors also plays an important role. Hence, the most important aspects of building a disease-specific knowledge graph lie in three parts: the disease-specific data sources, the building tools to extract specific entities and relations, and the help from the doctors.

The problem we are going to address in this paper is how to construct a knowledge graph for a specific disease and extend it to other diseases, based on prior medical knowledge, EMRs and doctors.

To solve this problem, we propose a knowledge graph building framework DEKGB that can be used to create a knowledge graph with many diseases. We use EMRs from hospitals and implement a toolset to help the doctors put forward professional knowledge, along with existing medical knowledge.

This paper is organized as follows. In Sect. 2 we introduce the related work. In Sect. 3 we present the framework and data flow of DEKGB. In Sects. 4 and 5 we show the construction of CKG and IKG for cardiovascular diseases in detail. In Sect. 6, we show the extension process to include a new disease in an existing health knowledge graph by using DEKGB. In the end, we summarize the paper and propose future work in Sect. 7.

2 Related Work

We investigate several knowledge graph building frameworks in health domain, such as cTAKES, pMineR, I-KAT and RDR. According to the three most important aspects to build disease-specific knowledge graphs in the introduction, the related works will be compared from 3 aspects, data sources, building tools adopted and the help from experts (Table 1).

In general, pMineR supports Processing Mining for clinical data from both administrative and clinical aspect. It provides automatically identification services for process discovery [4] and is currently exploited in Hospitals for supporting domain

Table 1. Comparisons of building frameworks.

Name	Data Sources	Building Tools						The help from experts	Extensibility
		Entity extraction	Relation extraction	Event Extraction	Entity alignment	ER/OWL mapping	Human		
cTAKES	UMLS	√	√		√			√	
pMineR	EMRs,...			√					
I-KAT	SNOMED CT,...					√	√	√	√
RDR							√		
DEKGB	UMLS, EMRs,...	√	√	√	√	√	√	√	√

experts in the analysis of the extracted knowledge models. cTAKES [5] is an open-source Natural Language Processing (NLP) system that extracts clinical information from EMRs. I-KAT provides a user-friendly environment to create Arden Syntax MLM (Medical Logic Module) as shareable knowledge rules for intelligent decision-making by CDSS [6].

2.1 Data Sources of Frameworks

The building frameworks listed above have different data sources. For example, cTAKES and I-KAT collect data from medical databases like UMLS, SNOMED CT and so on, while pMineR gathers data from open source EMRs. In general, the data sources of building frameworks in medical domain are mainly from public resources, including medical standards and clinical records.

2.2 Building Tools of Frameworks

Different frameworks adopt different measures to process massive medical knowledge or clinical data, on the purpose of meeting multiple requirements. The building tools listed above show the differences of building health knowledge graphs.

pMineR can encode clinical events by extracting processes under the form of directed graphs, which can calculate the real model of the processes. It also provides graphical comparison tool between different processes, allows doctors to model the adherence to a given clinical guidelines and to estimate performance together with the workload of the available resources in health care. cTAKES offers Natural Language Processing tools like annotation system to extract entities and relations from EMRs. I-KAT creates a knowledge base from MLMs using Arden Syntax to achieve share-ability, uses standard data models and terminologies to enhance interoperability, and reduces complexity by abstraction at the application layer to provide physician friendliness.

In DEKGB, multiple tools are adopted to construct the disease-specific knowledge graphs, including entity, relation and event extraction tool, normalization tool, ER-OWL mapping tool and doctor-involved tools. The tools we adopt support better knowledge extraction and knowledge graph construction.

2.3 The Help from Doctors

Experts offer their prior knowledge and demands to construct health knowledge graphs for different usages and applications. cTAKES offers the creation of a personalized dictionary from UMLS according to experts' demands, to process clinical notes and identify types of clinical named entities - drugs, diseases/disorders, signs/symptoms, anatomical sites and procedures; while I-KAT provides a user-friendly platform for doctors to create knowledge bases based on their prior knowledge and use standard syntax to share the knowledge.

DEKGB supports doctors to input personalized prior knowledge. At the same time, public medical standards will also be involved, to construct a disease-specific CKG, meeting experts' demands and covering comprehensive medical knowledge simultaneously. DEKGB also allows experts to propose extraction rules on professional medical records to form instance knowledge graphs that can exploit in-depth medical knowledge and their associations. What's more, for both CKG and IKG, DEKGB offers tools for experts setting different mapping rules to convert structured data to triples in knowledge graphs.

3 Framework of DEKGB

In this section, we will present the framework of DEKGB. The framework includes framework architecture and work flow of DEKGB in detail.

3.1 Architecture of DEKGB

DEKGB can build a disease-specific knowledge graph or can be applied to an existing disease-specific knowledge graph to extend the single disease to other diseases, such as extending from cardiovascular diseases to diabetes mellitus. It is suitable for expanding to all diseases incrementally. As shown in Fig. 1, based on the existing medical thesaurus, EMRs from hospitals in a specific disease and doctors in the study of that disease, the construction of a disease-specific knowledge graph could be implemented.

The building process of knowledge graphs using DEKGB can be divided into two modules:

1. CKG Building Module: construction of concept knowledge graphs from doctors' prior knowledge and medical standards like UMLS.
2. IKG Building Module: extraction of entities and relations from EMRs and fusion of concept nodes and instance nodes.

Specifically, DEKGB introduces doctor-involved tools into building modules, including doctor input tool, rule base tool and doctor annotation tool.

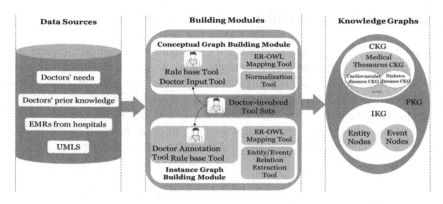

Fig. 1. The framework of DEKGB.

3.2   Work Flow

As shown in Fig. 2, three main problems that DEKGB needs to solve are data sources, building modules and the help from doctors.

The data sources of DEKGB are (1) EMRs from disease-specific Hospital: clinical data from professional hospitals specialized in a specific disease, (2) doctors in related diseases: leading doctors in the study of the specific disease and (3) medical thesaurus containing different medical standards like UMLS. To involve the doctors in DEKGB, we propose doctor-involved tools: doctor input tool, doctor annotation tool and rule base tool. Doctor input tool and rule base tool are used in the construction of CKG while doctor annotation tool and rule base tool are applied to build IKG. For building modules, the construction of CKG is based on doctors' prior knowledge and medical thesaurus and this module contains normalization tool, ER-OWL tool and doctor-involved tools. Meanwhile the building modules of IKG are divided into structured data conversion module (from ER model to RDF model) and unstructured data conversion module (extraction of entities, relationships and events). And the construction of IKG is based on EMRs from hospitals, extraction tools and doctor-involved tools. Finally, for different possible usages, DEKGB generates CKG and IKG.

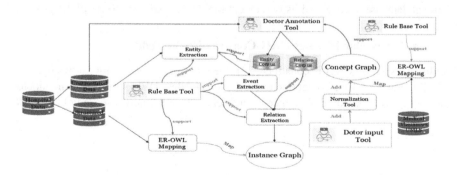

Fig. 2. The data sources and building workflow of DEKGB.

4   Building CKG for Cardiovascular Diseases

Conceptual knowledge graph integrates medical standards from medical thesaurus like UMLS and doctors' prior knowledge from the doctor input tool. Two steps are contained in the conceptual graph building module. The first step is the construction of medical thesaurus CKG and it will be conducted when DEKGB is firstly applied to construct a disease-specific knowledge graph. The second step is the construction of a disease-specific CKG when a new disease is going to be included in existing CKG. Here we take building CKG for cardiovascular diseases as an example (Fig. 3).

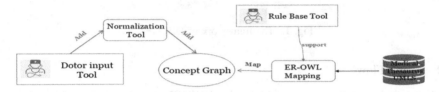

Fig. 3. Conceptual graph building module.

4.1   Medical Thesaurus CKG Construction Procedure

In DEKGB, the data source of Medical thesaurus CKG is UMLS. UMLS is the abbreviation of Unified Medical Language System, a set of files and software that brings together many health-related standards. The medical knowledge in ULMS is stored in ER databases. Hence, medical knowledge in UMLS needs to be mapped to nodes in CKG. For user-friendly purpose, DEKGB provides a mapping rule tool for doctors to decide the mapping format. The generated mapping rules in rule base is applied to convert the data from ER database to RDF graphs [7]. In specific, doctors set rules indicating which column (in ER databases) should convert to which concept node (in knowledge graphs).

At present, the conversion from ER to RDF includes direct mapping and custom mapping. Here we adopt a custom mapping method to better meet doctors' needs. The standards and tools that support this method are as follows: R2RML, Virtuoso, etc. In DEKGB, we use R2RML, a standard transformation language of converting a relational database to RDF and its implement tool D2R is adopted to fulfill the process.

4.2   Cardiovascular Diseases CKG Construction Procedure

The disease-specific CKG is constructed on the basis of doctors' prior knowledge and medical thesaurus CKG. To get doctors' prior knowledge, DEKGB provides the doctor input tool for doctors to define concepts and relations in the new disease field and add them into CKG. Here we take cardiovascular diseases for example. The steps to construct cardiovascular diseases CKG are as follows.

1. A group of doctors in cardiovascular diseases are invited to offer crucial medical knowledge through doctor input tool. The prior knowledge from doctors contains medical entities, relations and triples, which may be useful for diagnosis or other actual usage.
2. The knowledge from doctors are put into normalization tool. The process of normalization is divided into two kinds, depending on whether the concepts, relations or triples offered by doctors exist in medical thesaurus CKG or not. If the knowledge does not exist, it will be inserted into medical thesaurus CKG according to the encoding system of UMLS. Otherwise, standard medical knowledge encodes by UMLS will be used. Notice that for efficiency, the standard encoding is merely an attribute of the Disease-specific CKG nodes.

Hence, a comprehensive medical thesaurus spanning all kinds of diseases can be constructed incrementally. What's more, despite a universal medical thesaurus CKG, small scale of disease-specific conceptual knowledge graphs will be constructed individually, with which doctors' actual needs can be satisfied. Table 2 shows different normalization formats for different kinds of doctors' prior knowledge after knowledge normalization in cardiovascular diseases.

Table 2. Knowledge normalization in cardiovascular diseases.

Prior Knowledge	In medical thesaurus CKG or not	CUI (concept unique identifier)	LAT (language type)	...	AUI (atom unique identifier, may be various)	SAB (Source Abbreviation, may be various)	STR
unstable angina	√	C0002965	ENG	...	A22810054 A18571195 ...	SNOMEDCT_US CHV ...	Unstable angina
acute cerebral infarction	×	C010523	ENG	...	A999010523	Doc-Def	acute cerebral infarction
原发性高血压3 级（极高危）	×	C020379	CHN	...	A999020379	Doc-Def	原发性高血压 3级（极高危）

5   Building IKG for Cardiovascular Diseases

To build the IKG in an assigned disease field effectively, structured clinical data and unstructured clinical data should adopt different conversion procedures. The procedures include: (1) structured data to IKG and (2) unstructured data to IKG. Here we take the building of IKG for cardiovascular diseases for example (Fig. 4).

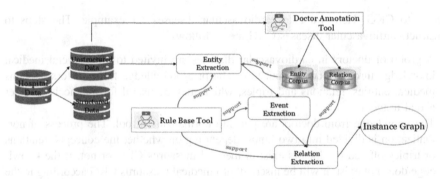

Fig. 4. Instance graph building module.

5.1 Structured Data Conversion Procedure

The main process of structured data transformation is mapping from structured data in ER databases to RDF/OWL instance knowledge graphs, supported by mapping rules from doctors setting through rule base tool. The detailed technology is introduced in the conversion of UMLS to medical thesaurus CKG in Sect. 4.1.

5.2 Unstructured Data Conversion Procedure

The key tools of unstructured data conversion procedure in DEKGB are as follows: entity extraction [8], event extraction and relation extraction shown in Fig. 5. The purpose of this procedure is to extract entities, events and relations in unstructured data and convert them to IKG. In extraction tasks, machine learning-based methods are widely used, but they may be so noisy as to provide many wrong results. So rule-based data integration and extraction approaches are adopted and it has better interpretability and effective interactive debugging [9]. Hence, for better extraction performance and the ability to process massive EMR data, DEKGB provides rule base tool and doctor annotation tool to involve doctors and adopt machine learning-based methods at the same time. Doctor Annotation Tool provides the annotation interface, with which doctors can annotate the unstructured data based on the concepts provided by the CKG. The annotated results will be stored in the entity corpus and relation corpus, used as training set to support entity and relation extractions with machine learning algorithms. The combination of doctors' annotation and machine learning methods can augment the performance of entity and relation extraction [10].

Entity Extraction Tool. The entity extraction tool in DEKGB is based on the sequence annotation method and the rule-based method. To implement the methods, rule base tool and entity corpus are adopted to support it (Table 3).

Sequence Annotation Method. Based on sequence annotation method, entities and relations can be extracted, and used as training set for machine learning method to extract entities and relations in a larger data set. Comparing the results and efficiency among different models, we use LSTM-CRF and CRF in our method [11, 12]. Here is an example of annotation-based entity extraction in cardiovascular diseases:

Table 3. Annotation-based entity extraction in cardiovascular diseases.

Input:
When the patient got up in a morning 1 week ago, he had **chest pain** with no obvious inducement, located in the **precordial region, radiating** to left **shoulder** and left **elbow joint,** accompanied by **sweating** and **palpitations**....
Output:
<chest pain, CUI, C0008031 >
<precordial region, CUI, C0230134>
<radiating, CUI, C0332301>
<shoulder, CUI, C0037004 >
<elbow joint, CUI, C0013770 >
<sweating, CUI, C0038990>
<palpitation, CUI, C0030252>

Pattern-Based Entity Extraction. Pattern-based entity extraction [13] can extract entity and relation at the same time, which will be described in relation extraction.

Relation Extraction. The relation extraction is composed of two parts: pattern-based module and supervised learning method-based module [14].

Pattern-based method consists of two steps: (1) recognition of medical entities and (2) identification of the correct semantic relation between each pair of entities. In DEKGB, patterns are defined by doctors in the rule base. For example, many EMRs in inpatient medical records have patterns like "The patient has symptoms such as ***" and "The patient was admitted because of ***". Such patterns can be applied to entity extraction and relation extraction. At the meantime, supervised learning method is adopted, which would improve the accuracy when data scale is larger (Table 4).

Here is an example of pattern extraction using DEKGB in cardiovascular diseases:

Table 4. Pattern extraction in cardiovascular diseases.

Input:
The patient had chest tightness after a physical activity 4 years ago, no chest pain, no abdominal pain or diarrhea, no nausea or vomiting, and was diagnosed as "coronary heart disease" in the local hospital. ....
PATTERN1: The patient/ He / She had + * (may split by ',') + after+ *
Output Entity:
{chest tightness}: C0232292, {physical activity}: C0026606
Output Relation:
Patient<has>chest tightness, chest tightness <after>activity
PATTERN2: no +*+ or + * + , (split by ',')
Output Entity:
{chest pain}: C0008031, {abdominal pain}: C0000737......
Output Relation:
Patient<no>chest pain, Patient<no>abdominal pain......

6   Extension to Include a New Disease

In addition to building disease-specific knowledge graphs, DEKGB is also extensible to include new diseases into current knowledge graphs. Except for the input of EMRs and doctors' prior knowledge in another disease, the building tools and the input of medical thesaurus can be reused. Hence, workload of building health knowledge graphs for a specific disease will be reduced and a health knowledge graph covering different kinds of diseases can be constructed incrementally. For example, when DEKGB is going to include diabetes mellitus into the existing cardiovascular diseases knowledge graph, the following steps need to be implemented:

Firstly, DEKGB needs EMRs and doctors specialized in diabetes mellitus. Specifically, doctors need to provide their prior knowledge from three aspects:

(1) Diabetes mellitus related concepts, relations and RDF triples, and Table 5 presents an example from doctors in C2 hospital;

Table 5. Concepts, relations and triples in diabetes mellitus.

	Doctors' Prior Knowledge
Concepts	Insulin-dependent diabetes mellitus、 Hyperglycemia、 Mumps virus、 Coronary heart disease、 Neuropathy、 Polyphagia、 Polyuria、 Polydipsia、 Insulin、 Vomit......
Relations	Has_sign_or_symptom、 Associated_disease、 Cause_of、 Diagnosed_by......
Triples	<Insulin-dependent diabetes mellitus, Cause_of, Hyperglycemia>; <Insulin-dependent diabetes mellitus, Associated_disease, Neuropathy>; <Insulin-dependent diabetes mellitus, Has_sign_or_symptom, Polyphagia>......

(2) Mapping rules from ER to RDF based on the structured data in EMRs;
(3) Entity and relation extraction rules based on the features of unstructured data in EMRs. Table 6 shows an example.

Comparing to cardiovascular diseases, the extraction patterns of diabetes mellitus have their own features, which also proves the necessity of doctors.

Secondly, CKG of diabetes mellitus will be constructed. After getting prior knowledge from doctors through doctor input tool, the concepts, relations and triples will be put into normalization tool for standardization, based on the existing medical thesaurus CKG. Afterwards, the CKG of diabetes mellitus will be implemented. Figure 5 shows a part of CKG of diabetes mellitus based on prior knowledge from doctors after the normalization process.

Finally, IKG of diabetes mellitus will be built. In this process, doctors firstly need to annotate the unstructured data based on the CKG and EMRs in diabetes mellitus. Then machine learning methods are adopted to process massive EMR data and generate entity and relation corpus. Afterwards, on the basis of extraction rules in rule base and automatic extraction methods, the medical knowledge in EMRs of diabetes mellitus will be extracted. Hence, the IKG of diabetes mellitus can be implemented.

Table 6. Pattern extraction in diabetes mellitus.

Input: The patient has found to have hyperglycemia for more than 3 years. ...... The patient was admitted in our department with "diabetes mellitus ". Since onset, the patient has polydipsia, polyphagia, polyuria and 3 kg loss in body weight.
PATTERN1: The patient/ He / She had symptoms such as + *, (split by ',') Output Entity: 　　{headache}: Concept node: C0018681 　　{dizziness}: Concept node: C0012833/ C0220870/C0012833 /C0149746 　　{thirst}: Concept node: C0039971 Output Relation: 　Patient<has>headache 　Patient<has>dizziness 　Patient<has>thirst
PATTERN2: Since onset, the patient has +*+ (split by ',') Output Entity: 　　{polydipsia}: Concept node: C0085602 　　{polyphagia}: Concept node: C0020505 　　{polyuria}: Concept node: C0032617 　　{body weight}: Concept node: C0005910

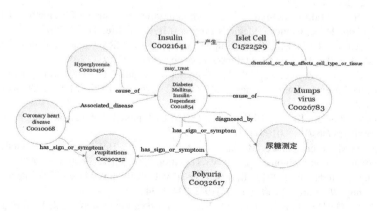

Fig. 5. CKG of diabetes mellitus.

7 Conclusion and Future Work

In this paper, we propose a disease-specific and extensible knowledge graph building framework named DEKGB. This framework can be used to construct a disease-specific knowledge graph or applied to extend the current health knowledge graph to include a new disease based on medical standards, doctors' prior knowledge and EMRs from a professional hospital. In order to augment the accuracy of knowledge and provide a user-friendlier application, we adopt doctor-involved tools in DEKGB.

In the future, we will gradually involve more medical knowledge from multiple international medical standards and from other channels other than hospitals, to enrich the knowledge graphs built by DEKGB and we will refine the tools we adopt to better fit the actual needs and augment the efficiency and accuracy.

Acknowledgements. This work was supported by NSFC (91646202), National Key R&D Program of China (2018YFB1404400, 2018YFB1402700).

References

1. Ehrlinger, L., Wöß, W.: Towards a definition of knowledge graphs. In: SEMANTiCS (Posters, Demos, SuCCESS) (2016)
2. Nickel, M., Murphy, K., Tresp, V., Gabrilovich, E.: A review of relational machine learning for knowledge graphs: from multi-relational link prediction to automated knowledge graph construction. CoRR abs/1503.00759 (2015)
3. Huang, Z., Yang, J., van Harmelen, F., Hu, Q.: Constructing disease-centric knowledge graphs: a case study for depression (short version). In: ten Teije, A., Popow, C., Holmes, John H., Sacchi, L. (eds.) AIME 2017. LNCS (LNAI), vol. 10259, pp. 48–52. Springer, Cham (2017). https://doi.org/10.1007/978-3-319-59758-4_5
4. Gatta, R., et al.: Generating and comparing knowledge graphs of medical processes using pMineR. In: Corcho, Ó., et al. (eds.) K-CAP, pp. 36:1–36:4. ACM (2017)
5. Savova, G.K., et al.: Mayo clinical text analysis and knowledge extraction system (cTAKES): architecture, component evaluation and applications. J. Am. Med. Inform. Assoc. **17**(5), 507–513 (2010)
6. Ali, T., et al.: Multi-model-based interactive authoring environment for creating shareable medical knowledge. Comput. Methods Programs Biomed. **150**, 41–72 (2017)
7. Unbehauen, J., Martin, M.: SPARQL update queries over R2RML mapped data sources. In: Eibl, M., Gaedke, M. (eds.) GI-Jahrestagung, pp. 1891–1901. GI (2017)
8. Zhang, Z., Tong, Z., Yu, Z., Yali, P.: Attention-based deep residual learning network for entity relation extraction in Chinese EMRs. BMC Med. Inf. Decis. Making **19–S**(2), 171–177 (2019)
9. Huang, Z., Wei, X., Kai, Y.: Bidirectional LSTM-CRF models for sequence tagging (2015). http://arxiv.org/abs/1508.01991
10. Yimam, S.M., Biemann, C., Majnaric, L., Šabanović, Š., Holzinger, A.: Interactive and iterative annotation for biomedical entity recognition. In: Guo, Y., Friston, K., Aldo, F., Hill, S., Peng, H. (eds.) BIH 2015. LNCS (LNAI), vol. 9250, pp. 347–357. Springer, Cham (2015). https://doi.org/10.1007/978-3-319-23344-4_34
11. Fan, J., Li, G.: Human-in-the-loop rule learning for data integration. IEEE Data Eng. Bull. **41**(2), 104–115 (2018)
12. Lample, G. Ballesteros, M., Subramanian, S., Kawakami, K., Dyer, C.: Neural architectures for named entity recognition. CoRR abs/1603.01360 (2016)
13. Chen, C., Liu, H., Wang, G., Ding, L., Yu, L.: Entity relationship extraction based on potential relationship pattern. In: Wang, F.L., Gong, Z., Luo, X., Lei, J. (eds.) WISM 2010. LNCS, vol. 6318, pp. 370–377. Springer, Heidelberg (2010). https://doi.org/10.1007/978-3-642-16515-3_46
14. Qu, M., Xiang, R., Yu, Z., Jiawei, H.: Weakly-supervised relation extraction by pattern-enhanced embedding learning. In: Champin, P.-A., et al. (eds.) WWW, pp. 1257–1266. ACM (2018)

Research on Three-Dimensional Reconstruction of Brain Image Features Based on Augmented Reality Technology

Long Lu[✉] and Wang Zhao

School of Information Management, Wuhan University, Wuhan, China
bioinfo@gmail.com, 199223263@qq.com

Abstract. With the application of artificial intelligence technology, automatic recognition of brain image features has reached the stage of application. At present, the results of automatic recognition and labeling of brain images are displayed in two-dimensional form, which is not easy for doctors to observe intuitively. In addition, in the real medical environment, it is necessary to combine the virtual and the real, and to display some additional information in the real environment. Augmented reality can meet the above practical business needs. This paper studies the process of feature extraction and three-dimensional reconstruction of brain image diseases, designs the function module of augmented reality, explores the application of augmented reality in three-dimensional reconstruction, and realizes the three-dimensional reconstruction and visualization of brain image features by programming with Unity tool.

Keywords: Augmented reality · Three-dimensional reconstruction · Unity · Visualization

1 Introduction

The rise of three-dimensional reconstruction technology was first proposed by Idesawa [1] in 1973. Hartley [2] and Faugras [3] described the complete reconstruction theory in 1992, which indicates that the three-dimensional reconstruction technology is beginning to mature and brings opportunities for the practical application of three-dimensional reconstruction technology in various fields. Three-dimensional reconstruction of medical images refers to the transformation of two-dimensional tomographic image sequences, such as ultrasound, CT, MRI, tissue and electron microscopy, into three-dimensional images with intuitive stereoscopic effect by means of computer image processing technology, showing the three-dimensional shape and spatial relationship of three-dimensional structures [4]. Three-dimensional reconstruction technology not only provides a complete three-dimensional model, but also interacts with three-dimensional images such as enlargement, reduction, rotation and contrast. It helps doctors to observe the region of interest in detail from multi-level and multi-directional perspectives. These new imaging technologies will continue to make up for the shortcomings of traditional diagnostic methods [5], thus greatly improving the efficiency and accuracy of doctor's diagnosis.

© Springer Nature Switzerland AG 2019
H. Chen et al. (Eds.): ICSH 2019, LNCS 11924, pp. 39–47, 2019.
https://doi.org/10.1007/978-3-030-34482-5_4

Brain is the control center of human body, its pathological changes will cause serious consequences for patients. At the same time, the brain is not suitable for invasive examination. Therefore, medical imaging plays an important role in the early diagnosis of common brain diseases. At present, the research progress of automatic recognition of brain image features is rapid, but the results of automatic recognition and marking of a large number of discrete two-dimensional brain images are not intuitive, which affects doctors' observation and understanding of the disease features of brain images. Three-dimensional reconstruction and augmented reality technology play an important role in providing diagnostic information for doctors, making up for the subjectivity and limitations of artificial diagnosis, and improving the accuracy of surgery. Therefore, how to scientifically and effectively process the recognition results of various brain image diseases, and how to carry out the three-dimensional reconstruction and visualization interaction of brain images, has become the current research hotspot.

Jie proposed the texture features of brain CT images and the three-dimensional reconstruction method [6]. Hou studied the precise segmentation and three-dimensional reconstruction of brain tumors [7]. Domestic scholars use relatively old tools for three-dimensional reconstruction of the brain, they do not use some of the latest technology, there is no realistic visualization effect. At present, doctors urgently need to increase the function of user interaction after three-dimensional reconstruction. They need better visual and simulation effects to improve user experience and practical application effect.

The innovation of this paper is to study the three-dimensional reconstruction and visualization methods of brain image disease characteristics from the perspective of visual human-computer interaction, combining image segmentation, image three-dimensional reconstruction, visual human-computer interaction and other theoretical methods. In addition, a software for three-dimensional reconstruction and visualization of brain image disease features is designed and developed by using augmented reality technology.

2   Feature Extraction and Three-Dimensional Reconstruction of Brain Imaging Diseases

Data processing and three-dimensional reconstruction process includes two processes, forming three files. The first process includes the processing of DICOM files of brain images, including data preprocessing, feature extraction, feature classification and feature marking. The second process includes the reconstruction of brain image features and 3D rendering. The original DICOM image file is processed by the first process and converted into a feature tag file. After the second process, the feature tag file is transformed into a 3D model file. Data processing and three-dimensional reconstruction are shown in Fig. 1.

Finally, using 3D model file and augmented reality tools, we can reconstruct the three-dimensional brain and display disease features in the three-dimensional model.

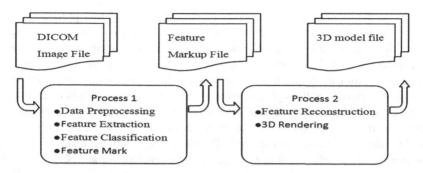

Fig. 1. Data processing and three-dimensional reconstruction

2.1　Feature Extraction of Brain Imaging Diseases

With the development of medical imaging technology, the technology of using computer technology to detect brain structural changes from MRI images to assist early diagnosis and treatment of diseases has been in the practical stage. The steps of feature extraction for brain imaging diseases are shown in Fig. 2.

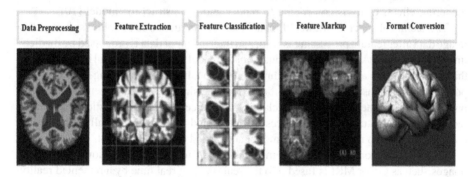

Fig. 2. Feature extraction procedures of brain imaging diseases

Because the results of feature extraction of brain image diseases are still stored in DICOM data format, it is necessary to use medical image development toolkit to transform the format, so as to carry out three-dimensional reconstruction in the next research.

2.2　Three-Dimensional Reconstruction of Brain Image

The existing research methods of three-dimensional reconstruction of medical images are mainly realized by ITK + VTK. It mainly deals with medical image data in DICOM format, recognizes the boundary of two-dimensional medical image, and redraws the three-dimensional image of tissue or organ. At present, three-dimensional reconstruction methods of medical images can be divided into three categories according to the different data description methods in the rendering process: surface rendering method, volume rendering method, and hybrid rendering method combining the two [8]. Among them, the basic idea of surface rendering method is to recognize and segment the boundary from a series of two-dimensional image data, extract the body surface information, and restore the object's three-dimensional model by using the rendering algorithm through illumination, shading, texture mapping and other algorithms. For example, contour reconstruction method based on fault boundary, Cuerille algorithm based on voxel isosurface reconstruction, Marching Cubes algorithm, Dividing Cubes algorithm, etc. [9]. The main idea of volume rendering method is not to produce isosurface, but to give each voxel a certain color and photoresistivity to project volume data directly to the image plane as a whole. For example, Ray-Casting algorithm in order of image space, Splatting algorithm in order of object space, Shear-Warp algorithm and so on. Surface rendering algorithm is superior to volume rendering algorithm in computational efficiency and real-time interactivity. The algorithm is simple and occupies less memory resources, but the image details are lost. Volume rendering algorithm contains more detailed information than surface rendering algorithm. Volume rendering algorithm is preferred because of the need for rich detail information in this study.

There are many tools in three-dimensional image rendering, such as OpenGL, Direct3D, Unity and so on. After considering the supporting format, rendering time and rendering effect, Unity is considered to render and reconstruct the model [10].

The technical scheme of three-dimensional reconstruction is as follows: firstly, the image data after feature processing is read, and then the input data is processed by medical image development kit ITK and VTK into. obj format of three-dimensional image data, so that it can be used as input data of three-dimensional image processing API Unity to preliminarily reconstruct the whole brain image using the three-dimensional image processing API. The next step is to classify and screen the characteristic brain slices, reconstruct the features of these slices in detail, and mark them. Finally, the texture mapping and stereo rendering of the model are carried out by Unity [11].

The virtual model obtained from three-dimensional reconstruction of medical images such as CT or MRI is fused into the real scene in real time by augmented reality technology. The doctor's visual system is enhanced, and the internal information of organs that can not be seen by the naked eye can be seen. At the same time, the accurate spatial information of organs relative to the patient's body can be obtained [12].

3 Augmented Reality Technology and its Function Modules

Augmented Reality (AR) is the latest visualization technology. It develops from virtual reality [13]. It superimposes the virtual world constructed by computers in the real world, strengthens users' understanding of reality, and increases various additional information of the real world.

Augmented reality, as the latest visualization technology and method, mainly exists in the form of system function module, and there is data exchange between it and resource database. The function modules of augmented reality system are shown in Fig. 3.

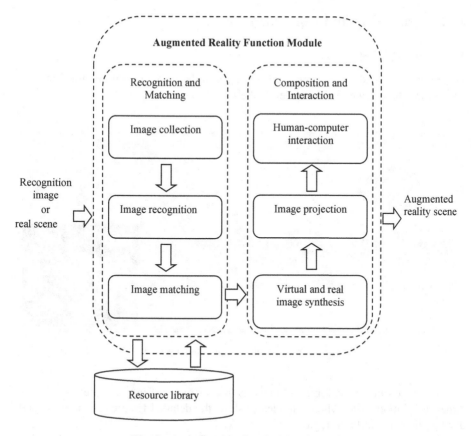

Fig. 3. Augmented reality function module

The functional modules of augmented reality system include recognition and matching program and synthesis and interaction program. The recognition and matching program includes three parts: image acquisition, image recognition and image matching. The image acquisition program mainly collects effective recognition images or scene maps, and provides them to image recognition programs for feature extraction. The recognition features are transmitted to image matching programs. The image matching programs retrieve the identical or similar resources from the repository according to the recognition features, and at the same time provide these resources to the synthesis and interaction programs. The synthesis and interaction program includes three parts: virtual and real image synthesis, image projection and human-computer interaction. Firstly, virtual and real image synthesis reads the image or knowledge that needs to be displayed in the resource database, and then fuses the image or knowledge with the real scene to form the target image. Through the image projection program, the target image is projected on the display device to form an augmented reality scene. Doctors and other users can perform various operations through human-computer interaction programs.

Augmented reality function module has good expansibility and stability. Augmented reality module can be used as standard modules for different medical systems or mobile devices.

4 Programming and Core Algorithms

4.1 Program Design

The software is made with Unity tool. Figure 4 is the development environment and loading the three-dimensional model of the brain.

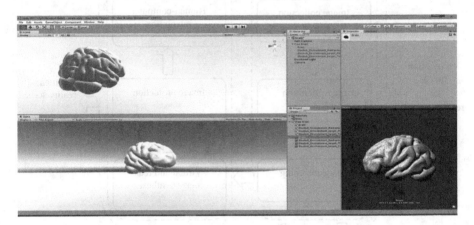

Fig. 4. Loading three-dimensional model

The three-dimensional brain model is reconstructed from the previous three-dimensional model file, which can clearly show the detailed features of the brain and display the relevant brain regions.

Figure 5 is the loading material for the model. Different materials can be selected to adjust the visual effect. The material can display information of brain area or the location of disease.

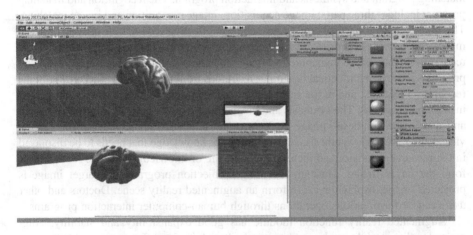

Fig. 5. Loading model material

Figure 6 is a program interface. The three-dimensional model of the brain can be controlled by mouse, including zooming, zooming and moving. Clicking on the brain can display the corresponding two-dimensional disease feature image file, which is convenient for doctors to observe from two-dimensional or three-dimensional perspective.

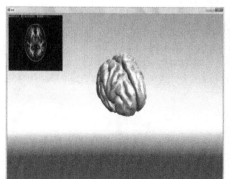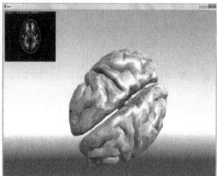

Fig. 6. Program interface

4.2 Core Algorithm

- Controlling Three-Dimensional Brain Model
  The human-computer interaction code for the three-dimensional brain model is as follows:

```
using System.Collections;
using System.Collections.Generic;
using UnityEngine;
public class braincontrol : MonoBehaviour
{   public float rotateSpeed = 10;
  private void RotateAndLookForward()
  {
    if (Input.GetMouseButton(0))
    { GetMouseXY();
  this.transform.RotateAround(targetTF.position,        Vec-
tor3.up, horizontal);
    this.transform.RotateAround(targetTF.position,        Vec-
tor3.right, -vertical);
    }
  }
}
```

- Augmented Reality Image Recognition

  Recognition image is the basic function of augmented reality. The algorithm is as follows:

```
Mat H12;
H12 = findHomography( Mat(points1), Mat(points2),
CV_RANSAC, ransacReprojThreshold );
vector<char> matchesMask( matches.size(), 0 );
Mat points1t;
perspectiveTransform(Mat(points1), points1t, H12);
for( size_t i1 = 0; i1 < points1.size(); i1++ )
    {                   if(          norm(points2[i1]          -
points1t.at<Point2f>((int)i1,0)) <= ransacReprojThreshold
)
    matchesMask[i1] = 1;
}
drawMatches(obj,obj_keypoints,scene,scene_keypoints,
matches,match_img2,matchesMas);
perspectiveTransform( obj_corners, scene_corners, H12);
```

5 Testing and Application

5.1 System Testing

This paper chooses personal computers and servers, as well as two different systems of mobile phones as the test environment, hardware and software environment as shown in Table 1.

Table 1. Testing environment

Testing equipment	Hardware environment	Software environment
OPPO R17 Mobile Phone	CPU: SDM670 RAM: 8 GB	Android
IPhone 8 Mobile Phone	CPU: A11 RAM: 2 GB	iOS
Personal Computer	CPU: Intel i7 RAM: 16 GB	Windows 10
Server	CPU: Intel W2133 RAM: 16 GB	Windows Server 2019

After testing, the response time of the software meets the requirements, the display effect is normal in different devices, and the user interaction experience is better.

5.2 Application Environment

Because the development tool Unity can release software versions suitable for different application environments, the software can be used in personal computers, servers, mobile phones and other devices, and has the advantages of cross-platform application and good stability.

6   Conclusion

Because of its practicability, augmented reality has important value in three-dimensional reconstruction of brain image features. In this paper, a three-dimensional brain reconstruction program based on augmented reality is preliminarily implemented. It also needs to be tested and applied in actual scenes, and the function of the program is improved and increased to solve the problem of displaying a large amount of medical information and data. Augmented reality technology can be used to visualize various medical knowledge. This paper will continue to study the application scenarios of augmented reality in the process of hospital information construction, promote the effect of medical information display and improve the effect of user experience.

Acknowledgements. This research has been possible thanks to the support of projects: National Natural Science Foundation of China (No. 61772375) and Independent Research Project of School of Information Management Wuhan University (No: 413100032).

References

1. Idesawa, M.A.: System to generate a solid figure from three view. Bull. JSME **16**(2), 216–225 (1973)
2. Hartley, R.I.: Estimation of relative camera positions for uncalibrated cameras. In: Sandini, G. (ed.) ECCV 1992. LNCS, vol. 588, pp. 579–587. Springer, Heidelberg (1992). https://doi.org/10.1007/3-540-55426-2_62
3. Faugeras, O.D.: What can be seen in three dimensions with an uncalibrated stereo rig? In: Sandini, G. (ed.) ECCV 1992. LNCS, vol. 588, pp. 563–578. Springer, Heidelberg (1992). https://doi.org/10.1007/3-540-55426-2_61
4. Rodriguez, J.A., Xu, R., Chen, C.C., et al.: Three-dimensional coherent X-ray diffractive imaging of whole frozen-hydrated cells. IUCrJ **2**(Pt 5), 575–583 (2015)
5. Wang, Y., Du, X., Zhao, S., et al.: Medical Image Processing, pp. 169–202. Tsinghua University Press, Beijing (2012)
6. Jie, Z., Gong, S., Long, W.: Three-dimensional reconstruction and texture characteristics of brain CT images. Laser Mag. **35**(06), 62–65 (2014)
7. Hou, D., Lu, Y., Wang, Y., Liu, W.: Segmentation and three-dimensional reconstruction of brain tumors on MRI. J. Appl. Sci. **36**(05), 808–818 (2018)
8. Wang, R., Zhang, J., Peng, K.: Algorithmic analysis of three-dimensional reconstruction of computer-aided medical images. Tissue Eng. Res. Clin. Rehabil. China **15**(04), 745–748 (2011)
9. Ping, X., Yun, Y.: Fast three-dimensional surface reconstruction algorithm based on isosurface points. Microcomput. Inf. **26**(14), 6–7 + 14 (2010)
10. Yuan, Y.: Research on three-dimensional reconstruction technology in augmented reality environment. University of Electronic Science and Technology (2009)
11. Li, C., Liu, S.: Brief analysis of several ways of introducing three-dimensional model formats into unity 3D. New Chin. Technol. Prod. **5**, 23–24 (2016)
12. Niu, Y.: Augmented Reality Technology in Surgical Navigation. Zhejiang University (2004)
13. Li, Q., Zhang, L.: An empirical study of mobile learning based on augmented reality. Audiov. Educ. China **01**, 116–120 (2013)

Towards an E-health Ecosystem for China

Xiangzhu Gao and Jun Xu[✉]

Southern Cross University, Lismore, NSW 2480, Australia
jun.xu@scu.edu.au

Abstract. E-health plays vital roles in tackling the challenges to China's healthcare system and providing opportunities for its development in a sustainable way, aiming at equal access to affordable and consumer-centric medical service and customized personal care and wellbeing. For these aims, the authors propose an e-health ecosystem based on an analysis of challenges that the Chinese healthcare is facing, and current status of e-health market in China. The outcome of the research is a conceptual framework for the ecosystem, which will assist Chinese government in making decisions on the Internet+ healthcare; healthcare professionals in establishing e-health system standards; and industry vendors in seeking opportunities in China's e-health market.

Keywords: Health system · E-health · Consumer needs · China · Ecosystem

1 Introduction

Digital technologies are impacting the wellbeing and economic growth worldwide [1]. The past decade has seen rapid development and adoption of technologies that change the way people live and will have a similarly transformative impact on health and care [2]. The Chinese government's Internet+ blueprint released in March 2015 offers a comprehensive assessment of China's digital capabilities [3]. The healthcare industry in China is experiencing a period of high-speed development, and e-health solutions are experiencing exponential growth [4]. However, these solutions are mainly developed by local technical companies based on their technical strengths, and the development is isolated from each other [5]. These task-specific solutions are not interactive and cannot be easily integrated with other existing healthcare services. Also the solutions developed in one environment do not work in a different environment [6].

The emerging markets are unlikely to adopt the traditional e-health models, and new e-health models will play a pivotal role in overcoming many of the challenges to the traditional models [7]. The authors propose an e-health ecosystem for sustainable growth of healthcare in China. In a guide for establishing holistic digital health ecosystems, SPDA [1] recommends that there is no one-size-fits-all solution for e-health, and establishment of a national digital health ecosystem should be based on an integrated framework appropriate for the health system, technologies and especially the healthcare consumers of the nation. Digital health information lays the foundation of new health models and associates other components [7]. In this research, the authors focus on a framework of the healthcare ecosystem, in which healthcare services or

H. Chen et al. (Eds.): ICSH 2019, LNCS 11924, pp. 48–60, 2019.
https://doi.org/10.1007/978-3-030-34482-5_5

solutions interoperate with others via health data interaction while engaging healthcare consumers or individuals.

Global experience suggests that a focused approach that delivers early benefits to core actor groups is essential. An e-health ecosystem should be built on low-hanging fruits and early benefits for healthcare delivery to integrate what is already there [1]. The authors also summarise the benefits for healthcare consumers available from the existing or planned e-health solutions in the Chinese market, analyse their roles in term of addressing the challenges that the Chinese healthcare is facing. The analysis will contribute to a prototype of the ecosystem.

2 Available E-health Solutions

E-health refers the use of the Internet and relevant technologies in healthcare and related fields. E-health encompasses products, systems and services, involving health authorities, professionals and consumers or individuals. China's technology companies, especially the Internet giants including Baidu, Alibaba and Tencent (BAT), are entering the healthcare markets [8] with Artificial Intelligence (AI), E-commerce, Cloud Technology, Mobile Technology, Data Mining, Internet of Things (IoT), etc. [9–12]. The BAT has built strong market positions in e-health industry [10]. The authors investigated e-health solutions based on industry or trade magazines, media news, professional blogs, organisational white papers, and technical solutions accessible on the Web, company websites, and research publications as well. In this section, e-health solutions in the Chinese market are summarised with respect to their supporting Internet technologies.

Local Area Network (LAN) is mainly used by hospitals for Electronic Medical Record (EMR) or Electronic Health Record (EHR) systems [13], which are not accessible and sharable by other organisations, services or devices [14, 15]. The EHR was rarely integrated with delivery of clinical care [16], and a few people know that they have their EHRs [17]. Also the Chinese medical data standards lack support for different data types [18], especially images, which cannot be included in the systems. Source of data in EHR is an issue, as the EHR standard lacks support for easy additions and extensions to various medical domains and organizations [18]. Although EMR focuses on clinical information and EHR focuses on health information, there is an overlap of information between them. Health data and clinical data are often combined to get information for medication, treatment or care plans. In 2011, the Ministry of Health (MOH) began to develop the *Resident Health Card* to link individual's EHR and EMR for cross-institutional and trans-regional data sharing. However, it is not successful, and nationwide data sharing is still far away [19].

Cloud Technology has been applied in healthcare sector mainly for imaging services supported by AI [8]. The main players are Alibaba [20–22], Tencent [23] and collaboration of Philips and Digital Health China [24]. In 2016, Baidu, launched the project of *Baidu Medical Brain* system, which learns from big data by means of AI. Patients can learn more about their health status through online interactions with the system on the Cloud [25].

IoT extends healthcare services outside of medical institutions and provides opportunities for rehabilitation and chronic disease management. Medical Internet of Things (MIoT) have emerged in response to the changing needs and conditions [26]. In the Chinese market, MIoT products collect and analyse user's vitals and other measures, and report the analysis results [27, 28]; and monitor activities and life signs and send the information to doctors or family members [23, 29]. Some MIoT products are developed for rehabilitation [30], healthy lifestyle [31] and assistance for impaired people [32, 33].

Website Platforms mainly apply e-commerce models in outpatient service for performance improvement, cost reduction, customer relationship management, and marketing. Some platforms are click-and-mortar for referral, booking, payment, checking test results, and drug sales [28, 34] while some others are pure online players with limited services of consultation or diagnosis [35–39]. Their common role is to connect the involved stakeholders. Some platforms also provide additional values by including such functions as health information search, access to a health community forum, medical insurance, and drug supervision [28, 40, 41].

Application Software has been developed in China for computers and smart phones. However, most health applications (apps) have failed to generate significant numbers of active users [42]. These apps normally offer opportunities for access to health information and self-diagnosis supported by remote platforms or AI technology based on Big Data [32, 43, 44]. Besides monitoring and tracking purposes, smart phone apps are used for fitness and wellbeing [30, 45].

Blockchain Technology could be the solutions for many problems with the current services of the above technologies. It has been used to address the issue of health data security and information privacy [46–48]. The Peer to Peer (P2P) network of blockchain is appropriate for the MIoT to link the distributed devices. Technical solution providers in China are applying blockchain technologies in the areas such as pharmaceutical logistics for drug traceability, and in medication for prevention of tampered prescription [49–53].

E-health holds tremendous opportunities in China to help improve healthcare [38]. Well-capitalized BAT are providing variety of e-health solutions, which are now growing beyond them [10], although international vendors are seeking opportunities in Chinese e-health market [34]. Many (if not most) e-health solutions are not interactive and have difficulties integrating with other existing healthcare services.

Medical and health data are segregated in data 'islands' of EMR system or EHR system within each hospital or healthcare institution [10]. Data are not consistent between EMR systems as there is not a unified data standard for different vendors, and data in EHR are not accurate as they are not collected in professional ways [17]. Many e-health solutions need and/or generate medical/health data, however they don't share the data with other solutions including EMR and EHR.

The blockchain technology has been applied for health data security and drug traceability. It has great potentials for e-health. Blockchain technology has the potential to transform healthcare [54].

3   E-health Ecosystem for China

In China, e-health is still at its early stage [12]. A few, if any, e-health companies have been successful [44]. Many digital technologies discussed in Sect. 2 are not commonly accepted or used by users [55, 56]. Some main obstacles hinder the e-health in achieving their original goals to provide needed healthcare in cost effective ways equally to all the consumers. These obstacles include: (1) different vendors developed monolithic and proprietary software systems, and many e-health projects do not layout a long-term plan; (2) interoperability of the solutions is poor; and (3) individuals' health information is not shared by different solutions [1, 10, 16].

Xu et al. [57] proposed a Value Added EHR System (VAEHRS) based on their study on Australia's Personally Controlled Electronic Health Record (PCEHR) system, which was not actively accepted by Australian individuals because of its limited benefits for individuals. To increase the benefits or usefulness, the VAEHRS is an integration of e-health solutions based on the PCEHR system, from which health data can be retrieved for information needed by other e-health solutions.

Based on the concepts of the VAEHRS, the authors propose an e-health ecosystem for China, which consists of health services and technologies for the healthcare needs of the consumers and involves multiple stakeholders in healthcare system. Each node of the ecosystem is a module of services enabled by specific technologies on a computer including a smartphone or a device, with which a user accesses the services. A node not only provides services to users but also provides values to other nodes. The basic requirements for the ecosystem are described as follows.

The ecosystem is individual centric for both patients and healthy consumers [58]. To a user, the ecosystem is used as an interconnected environment around an individual [37]. The real force for change in healthcare is the power of the patient or consumer to engage and participate across the continuum of care and the lifespan [37]. Consumers demand personalised services, transforming healthcare from its predominant one-size-fits-all approach to a more customer-centric tailored approach [35]. End users must be central to the design [1]. Personalisation shifts the healthcare focus toward tailored patient engagement [2, 12].

1. The proposed ecosystem should serve the needs of consumers in China and evolve to reflect the needs [37]. A successful product or service that meets the needs of existing consumers will fail if it does not evolve [59]. The ecosystem requires open standards to ensure a plug-and-play architecture, where any modules can be swapped out without affecting the integrity of the ecosystem, and allow e-health services to be built across organisational boundaries [60].
2. The ecosystem is data-driven for interoperability. In a digitising environment, value is data [34]. Data is the flesh and interoperability is the spine of e-health [61]. In the ecosystem, a node is able to find data needed for the services from other nodes, and allow other nodes to share its data with the constraints of meaningful use: agreement on which node needs what data in what format in what situation for what purpose [1, 12]. Data standards, including vocabulary, structures and protocols are determined based on the legacy *Resident Health Records System*, a national database that records the data of common chronic non-communicable diseases and the relevant treatment of individuals [17].

3. The ecosystem is essentially a P2P network. Data mobilisation between nodes of the ecosystem comes with security risks. The blockchain technology is also based on P2P networks and have been used by *Ali Health* [47] and *BlocHIE* [48] to secure health data transmission between different sources. Blockchain technology is an enabler of nationwide interoperability, allowing secured data mobilisation, and addressing the current issues of complexity and trustless collaboration [54].

As quoted in Patientcaresolutions [36], "Data changes everything". The EHR remains a cornerstone [12] in the proposed e-health ecosystem, which enables the changes from providers to consumers, from holistic services to personalised services and from doctors to data, and provides needed healthcare in cost effective ways equally to all the consumers. China has the 'Saudi Arabia of data', providing massive amounts of rich information for new algorithms to experiment with [8]. The ecosystem is sustainable, allowing growth and evolution in terms of size and the combination of physical and virtual innovation [10]. The ecosystem will last throughout an individual user's lifetime.

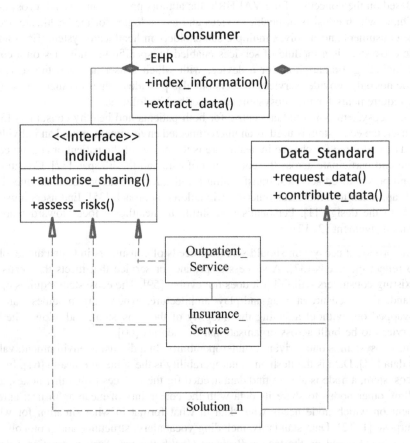

Fig. 1. Class diagram for the concept of the e-health ecosystem

Figure 1 illustrates the structure of a node of the ecosystem in terms of unified modelling language. Compared with the VAEHRS, which is EHR system centric, the ecosystem is consumer centric. In the ecosystem, EHR is the attributes of the conceptual Consumer, and the 'Index Information' and 'Extract Data' become operations of the Consumer. The Consumer is encapsulated with the Interface, where the individual user authorises an e-health service/solution to share data with the assistance of an operation to assess risks to data security and personal privacy. Beside the Interface, the Consumer has another part Data Standard, which all the services and solutions must comply with. A service or solution uses the language determined in the Data Standard to request needed data from, or contribute their generated data to, the Consumer. In practice, one service/solution may be associated with another service/solution, for example there is an association relationship between outpatient service and insurance service.

The success of this ecosystem relies on multiple dimensions involving different stakeholders including government laws, medical and health professional's data standards, medical and social professional's rules of meaningful use, healthcare providers' services, vendors' technical solutions, and especially individuals' acceptance. Section 4 investigates e-health services and solutions for the ecosystem with respect to two non-technical dimensions: their potentials to address the issues in Chinese healthcare system and user acceptance in practice.

4 Services and Solutions for the Ecosystem

Technologies continues to innovate at great speeds with enormous potential to change the Chinese healthcare landscape [12]. The young Chinese market is enabling rapid commercialization of digital models on a large scale [10]. There remains a great growth potential in China's healthcare market [12]. Existing e-health solutions may be one component of the ecosystem, while new solutions will be development. In any case, an e-health solution must address the issues in Chinese healthcare system and meet the consumers' needs.

The current healthcare system in China faces a range of challenges, and digital technologies can help to address them [10, 62]. The authors reviewed the healthcare system in China based on government documents, organisational reports and research publications, and identified the following challenges: (1) disparities and inequities, (2) difficult access to healthcare services, (3) tensional hospital and patient relationship, (4) resources abuse and misallocation, and (5) low level of health literacy. The Chinese government encourages technical players to experiment upon success [10, 63]. The strong governmental boost allows to test and implement e-health innovation [64]. Section 2 summaries e-health solutions in the Chinese market. In this section, these solutions are classified in terms of the above challenges. As shown in Table 1, one solution may address two or more challenges. For example individuals in remote areas may not have medical records in hospitals, and therefore their electronic Resident Health Record is needed when they seek medical services in hospitals. The health record has potentials to address many other issues. In the table, the numbers in brackets are used to associate with the challenges that the solutions can or have potential to address.

Table 1. Healthcare challenges in China and corresponding E-health solutions

Challenges	Solutions
(1). Inequities relate to residence and employment. Needed healthcare is not accessible for remote areas. Medical insurance policies are different between provinces or cities, and employment and unemployment	• electronic Resident Health Record (for health data mobilisation) (1, 2, 3, 5, 6) • online guide to the right hospitals or doctors according to the individual's location, medical insurance, symptom etc. (1, 2, 3) • online clinical diagnosis or consultation (1, 2) • online simultaneous speech-to-text transcribing tool (1)
(2). Difficult access to healthcare services refers to the difficulties in the cycle of an outpatient service	• online service booking or appointment (1, 2) • electronic prescription (1, 2) • online pharmacy (1, 2) • online checking test results (1,2) • online imaging diagnosis tools (1, 2) • electronic medical payment (1,2) • online fees reimbursement (1,2) • messaging alert or reminder for booked services, medications, etc. (1, 2) • online guide to high-end customized services (2, 4)
(3). Resources abuse and misallocation include bypass of primary care, unnecessary inpatient care, overmedication, unnecessary or repeated tests	• electronic Resident Health Record (for health data mobilisation) (1, 2, 3, 5, 6) • online guide to the right hospitals or doctors according to the individual's location, medical insurance, symptom etc. (1, 2, 3)
(4). Tensional hospital and patient relationship refers to unsatisfactory services, lack of trust, in-transparency in drug sale	• access to online consumer comment platform (4) • tools for post-treatment communication with doctors/nurses (4, 5) • app for bidding by local retail pharmacies (4) • authoritative information push for traceability of the prescription (4), including manufacturer, manufacture date, expiry, logistics, side-effects, allergies, undesirable consequences, etc.
(5). Low level of health literacy is the obstacle to personally engaged healthcare. Relevant issues include difficulty in searching the right care, stress and misunderstanding in medical process, and inability in preparation for care services	• applications for searching health information (5, 6), including guide for healthy life, health metrics, safety of drug use, medical advice etc. • access to platforms for health education (5, 6) • access to social media for care experience and advices (5, 6) • applications for customized care plan (5, 6) • applications for personal health assessment (5, 6)

(continued)

Table 1. (*continued*)

Challenges	Solutions
(6). Social health and wellbeing regards turning environmental health, food safety, wellness, fitness, independent living of aged people, etc. towards society to reduce the demand on hospital-based services	• smart devices/apps for self-diagnostics by, for example, monitoring vital signs or biomarkers, and providing personal health status (6) • smart devices/apps for rehabilitation by, for example, monitoring activities and keeping the user on the right track (6) • smart devices/apps for chronic disease management by, for example, monitoring patient metrics and providing actionable insights (6) • smart devices/apps for fitness by, for example, monitoring exercise routine, dietary intake, calculating calorie and providing stats (6) • online wellness programs, which, for example, include health/wellness agenda for participants, who will gain points for insurance premium on successful completion of the agenda (6)

Table 1 shows that there are not e-health solutions to directly address the challenge of resource abuse and misallocation. Although EHR can help address the issue, it cannot be a complete solution. Table 1 also shows that many mobile solutions are developed for social health and wellbeing, which is not included in the Chinese healthcare system. Thousands of e-health start-ups keep growing but a few have succeeded [44, 65]. Available e-health systems are not widely used [66], especially for primary healthcare [56]. E-health appears to be at a crossroads in China [30].

China is designing its own way, leveraging the power of digitization to achieve its health objectives [34]. Fast-moving players disrupt the market using technologies to offer cheaper and better products [37]. In the next few years e-health industry is set to enter its next stage of development, where only the fittest will survive [30]. Many e-health solutions have come from technologies and engineers who are excited by the technology and do not start with the true consumer needs [1, 66]. However, the adoption and use of the products depend on the needs of the consumers for the involved services or functions of the products. It is necessary to examine the needs and wants that exist in various patient and consumer segments [58].

Similarly an ecosystem must address the needs of Chinese consumers' demand for e-health products and services. China is largely a consumer-driven market and consumers' problems are opportunities for innovators [10]. Based on their technical advantages and in their own perspective, solution vendors developed e-health solutions for the needs of consumers. Future work is needed to determine the needs in user perspective.

5 Summary

Based on the review of e-health market in China, the authors identified three major obstacles that hinder the success of e-health solutions in achieving their original goals to address issues in Chinese healthcare system and provide needed healthcare in cost effective ways equally to all the consumers. To remove the obstacles, the authors proposed an e-health ecosystem based on the authors' previous research on Australia's PCEHR system. Compared with the existing e-health services and solutions, the ecosystem is consumer centric, enabling the changes from care providers to consumers, from holistic services to personalised services and from doctors to data. Also the open structure of the ecosystem allows sustainable system development and evolution.

The authors determined two major non-technical dimensions for the success of the ecosystem, and analysed the e-health solutions available on Chinese market with respect to each of the dimension: resolving challenges to Chinese healthcare systems and meeting consumers' needs. While many solutions resolve similar issues, there are a few that can resolve some other issues. Many mobile solutions are developed for social health and wellbeing, which is not included in the healthcare system of China. In China, most of the action is happening on the consumer side [44]. Recognition of individual needs and acceptance is the beginning stage [67] of the ecosystem development. Future work is needed to understand consumer needs, and determine candidate healthcare services/solutions for the (prototype) of the ecosystem.

China's digital globalisation is just getting started, and is likely to have a major impact on the world economy [10]. The concepts of the ecosystem would be of international reference significance for e-health systems. Table 1 provides domestic and international vendors with clues to business opportunities and competitive advantages on Chinese market.

References

1. SPDA: Digital Health Ecosystem for African countries: A Guide for Public and Private Actors for establishing holistic Digital Health Ecosystems in Africa (2018). https://www.bmz.de/en/publications/topics/health/Materilie345_digital_health_africa.pdf. Accessed 08 Feb 2019
2. NSW Health: eHealth Strategy for NSW Health 2016–2026 (2016). https://www.health.nsw.gov.au/ehealth/documents/ehealth-strategy-for-nsw-health-2016-2026.pdf. Accessed 08 June 2019
3. Keane, M.: Internet+ China: unleashing the innovative nation strategy. Int. J. Cult. Creative Ind. 3(2), 68–74 (2016)
4. Milcent, C.: Healthcare in China: From Violence to Digital Healthcare. Springer, Cham (2018). https://doi.org/10.1007/978-3-319-69736-9
5. Jolly, R.: The e health revolution - easier said than done, Research paper No. 3 (2011)
6. Zhou, X.: IT Choices for the Cloud, ICT Insights, Issue 11 (2014). https://e.huawei.com/mediafiles/Publication/Publications/hw_376150.pdf. Accessed 8 June 2019
7. McKeering, D., Norton, C., Gulati, A.: The Digital Healthcare Leap, Digital health in emerging markets, February 2017. https://www.pwc.com/gx/en/issues/high-growth-markets/assets/the-digital-healthcare-leap.pdf. Accessed 13 Apr 2019

8. Deloitte: 2018 Global health care outlook: The evolution of smart health care (2018). https://www2.deloitte.com/content/dam/Deloitte/global/Documents/Life-Sciences-Health-Care/gx-lshc-hc-outlook-2018.pdf. Accessed 8 June 2019

9. Accenture: Future Agenda: Ope Foresight (2018). https://www.accenture.com/_acnmedia/PDF-78/Accenture-Health-Future-of-Patient-Data-2018.pdf. Accessed 14 Apr 2019

10. McKinsey Global Institute: Digital China: Powering the Economy to Global Competitiveness (2017). http://www.iberchina.org/files/2017/MGI-Digital-China.pdf. Accessed 8 June 2019

11. Rapp, J: China health tech (2018). https://www.jwtintelligence.com/2018/10/china-health-tech/. Accessed 14 Apr 2019

12. PWC: The Evolution of the EMR in the Internet Era (2016). https://www.pwchk.com/en/healthcare/healthcare-emr-dec2016.pdf. Accessed 14 Apr 2019

13. Xu, Y., et al.: Development and validation of method for defining conditions using Chinese electronic medical record. BMC Med. Inform. Decis. Making **16**, 110 (2016)

14. Oracle: Building the Healthcare System of the Future, Oracle White paper (2017). http://www.oracle.com/us/industries/financial-services/healthcare-system-future-wp-2392577.pdf. Accessed 8 June 2019

15. Woetzel, J., Seong, J., Wang, K.W., Manyika, J., Chui, M., Wong, W.: Digital China: Powering the Economy to Global Competitiveness, MGI Report (2017). https://www.mckinsey.com/featured-insights/china/digital-china-powering-the-economy-to-global-competitiveness. Accessed 8 June 2019

16. Li, P., et al.: Promoting secondary analysis of electronic medical records in China: summary of the PLAGH-MIT critical data conference and health datathon. JMIR Med. Inform. 5(4), e43 (2017)

17. Gao, X., Xu, J., Sorwar, G., Croll, P.: Implementation of E-health record systems and E-medical record systems in China. Int. Technol. Manage. Rev. 3(2), 127–139 (2013)

18. Xu, W., Guan, Z., Cao, H., Zhang, H., Lu, M., Li, T.: Analysis and evaluation of the electronic health record standard in China: a comparison with the American national standard ASTM E 1384. Int. J. Med. Inform. **80**, 555–561 (2011)

19. Sun, Y., Gregersen, H., Yuan, W.: Chinese health care system and clinical epidemiology. Clin. Epidemiol. **9**, 167–178 (2017). https://doi.org/10.2147/CLEP.S106258

20. Harris, S.: China – The Market Maker for AI in Medical Imaging? (2017). https://www.signifyresearch.net/medical-imaging/china-the-market-maker-for-ai-in-medical-imaging/. Accessed 8 June 2019

21. Ge, C.: Alibaba, Tencent see AI as solution to China's acute shortage of doctors (2018). https://www.scmp.com/business/china-business/article/2102371/alibaba-tencent-see-ai-solution-chinas-acute-shortage. Accessed 8 June 2019

22. Rochester, N.Y.: Carestream Health and Alibaba Health Sign Agreement to Create Medical Image Management Cloud Platform in China (2016). https://www.businesswire.com/news/home/20160225005268/en/Carestream-Health-Alibaba-Health-Sign-Agreement-Create. Accessed 8 June 2019

23. Lew, L.: How Tencent's medical ecosystem is shaping the future of China's healthcare (2018). https://technode.com/2018/02/11/tencent-medical-ecosystem/. Accessed 8 June 2019

24. Royal Philips and Digital China Health: Philips and Digital China Health launch tele-radiology services in China (2018). https://www.philips.com/a-w/about/news/archive/standard/news/press/2018/20180412-philips-and-digital-china-health-launch-tele-radiology-services-in-china.html. Accessed 1 Mar 2019

25. Chinabrand: Baidu Develops "Medical Brain" for Computer-aided Diagnostics (2016). https://en.blog.chinabrand.de/2016/11/30/baidu-develops-medical-brain-for-computer-aided-diagnostics/. Accessed 8 June 2019

26. Bai, C.: E-health in China. In: Thuemmler, C., Bai, C. (eds.) Health 4.0: How Virtualization and Big Data are Revolutionizing Healthcare, pp. 155–185. Springer, Cham (2017). https://doi.org/10.1007/978-3-319-47617-9_8

27. News Medical: Dnurse Glucose Meter and Dnurse app gain CE approval (2016). https://www.news-medical.net/news/20160208/Dnurse-Glucose-Meter-and-Dnurse-app-gain-CE-approval.aspx. Accessed 1 Mar 2019

28. Xia, M., Poon, L., Choy, M., Wong, J.: China's Digital Health-Care Revolution, BCG Report (2015). https://www.bcg.com/en-au/publications/2015/biopharmaceuticals-medical-devices-technology-chinas-digital-health-care-revolution.aspx. Accessed 8 June 2019

29. Li, J., Seale, H., Ray, P.: e-Health preparedness assessment in the context of an influenza pandemic: a qualitative study in China. BMJOpen **3**, e002293 (2013). https://doi.org/10.1136/bmjopen-2012-002293

30. Wu, Y., Ding, A.: Online Medicine at a Crossroads, Deloitte Perspective (2017). https://www2.deloitte.com/content/dam/Deloitte/cn/Documents/about-deloitte/dttp/deloitte-cn-dttp-vol5-chapter4-en.pdf. Accessed 8 June 2019

31. Arnautova, Y.: Top Healthcare Industry Trends to Watch in 2018 and Beyond (2018). https://www.globallogic.com/blogs/top-healthcare-industry-trends-to-watch-in-2018-and-beyond/. Accessed 8 June 2019

32. Assenmacher, A.: Artificial Intelligence, China's Newest Technology Temptress (2017). https://globalhealthi.com/2017/05/10/artificial-intelligence-china/. Accessed 4 Mar 2019

33. Bai, J., Lian, S.: Smart guiding glasses for visually impaired people in indoor environment. IEEE Trans. Consum. Electron. **63**(3) (2017). https://doi.org/10.1109/tce.2017.014980

34. Legrand, J.: How to navigate digitization in healthcare in China, Paris Innovation Review (2016). http://parisinnovationreview.com/articles-en/how-to-navigate-digitization-in-health care-in-china. Accessed 8 June 2019

35. Deloitte: A journey towards smart health: The impact of digitalization on patient experience (2018). https://www2.deloitte.com/content/dam/Deloitte/lu/Documents/life-sciences-health-care/lu_journey-smart-health-digitalisation.pdf. Accessed 8 June 2019

36. Patientcaresolutions: 5 Ways Interactive Patient Systems Activate and Comfort (2016). http://www.patientcaresolutions.eu/nl/blog/artikel/item/5-ways-interactive-patient-systems-activate-and-comfort.html. Accessed 8 June 2019

37. Roberts, D., et al.: Health care: the cross-currents of convergence deliver participatory health (2017). https://www.ey.com/Publication/vwLUAssets/EY-healthcare-the-cross-currents-of-convergence-deliver-participatory-health/$FILE/EY-healthcare-the-cross-currents-of-convergence-deliver-participatory-health.pdf. Accessed 4 Mar 2019

38. Frick, J.: Panel Discussion: China's evolving Digital-health Landscape, Clearstate, The Economist, Intelligence Unit (2017). https://www.clearstate.com/wp-content/uploads/2017/05/Digital-Health-China.pdf. Accessed 8 June 2019

39. CSIRO: A powerful audio-video platform developed by CSIRO's Data61 has the potential to raise the standard in the delivery of medical services internationally (2018). https://www.csiro.au/en/News/News-releases/2016/Data61s-Coviu-platform-to-help-drive-medical-tourism-growth. Accessed 8 June 2019

40. Najberg, A.: Alibaba Health, Merck Team Up on China Healthcare Services (2018). https://www.alizila.com/alibaba-health-merck-china/. Accessed 8 June 2019

41. CN-Healthcare: The Golden era of UK-CHINA collaborations will determine the future of medicine (2018). https://www.cn-healthcare.com/article/20180206/content-500090.html. Accessed 8 June 2019

42. Towson J: Why Chinese healthcare apps are struggling. Asian Rev. (2016). https://asia.nikkei.com/Viewpoints-archive/Viewpoints/Jeffrey-Towson-Why-Chinese-healthcare-apps-are-struggling. Accessed 8 June 2019

43. Digital Health: Babylon expands its AI technology to mainland China (2018). https://www.digitalhealth.net/2018/04/babylon-ai-technology-china-tencent/. Accessed 4 Mar 2019
44. Towson, J.: The Solution to China's Digital Health Problems? Go Direct to Consumers (2017). http://jefftowson.com/2017/08/the-solution-to-chinas-digital-health-problems-go-direct-to-consumers/. Accessed 8 June 2019
45. Roese, J.: ICT: The Convergence of Consumer, Enterprise, and Carrier Technologies, ICT Insights, Issue 2 (2012). https://e.huawei.com/se/publications/global/ict_insights/hw_133629/feature%20story/HW_134495. Accessed 8 June 2019
46. Makridakis, S., Polemitis, A., Giaglis, G., Louca, S.: Blockchain: the next breakthrough in the rapid progress of AI. Robot. Autom. Eng. J. **2**(4) (2018). RAEJ.MS.ID.5555892
47. Suberg: Alibaba Deploys Blockchain to Secure Health Data in Chinese First (2017). https://cointelegraph.com/news/alibaba-deploys-blockchain-to-secure-health-data-in-chinese-first. Accessed 5 Mar 2019
48. Jiang, S., Cao, J., Wu, H., Yang, Y., Ma, M., He, J.: BlockHIE: a BLOCkchain-based platform for healthcare information exchange. In: 2018 IEEE International Conference on Smart Computing (SMARTCOMP), 18–20 June 2018, Taormina, Italy (2018)
49. Bell, L., Buchanan, W., Cameron, J., Lo, O.: Applications of blockchain within healthcare. Blockchain Healthc. Today **1** (2018). https://doi.org/10.30953/bhty.v1.8
50. COCIR: Beyond the Hype of Blockchain in Healthcare (2017). https://www.cocir.org/uploads/media/17069_COC_Blockchain_paper_web.pdf. Accessed 5 Mar 2019
51. Zuckerman, M.J.: Alibaba-Founded Insurtech Firm Promotes Blockchain Use in Healthcare Industry (2018). https://cointelegraph.com/news/alibaba-founded-insurtech-firm-promotes-blockchain-use-in-healthcare-industry. Accessed 5 Mar 2019
52. Shen, M.: A Solution to China's Pharma Woes Might Be a Blockchain Away (2018). https://www.coindesk.com/a-solution-to-chinas-pharma-woes-might-be-a-blockchain-away. Accessed 5 Mar 2019
53. Vayyapuri, R.: Tencent introduced blockchain medical prescription: shaping the future of China's healthcare (2018). https://bcfocus.com/news/tencents-introduced-blockchain-medical-prescription-shaping-the-future-of-chinas-healthcare/6186/. Accessed 8 June 2019
54. Krawiec, R.J., et al.: Blockchain: Opportunities for Health Care, Deloitte White Paper (2016). https://www2.deloitte.com/us/en/pages/public-sector/articles/blockchain-opportunities-for-health-care.html. Accessed 14 Apr 2019
55. Wickramasinghe, N., Schaffer, J.L.: Realizing Value Driven e-Health Solutions, IBM Center for The Business of Government (2010). https://www.epworth.org.au/about-us/documents/ibm_wickramasinghe_v12-final.pdf. Accessed 8 June 2019
56. Li, X., et al.: The primary health-care system in China. Lancet **390**(10112), 2584–2594 (2017). https://doi.org/10.1016/S0140-6736(17)33109-4
57. Xu, J., Gao, X., Sorwar, S., Croll, P.: Implementation of E-health record systems in Australia. Int. Technol. Manage. Rev. **3**(2), 92–104 (2013)
58. Hew, C.: Executive Summary: Digital Health China Breakfast Meeting, Clearstate, The Economist, Intelligence Unit (2017). https://www.clearstate.com/wp-content/uploads/2017/05/Digital-Health-China.pdf. Accessed 8 June 2019
59. Tiwana, A.: Platform Ecosystems: Aligning Architecture, Governance, and Strategy. Elsevier (2014). https://doi.org/10.1016/C2012-0-06625-2. Accessed 8 June 2019
60. Crouch, H.: Hancock's 'tech revolution' to include mandatory open standards (2018). https://www.digitalhealth.net/2018/10/hancock-tech-revolution-mandatory-open-standards/. Accessed 10 Mar 2019
61. HISA: The Future of Healthcare is Digital 2018 HIC Handbook (2018). https://www.hisa.org.au/wp-content/uploads/2018/08/180814_LIVE_BOOK_FINAL.pdf. Accessed 8 June 2019

62. Milcent, C.: Evolution of the Health System: Inefficiency, Violence, and Digital Healthcare, China Perspectives, pp. 39–50 (2016). https://journals.openedition.org/chinaperspectives/7112. Accessed 8 June 2019

63. Li, X., Huang, J., Zhang, H.: An analysis of hospital preparedness capacity for public health emergency in four regions of China: Beijing, Shandong, Guangxi, and Hainan. BMC Public Health **8**, 319 (2008). https://doi.org/10.1186/1471-2458-8-319

64. The Medical Futurist: China Is Building The Ultimate Technological Health Paradise. Or Is It? (2019). https://medicalfuturist.com/china-digital-health. Accessed 11 Mar 2019

65. Zhao, Q.: Reformation of China's Healthcare (2018). https://theeconreview.com/2018/08/15/reformation-of-chinas-healthcare/. Accessed 8 June 2019

66. Taylor, P.D.: Patient reported outcomes – what we can learn from our European colleagues (2018). https://www.vitalhealthsoftware.com/vitalblog/vitalblog-us/2018/07/26/patient-reported-outcomes-what-we-can-learn-from-our-european-colleagues. Accessed 8 Mar 2019

67. Taherdoost, H.: A review of technology acceptance and adoption models and theories. In: 11th International Conference Interdisciplinarity in Engineering, INTER-ENG 2017, 5–6 October 2017, Tirgu-Mures, Romania (2018)

Using Deep Learning and Smartphone for Automatic Detection of Fall and Daily Activities

Xiaodan Wu[1], Lingyu Cheng[1], Chao-Hsien Chu[2(✉)],
and Jungyoon Kim[3]

[1] Hebei University of Technology, Tianjin 300130, People's Republic of China
xwu@hebut.edu.cn, clybah@163.com
[2] The Pennsylvania State University, University Park, PA 16802, USA
chu@ist.psu.edu
[3] Kent State University, Kent, OH 44242, USA
jykim2@kent.edu

Abstract. The rapid growth of elderly population makes the health of the elderly one of the major social concerns. The elderly is often facing with several physical and mental healthcare related problems, among those, instance of fall and injuries ranked at the top. If people fall unexpectedly and without timely assistance, it is easy to cause irreparable harm. Therefore, how to automatically detect fall and alert for care/attention using advanced assisted technologies is a hot area of research. In this paper, we examine six machine learning-based methods and propose and carefully configure two novel deep learning-based architectures for fall detection. We compare the relative performance of these methods using an open source dataset, MobiAct, which was collected with four simulated fall types and nine daily living activities using smartphones. Our experimental results show that the proposed long short-term memory (LSTM) deep learning model is quite effective for the fall detection classification; its accuracy reaches 98.83%, the specificity is 99.38%, the sensitivity is 90.57% and the F1 score is 90.33%. These results are better than existing machine learning methods in all types of fall and most of daily activities.

Keywords: Fall detection · Deep learning · LSTM · Wearables devices · Machine learning

1 Introduction

A good living environment and comprehensive medical care services have extended people's lives, which led to an increasing number of elderly people around the world. Ageing population is a worldwide trend. The rapid growth of the elderly population makes the physical and mental health of the elderly the major social concerns. Most elderly are often facing with several healthcare related problems, such as fall, depression, stress, Alzheimer, and chronical diseases. Among those problems, the rate of fall injuries ranked among the highest. According to the World Health Organization statistics [1], falls are the second leading cause of accidental or unintentional injury

© Springer Nature Switzerland AG 2019
H. Chen et al. (Eds.): ICSH 2019, LNCS 11924, pp. 61–74, 2019.
https://doi.org/10.1007/978-3-030-34482-5_6

deaths around the world, and about 23–40% of injury-related deaths among the elderly are caused by falls.

After the accidental fall, if the person cannot be identified and treated within a short period of time, it may cause paralysis or even death. Therefore, using advanced sensing and analytics technologies to monitor and automatically detect the incidence and call for assistance and treatment timely become the consensus of academic and healthcare community.

In general, fall detection sensors and technologies can be divided into three main categories, external sensors, video-based sensors and wearable devices with sensors [2–4]. For example, external environmental sensors (e.g., motion sensors) and video camera and sound devices [5, 6] were used to monitor and capture motions of the elderly, and then algorithms were used to recognize the daily activities and falls based on the perceived information. This setting is limited in a fixed location such as home and they are personal privacy concerns too. Recently researchers have proposed to use mobile and wearable devices [7, 8] to monitor daily activities and detect falls based on the collected activity information. These devices typically have various sensors such as camera, microphone, accelerometer, gyroscopes, magnetometers, etc. built in that they can be used to sense the environment and comprehensively collect various behavior data to identify the activity state of the human. Using wearable device for healthcare has the advantages of low cost and good portability/mobility, which has become a popular choice for fall detection and other healthcare related research (e.g., sleep disorder, heart failure, hypertension etc.).

In the past, fall detection research used threshold-based methods and machine learning algorithms [2–6, 10]. Threshold-based methods [10, 21] detect fall based on fixed interval values for selected attributes such as acceleration speed, sensor orientation and impact forces for all users. These approaches have certain limitations as different people's fall peaks will be affected by gender, height, weight and other factors. In addition, setting the threshold interval only by experience does not work well for different people (i.e., personalization issue). When using machine learning methods for fall detection, first of all, it is necessary to extract signal features based on professional domain knowledge and experience. Secondly, according to human expertise, only shallow features can be extracted. These features usually refer to some statistical information, such as mean, variance, frequency and amplitude. They can only be used to identify low-level activities such as walking or running, and it is difficult to infer advanced activities such as complicated falls. In recent years, deep learning [11–14] has become the technology of choice for many human related tasks, such as speech, natural language, vision and games. When using deep learning, tedious feature engineering tasks are not required, as raw data can usually be used by simply passing directly to the network. This completely eliminates the cumbersome and challenging feature engineering phase of the entire process.

The main purpose of this study is to examine how effective of using advanced technologies such as machine learning and deep learning for automatic detection on fall and daily activities using smartphones or wearable devices. Two deep learning models, Convolutional Neural Network (CNN) and Long Short Time Memory (LSTM) model were used for exploration and comparison. We use an open source data set, MobiAct, collected by using smartphones [2] for evaluation. Nine daily living activities and four fall activities were included in the experiment. Performance metrics considered include accuracy, precision, sensitivity (also known as recall), and specificity, and aggregated measure such as F1 score was used to deal with data imbalance issues. Deep learning models need to properly design, configure and tune in order to automatically learn deep features to achieve good prediction performance. Therefore, key contributions of this study lie in two-fold: (1) adopt, configure and tune deep learning models for automatic learn data features for fall detection and (2) design comprehensive experiments to evaluate and analyze the relative performance of six machine learning algorithms and two deep learning models.

2   Related Works

The wearable fall detection system can collect data such as acceleration, inclination, multi-degree of freedom motion, etc. of the human body by wearing micro-miniature electronic sensors, and then analyzes the collected data to make a fall judgment. With the introduction of mobile phones and other wearable devices, inertial sensor data uses data from mobile or wearable embedded sensors located at different body locations to infer human activity details and the way of movement. Many scholars have proposed alternative solutions/systems over the past decades for automatic fall detection [3, 4]. The algorithms used to classify activities can be divided into three categories – heuristics, machine learning and deep learning.

2.1   Heuristic and Machine Learning Approaches

Currently, the most widely used wearable fall detection systems are based primarily on pressure sensors, acceleration sensors, and gyro sensors. The final judgment of the fall is achieved in two ways: (1) threshold-based methods and (2) machine learning methods. Threshold-based methods determine that a fall is caused when the acceleration or other shape change reaches a predetermined threshold. Bagalà [7] evaluated 13 existing threshold methods to detect falls in an actual environment. Their results shown that the methods of Chen and Bourke3 are the more effective ones. In [8, 9], the threshold technique which relies on the magnitude of the acceleration and its standard deviation is used to detect the falls.

The use of machine learning algorithms requires users to acquire data and extract features in advanced before data classification. Aziz [10] compared five threshold methods (including Chen and Bourke's) and five machine learning methods (including logical regression, Bayesian algorithm, K-nearest neighbor algorithm, decision tree and support vector machine) for fall detection. They show that machine learning methods, especially support vector machines, performed better than threshold methods in fall detection. Although the machine learning algorithms have achieved good results in classification, the feature extraction and selection work are tedious and require human expertise to obtain satisfactory performance. Deep learning can learn deeper features to alleviate this cumbersome process.

2.2 Deep Learning Approaches

Recently, various neural network models for simulating human activity recognition have emerged. Yang [11] used a multi-layer convolutional neural network (CNN) model to demonstrate good recognition on both Opportunity and Hand Gesture datasets, and was significantly better than machine learning algorithms such as SVM. Ordóñez and Roggen [12] used deep learning techniques to detect falls. The architecture they used consists of two parts: a CNN and a cyclic neural network. The former is used to automatically extract features from sensor signals, while the latter defines the temporal relationship between samples. Chen et al. [13] proposed a LSTM model, using the open WISDM database, to extract the data features and then classify the activities using the LSTM architecture, and achieving a classification accuracy of 95.1%. Although the recognition works well, the model was only verified using small sample sizes. Hammerla [14] examined the effects of CNN and RNN on the three activity identification datasets, Opportunity dataset, PAMAP2 dataset and Daphnet Gait dataset. Their results shown that the LSTM model is significantly better than the CNN model on the activity identification dataset. Musci et al. [15] used the SisFall dataset to verify the proposed multi-layer LSTM model, which achieved higher accuracy in both fall and non-fall activity recognition. Edel et al. [16] proposed an optimized two-way LSTM for human activity recognition for mobile and wearable device data.

Human activity is a classic time series classification problem consisting of complex movements, and the categories of activities vary over time. Capturing temporal dynamic continuous correlation in motion patterns will help simulate complex activity details and improve the performance of the recognition algorithms. CNN can only extract translationally invariant local features but become ineffective when modeling global time dependencies in sensor data. On the other hands, the RNN can solve this problem [14]. The results of DNN, CNN and RNN were verified by 4000 experiments on some public HAR datasets. Some conclusions are drawn through experiments as follows: RNN and LSTM can identify short activities with natural order, while CNN can better infer long-term repetitive activities [14, 17]. In the current applications [18], CNN are observed to better use for the relationship between activity and sleep patterns, and the performance of complex activity details is not good. LSTM is better used to simulate the daily activities of the elderly, mode, detection of activity levels, and detection of falls. We adopt and carefully configure deep learning model further validate the results in this study.

3 Materials and Methods

3.1 Data Set

We use a publicly available dataset MobiAct [2] to evaluate the relative performance of six existing machine learning algorithms and our proposed deep learning models for fall detection. The data set was captured using a Samsung Galaxy S3 device with the LSM330DLC inertial module (3D accelerometer and gyroscope). The gyroscope was calibrated prior to the recordings using the device's integrated tool. For the purpose of data capture, an Android application was developed that records raw data for acceleration, angular velocity and orientation with the enabled parameter "Sensor_Delay_Fastest." This provides the highest possible sampling rate. The dataset was captured based on a scenario of daily living, which includes four different types of falls and 9 different activities of daily living (ADLs). A total of 57 subjects with more than 2500 trials, all captured by a smartphone. Please refer to [2] for details on how this simulated data set was captured and recorded.

3.2 Data Pre-processing

Since the LSTM model requires a fixed length time series as input, we pre-processed the raw data in advance. First, we set up labels for each piece of data in the dataset to facilitate model training. In order to improve the accuracy of the data, the value of the signal point is expanded to a section containing the point, and the interval of window is used to judge. We use a 300-length time window (about 3.45 s) to preprocess the signal. Each generated sequence contains 300 training examples. Our training dataset has drastically reduced in size after the transformation. Similarly, in order to maintain the global feature of the time series signal, we also do a corresponding sliding time window processing on the test set to ensure the timing of the short-term signal. When the model detects that the category label is falling within the time window, it is determined that a fall has occurred.

3.3 Feature Extraction

In this study we compare the performance of our proposed deep learning models with six machine learning algorithms, K-nearest neighbor algorithm (KNN), Naive Bayesian algorithm (NB), J48 decision tree (J48), random forest (RF), Adaboost algorithm, and support vector machine (SVM). These methods require the key features are extracted first, and the selected feature sequences are then classified. The features were automatically selected for activity recognition using WEKA's implemented attribute evaluator "CfsSubsetEval," using the "BestFirst" search method [20]. The twelve features selected are: median and standard deviation in the z axis, mean and minimum in the y axis, skew (a measure of the direction and extent of statistical data skew, and is a numerical feature of the degree of asymmetry in statistical data distribution) in the x axis, median and skew around the z axis, mean or the rotation rate around the x and y axes, kurtosis (characterizing the number of peaks at which the probability density distribution curve peaks at the mean. Intuitively, the kurtosis reflects the sharpness of the peak around the x axis, as well as EEB (entropy of the energy in 10 equal sized blocks and spectral flux (The envelope area of the signal spectrum, which reflects the sum of the energy of the components of each band in the signal).

3.4 Model Construction

Two deep learning models, CNN and LSTM, were examined and analyzed for fall detection.

Convolutional Neural Networks (CNN). CNN is a variation of feedforward neural network with convolutional computation and deep structure. It is one of the most popular and representative algorithms of deep learning. The hidden layer of the CNN consists of convolutional, pooling and fully connected layers. The CNN model we built for fall detection (as shown in Fig. 1) contains seven layers, input layer, two convolutional layers, two pooling layers, one fully connected layer and output layer.

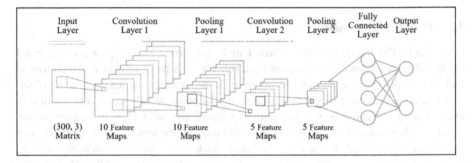

Fig. 1. The CNN model for fall detection

Input Layer. The input is a 3D accelerated data acquired by the smartphone. X is the x-axis direction acceleration measured by the mobile phone accelerometer. Y is the y direction and Z is the z direction. We combine the acceleration data in three directions into a three-dimensional matrix of sliding windows with a length of 300 values. Therefore, the input data of the model is time series data of a three-dimensional matrix.

Convolutional Layers. Feature learning of the raw data is performed through the convolutional layer. We use two 3 * 3 convolution kernels to calculate. Set the step size to 1, that is, slide one unit to the right with a fixed window of 3 * 3. The first layer of input data is subjected to a convolution operation to obtain a second feature map with a depth of 10.

Pooling Layers. The second layer of the feature map is pooled to obtain a third layer having a depth of 10 by 3 * 3 window. Repeat the above operations with a 2 * 2 window to get the feature map with the fifth layer depth of 5. Finally, the five feature maps, that is, the five matrices, are expanded into row by row.

Fully Connected and Output Layers. These layers form a backpropagation (BP) neural network with full connectivity. All neurons in these layers are fully connected. The output layer contains two binary neurons serving as "Yes" or "No".

The Long and Short-Term Memory (LSTM) Model. LSTM is a variation of recurrent neural network (RNN) structure proposed by Hochreiter and Schmidhuber in 1997 [19]. Like most RNNs, the LSTM network is generic, and given enough network elements, which can compute anything that a regular computer can compute, provided it has an appropriate weight matrix that can be considered its program. For non-traditional RNNs, the LSTM network is well-suited for learning from experience so that time series can be classified, processed, and predicted with very long unknown time lags between important events. This is one of the main reasons why LSTM performs many alternatives to traditional RNN and hidden Markov models and other sequential learning methods in many applications. The LSTM model we built for fall detection (as shown in Fig. 2) contains seven layers, input layer, two LSTM layers, two dropout layers, one fully connected dense layer and output layer.

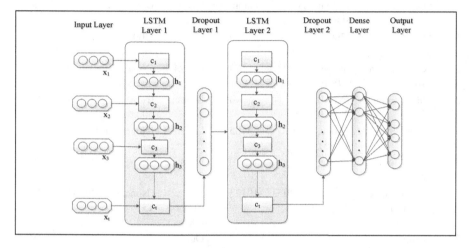

Fig. 2. The LSTM model for fall detection

In order to form a richer data representation, our model uses two LSTM layers for feature learning. The setting of the model requires fewer parameters to be optimized and thus, the detection can ensure real-time performance. The first layer of LSTM learns the features for effective discriminative power in the signal. The second layer of LSTM splice the features learned in the previous layer to form high-level features for classification. The number of neurons and the setting of the batch size have been experimentally verified and the values are optimized. The dropout layer not only prevents over-fitting of the data during the model training process, but also sets the dropout rate to 0.3, and only randomly proposes a few neurons to ensure the validity of the model.

The activation function of the CNN layer uses the ReLU, which reduces the computational complexity of the whole process. ReLU will make the output of a part of the neurons 0, which causes the sparseness of the network and reduces the interdependence of parameters and eases the occurrence of overfitting problems. However, using the ReLU in the LSTM layer will result in instability of the model training process, so we choose the Tanh function to avoid the gradient explosion problem. In the fully connected layer, the Sigmoid and Softmax functions and their combinations usually work better when they were used in a classifier. However, the Sigmoid function is usually only used for binary classification tasks, and it is easy to generate the gradient disappearance problem. In order to avoid these problems, we choose the Softmax function as the activation function.

We conduct pilot tests to determine the setting of these parameters. Table 1 lists the parameters and their corresponding setting for both CNN and LSTM models. The models were trained for 50 epochs.

Table 1. Parameters used in CNN and LSTM models

Layer	CNN model				LSTM model			
	Layer type	Output shape	Act.	Parameter	Layer type	Output shape	Act.	Parameter
1	Input	(300, 3)	–	0	Input	(300, 3)	–	0
2	Convolution 1d	(None, 298,10)	ReLU	100	LSTM 1	(None, 300,64)	Tanh	17408
3	Max_pooling 1	(None, 296,10)	–	0	Dropout 1	(None, 300,64)	–	0
4	Convoltion_2d	(None, 295,5)	ReLU	105	LSTM 2	(None, 64)	Tanh	33024
5	Max_pooling 2	(None, 294,5)	–	0	Dropout 2	(None, 64)	–	0
6	Full Connect (Dense)	(None, 13)	Softmax	19123	Full Connect (Dense)	(None, 13)	Softmax	845
7	Output	(None, 13)	–	0	Output	(None, 13)	–	0

Act: Activation function; –: Not Available

4   Performance Evaluation

4.1   Data Splitting

We select a complete data of 15 subjects for 13 kinds of activity. Since the WAL and STN activities lasted longer during data collection, which affect the balance of the data, we increase the amount of data for other types of activities, the remaining 11 kinds of data we take 20 subjects. A total of 218,435 data were obtained. Among them, there were a total of 42,651 falls, and a total of 27,876 other daily activities. There are no missing values. The data set was randomly divided into two parts, 80% of which were used for training and 20% for testing in one run. The proportion of various types of activity data is shown in Table 2. We repeat the process for 10 times and use their average results for analysis.

4.2   Performance Evaluation Criteria

Fall detection is a typical classification problem. In classification problems, an instance may be judged to be one of the following four types: True Positive, False Positive, False Negative and True Negative. From this, a confusion matrix can be composed.

Table 2. Number of activity data

Number	Activity	Training data	Test data
1	BSC	10256	2051
2	CSI	10815	2163
3	CSO	10705	2141
4	FKL	9723	1945
5	FOL	10401	2080
6	JOG	13771	2754
7	JUM	13399	2680
8	SCH	9677	1935
9	SDL	12271	2454
10	STD	27879	5576
11	STN	12608	2522
12	STU	12660	2532
13	WAL	27864	5573
Total		182029	36406

We use five quality performance metrics, sensitivity (also called recall), specificity, positive predictivity, accuracy, and F1 score to evaluate and compare the relative performance of our selected models. These metrics are commonly employed in data mining and can be obtained from confusion matrix.

4.3 Experimental Environment

We use the Keras with the TensorFlow backend to construct and test the CNN and LSTM models. To avoid gradient dissipation, we use the categorical cross entropy as the loss function. Moreover, we use the Adam optimization [22] to update the algorithm, because it has stronger convergence and the parameters were pilot tested and set as follows: learning rate = 0.0025, $\beta_1 = 0.9$, $\beta_2 = 0.999$. The classification test for machine learning was performed using WEKA.3.9 [23]. All training and tests were performed on a PC equipped with a 2.50 GHz i5-4200M CPU and 4G RAM.

5 Results and Analyses

Table 3 summarizes the average computational results and computational times for (a) all falls and (b) other activities of daily living.

5.1 Relative Performance of Algorithms

As shown in Table 3, overall, LSTM model has the best performance, the average accuracy and F1 score for all fall activities are 98.96% and 91.26% and are 98.78% and 89.91% for other activities of daily living. In contrast, although the performance of CNN model for detecting other ADL is acceptable (with 97.63% accuracy and 80.62%

Table 3. Summary of average results (NA: Not Available)

(a) All falls

Methods	Sensitivity	Specificity	Accuracy	Precision	F1 score	Training time	Test time
Adaboost [20]	25.00%	87.00%	81.08%	NA	NA	1.13 s	0.62 s
RF [20]	77.38%	98.93%	97.65%	82.05%	79.64%	10.23 s	3.11 s
KNN [20]	*81.11%*	*98.79%*	*97.75%*	*80.63%*	*80.86%*	*922.59 s*	*0.07 s*
NB [20]	36.57%	94.36%	91.08%	29.13%	30.58%	4.60 s	0.52 s
SVM [20]	22.02%	94.35%	90.28%	24.08%	15.06%	199.45 s	0.92 s
J48 [20]	70.43%	98.33%	96.69%	72.31%	71.34%	110.30 s	1.69 s
CNN	56.41%	97.01%	94.55%	54.69%	55.43%	877.53 s	0.002 s
LSTM	**91.69%**	**99.42%**	**98.96%**	**90.91%**	**91.26%**	**14948.52 s**	**0.28 s**

(b) Other activities of daily living

Methods	Sensitivity	Specificity	Accuracy	Precision	F1 score	Training time	Test time
Adaboost [20]	11.11%	96.98%	93.46%	NA	NA	1.13 s	0.62 s
RF [20]	65.76%	97.10%	94.92%	66.49%	65.92%	10.23 s	3.11 s
KNN [20]	64.24%	96.98%	94.49%	64.26%	64.23%	922.59 s	*0.07 s*
NB [20]	32.82%	95.50%	91.34%	39.82%	33.25%	4.60 s	0.52 s
SVM [20]	25.04%	94.01%	89.27%	33.62%	22.96%	199.45 s	0.92 s
J48 [20]	51.40%	95.93%	92.70%	51.34%	51.23%	110.30 s	1.69 s
CNN	*80.08%*	*98.77%*	*97.63%*	*81.56%*	*80.62%*	877.53 s	0.002 s
LSTM	**90.08%**	**99.36%**	**98.78%**	**90.06%**	**89.91%**	**14948.52 s**	**0.28 s**

F1 score), its performance on detecting fall activities is unacceptable (with 94.55% accuracy and 55.43% F1 score). The performance of CNN model on fall detection is even worse than the machine learning KNN algorithm, which has 97.75% accuracy and 80.86% F1 score. These indicate that (1) the LSTM model of deep learning outperforms other models/algorithms for all activities (fall and ADL); it performs better than CNN model for fall detection as the former takes special consideration on time series effect of fall data; (2) most machine learning algorithms except KNN did not perform well on detecting falls and ADLs, as machine learning must rely on a good feature extractions, which is difficult and tedious to do; (3) the deep learning model CNN is not necessarily guarantee to perform better than machine learning methods. There is a need to carefully configure the CNN models in order to get good results. (4) The adaboost algorithm does not seem to be suitable for the identification of time series data. It only recognizes one of the fall activities (SDL) and one of the daily activities (STD), and the effect is not very good, which leads to the average of the precision and F1 cannot be calculated. (5) It should be noted that due to the hardware requirements, using the RF classifier needs processing, we downsample the data samples, so the training time and test time are shorter than other machine learning methods.

In terms of the computational times, we can see that the two deep learning model, CNN and LSTM, take much longer to train the model, especially the LSTM model, but in the test stage, they nearly the same time as those of machine learning, which ensure the practical usage of deep learning for real-time recognition.

5.2 In-Depth Analysis on the Performance of LSTM Model

To better understand the behavior of LSTM model, we plot the converged process of LSTM in terms of loss function and accuracy it achieved. As shown in Fig. 3, our proposed LSTM model seems to learn well after 38 epochs with accuracy reaching above 98% and loss hovering at around 0.25. We also observed that at the beginning (about 8 epochs), the converge curves on both accuracy and loss functions are not smooth but later they were converged eventually. This may be because our training data is not adequate and the distribution is not very uniform. If we use larger amount of data, we will get a smoother blue line (test accuracy curve). The results show that the model used in this paper requires stronger regularization or fewer model parameters.

Welhenge and Taparugssanagorn [24] used four features such as SMAs and zero crossing rates as input to the LSTM model. They classified five activities namely standing, climbing stairs, jogging, jumping, and walking from MobiAct Dataset and achieved 90% accuracy. Chen et al. [13]. also used LSTM to classify activities and achieved an accuracy of 92%; however, they used the entire acceleration signal as the input. In this study, we analyze the data from 13 activities in the dataset as input and obtain higher results than previous research. In short, our proposed method outperforms some other methods proposed in the mentioned literature.

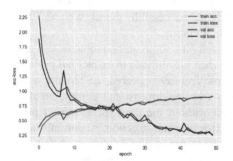

Fig. 3. Model training accuracy curve

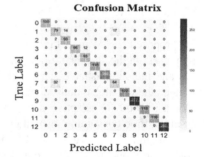

Fig. 4. LSTM classification confusion matrix

To further analyze the results in more details, we plot the confusion matrix of LSTM for the test data set (See Fig. 4). As shown, the model has a good recognition ability in all falls, especially in BSC and SDL, reaching 91.32% and 97.21% F1 score respectively, indicating that the model has a lower rate of missed detection in the identification of these two types of falls, and the rate of diagnosis is high. In the other two types of falls, it seems that the recognition effect is relatively poor (yet acceptable), which reaching 88.37% and 88.15% F1 score respectively.

In the identification of 9 types of daily living activities, the proposed LSTM model has significant recognition results on complex activities such as JUM, JOG, STU and STD, and also has good recognition results on simple activities such as WAL and STN. The confusion matrix indicates that many prediction errors are due to confusion between CSI and SCH activities. This is because these two activities are relatively similar.

6   Conclusion

Falls are a leading cause of accidental or unintentional injury deaths around the world. Many scholars and practitioners have conducted research to examine the use of analytics and sensors to detect falls. Several machine learning methods such as Gaussian mixture model, Bayesian net, SVM and neural network have been examined and evaluated, but the results are mixed (some show reasonable accuracy and others have low accuracy). Several deep learning models have been introduced and used, the results shown seem better, but the results shown on in one or two metrics and with average aggregated results for falls. In this paper, we propose to examine six popular machine learning algorithms (KNN, NB, SVM, RF, Adaboost and J48) and two deep learning architectures (CNN and LSTM) for fall detection.

According to our computational results, LSTM and KNN are the only two models that achieved more than 80% F1 scores for all four fall types detection, with the highest of 97.21% for SDL fall detection. LSTM is the only model that can successfully detect seven of the nine ADLs with F1 scores higher than 90% (the highest is 99.82%). Among the fall types, FKL and FOL are more difficult to detect (with 88.37% and 88.15% F1 score, respectively) as these two types of falls are similar to each other. CSI and SCH are the two ADLs that LSTM model cannot successfully detect (with 68.70% and 67.02% F1 scores) again due for their high similarity.

The proposed LSTM model is designed to overcome some of the problems that are usually present in the deep learning framework when it is difficult to extract fall posture features and indistinguishable static and dynamic features appeared. LSTM not only utilizes the inherent global dependence of time-series one-dimensional signals, but also provides a method for adaptive data extraction without the need for advanced pre-processing or time-consuming manual feature extraction and selection. At current stage we are examining how to adopt the LSTM model to run at mobile phones so that we can use smartphone to achieve our goal of using smartphone for automatic fall detection.

Acknowledgement. This project was supported in part by the National Social Science Foundation of China (No. 17BGL087). Our deepest gratitude goes to the anonymous reviewers for their careful review, comments and thoughtful suggestions that have helped improve this paper substantially.

References

1. World Health Organization, Global report on ageing and health (2015)
2. Vavoulas, G., Chatzaki, C., Malliotakis, T., Pediaditis, M., Tsiknakis, M.: The MobiAct dataset: recognition of activities of daily living using smartphones, pp. 143–151 (2016). https://doi.org/10.5220/0005792401430151
3. Igual, R., Medrano, C., Plaza, I.: Challenges, issues and trends in fall detection systems. BioMed. Eng. Online **12**, 66 (2013)
4. Mubashir, M., Shao, L., Seed, L.: A survey on fall detection: Principles and approaches. Neurocomputing **100**, 144–152 (2013)
5. Zhang, C., Tian, Y., Capezuti, E.: Privacy preserving automatic fall detection for elderly using RGBD cameras. In: Miesenberger, K., Karshmer, A., Penaz, P., Zagler, W. (eds.) ICCHP 2012. LNCS, vol. 7382, pp. 625–633. Springer, Heidelberg (2012). https://doi.org/10.1007/978-3-642-31522-0_95
6. Wang, S., Chen, L., Zhou, Z., et al.: Human fall detection in surveillance video based on PCANet. Multimedia Tools Appl. **75**(19), 11603–11613 (2016)
7. Bagalà, F., Becker, C., Cappello, A., et al.: Evaluation of accelerometer-based fall detection algorithms on real-world falls. PLOS One **7**, e37062 (2012)
8. Vilarinho, T., Farshchian, B., Bajer, D.G., et al.: A combined smartphone and smartwatch fall detection system. In: IEEE International Conference on Computer & Information Technology; Ubiquitous Computing & Communications; Dependable (2015)
9. Sucerquia, A., López, J.D., Vargas-Bonilla, J.F.: SisFall: a fall and movement dataset. Sensors **17**(1), 198 (2017)
10. Aziz, O., Musngi, M., Park, E.J., et al.: A comparison of accuracy of fall detection algorithms (threshold-based vs. machine learning) using waist-mounted tri-axial accelerometer signals from a comprehensive set of falls and non-fall trials. Med. Biol. Eng. Comput. **55**(1), 45–55 (2017)
11. Yang, J.B., Nguyen, M.N., San, P.P., et al.: Deep convolutional neural networks on multichannel time series for human activity recognition. In: Proceedings of IJCAI. AAAI Press (2015)
12. Ordóñez, F.J., Roggen, D.: Deep convolutional and LSTM recurrent neural networks for multimodal wearable activity recognition. Sensors **16**(1), 115 (2016)
13. Chen, Y., Zhong, K., Zhang, J., et al.: LSTM networks for mobile human activity recognition. In: International Conference on Artificial Intelligence: Technologies and Applications (2016)
14. Hammerla, N.Y., Halloran, S., Ploetz, T.: Deep, convolutional, and recurrent models for human activity recognition using wearables. J. Sci. Comput. **61**(2), 454–476 (2016)
15. Musci, M., De Martini, D., Blago, N., et al.: Online fall detection using recurrent neural networks (2018). https://arxiv.org/abs/1804.04976
16. Edel, M., Köppe, E.: Binarized-BLSTM-RNN based human activity recognition. In: IEEE International Conference on Indoor Positioning and Indoor Navigation, pp. 1–7 (2016)
17. Wang, J., Chen, Y., Hao, S., et al.: Deep learning for sensor-based activity recognition: a survey. Pattern Recogn. Lett. **119**, 3–11 (2018). S016786551830045X
18. Nweke, H.F., Teh, Y.W., Al-Garadi, M.A., et al.: Deep learning algorithms for human activity recognition using mobile and wearable sensor networks: state of the art and research challenges. Expert Syst. Appl. **105**, 233–261 (2018). S0957417418302136
19. Hochreiter, S., Schmidhuber, J.: Long short–term memory. Neural Comput. **9**(8), 1735–1780 (1997)

20. Vavoulas, G., Pediaditis, M., Chatzaki, C., et al.: The MobiFall dataset: fall detection and classification with a smartphone. Int. J. Monit. Surveill. Technol. Res. **2**(1), 44–56 (2014)
21. Vavoulas, G., Pediaditis, M., Spanakis, E.G., et al.: The MobiFall dataset: an initial evaluation of fall detection algorithms using smartphones. In: 13th IEEE International Conference on BioInformatics and BioEngineering (2014)
22. Kingma, D., Ba, J.: Adam: a method for stochastic optimization. Comput. Sci. (2014)
23. Hall, M., Frank, E., Holmes, G., Pfahringer, B., Reutemann, P., Witten, I.H.: The WEKA data mining software: an update. ACM SIGKDD Explor. Newslett. **11**(1), 10–18 (2009)
24. Welhenge, A.M., Taparugssanagorn, A.: Human activity classification using long short-term memory network. Signal, Image Video Process. (SIViP) **13**, 1–6 (2018)

Imbalanced Cardiotocography Multi-classification for Antenatal Fetal Monitoring Using Weighted Random Forest

Jia-ying Chen[1], Xiao-cong Liu[1,2], Hang Wei[1(✉)], Qin-qun Chen[1],
Jia-ming Hong[1], Qiong-na Li[3,4], and Zhi-feng Hao[5]

[1] School of Medical Information Engineering,
Guangzhou University of Chinese Medicine, Guangzhou, China
crwei@gzucm.edu.cn
[2] School of Computer Science and Technology,
Huaqiao University, Quanzhou, China
[3] Guangzhou Dongren Hospital, Guangzhou, China
[4] Guangzhou Sunray Medical Apparatus Co. Ltd, Guangzhou, China
[5] School of Mathematics and Big Data, Foshan University, Foshan, China

Abstract. In non-stress tests (NST) of antenatal fetal monitoring, the computerized cardiotocography (CTG) interpretation plays an important role. The digital CTG data are widely available, however, the number of abnormal cases is quite lower than that of the suspicious or normal cases. This phenomenon is referred to as imbalanced multi-classification, which has brought great challenge for machine learning to assess fetuses' health status. Therefore, in this paper we aim to establish an intelligent evaluation model using imbalanced CTG data for monitoring fetuses' growth. After data exploration, a weighted random forest (WRF) model was established by adjusting category weights to fulfill cost-sensitive learning. The efficiency of the proposed model was tested on the antenatal CTG dataset from the UCI repository. The WRF model achieved an average area under the receiver operating characteristic curve (ROC) of 0.99. Meanwhile, the average F1 score for the WRF (97.56%) exceeded that of the existing state-of-the-art models. The experimental results showed that the proposed model was promising for intelligent evaluating antenatal fetal health status using seriously imbalanced CTG data.

Keywords: Cardiotocography · Antenatal fetal monitoring · Imbalanced Multi-classification · Weighted random forest · Cost sensitive

1 Introduction

Cardiotocography (CTG) is an effective measure to evaluate antenatal fetal growth in Non-stress test (NST) [1]. Due to low cost and non-invasion, NST is widely used in antenatal fetal monitoring [2]. The demand for antenatal fetal monitoring becomes increasing dramatically. However, most pregnant women cannot enjoy convenient, timely and accurate fetal monitoring services, because of a serious shortage of fetal monitoring medical staff, especially in rural hospitals [3]. Furthermore, existing

© Springer Nature Switzerland AG 2019
H. Chen et al. (Eds.): ICSH 2019, LNCS 11924, pp. 75–85, 2019.
https://doi.org/10.1007/978-3-030-34482-5_7

antenatal fetal monitoring machine learning has not yet reached the level of intelligence due to seriously imbalanced CTG data, which means amount of abnormal cases in practical clinic [4–14].

In CTG interpretation, fetuses' health status is assessed as normal, suspicious or abnormal according to antenatal fetal monitoring guidelines [4]. The digital CTG data are widely available, however, the number of abnormal cases is quite lower than that of the suspicious or normal cases. This phenomenon is referred to as imbalanced multi-classification. Meanwhile, the existing models based on machine learning for fetal monitoring, mostly ignored the problem of imbalanced CTG data [5–14]. Hence, the cases tended to be classified as normal in existing algorithms based on sample distribution balance and classification longitude maximization. For example, in UCI antenatal CTG dataset [9], the amount of the normal, suspicious and abnormal accounts for 72%, 20% and 8% of the 2126 CTG records, respectively. The accuracy values of the suspicious and abnormal cases based on the existing models mostly ranged in 45%–84% and 66%–97%, respectively [7–14]. The mainly reason for the poor performance is neglecting the imbalanced multi-classification problem. To solve this problem, some studies directly transformed multi-classification to bi-classification by omitting the suspicious cases [5, 6]. Hence, the existing models based on machine learning cannot satisfy practical demand of fetal monitoring, for their low sensitivity, which will result in missing the best treatment timing. It is extremely risky and harmful to the health of both fetus and pregnant women [4].

In this paper, we designed a weighted random forest (WRF) model to improve the classification performance using the imbalanced CTG data. After data exploration and experiment, we found that the imbalance of CTG sample distribution will reduce the classification performance of the model. In the proposed WRF model, the classes' weights were adjusted to the inverse of the input frequency based on the labels. Therefore, the RF were more sensitive to suspicious and abnormal cases. In order to validate the effect of WRF on intelligent evaluation of antenatal fetal monitoring, the UCI antenatal CTG standard data set was used as an example to test. The simulation results showed that: in the normal, suspicious and abnormal class, the classification accuracy of the proposed model was 99.75%, 97.68% and 95.24%, respectively. WRF achieved high sensitivity (0.9978) and specificity (0.9836). And the average F1 score for the WRF (97.56%) exceeded that of the existing state-of-the-art models. Meanwhile, ten important features had been found in WRF. The experimental results showed that the proposed model was promising for intelligent evaluating antenatal fetal health status using seriously imbalanced CTG data. It can better assist obstetricians in making clinical decisions and be contributed to realizing intelligent assessment of CTG.

2   Related Works

2.1   CTG and Its Interpretations in Antenatal Fetal Monitoring

During antenatal fetal monitoring, it is necessary to record cardiotocography (CTG), including fetal heart rate (FHR) and uterine contraction (UC) [17, 18]. Obstetricians usually assess fetal health status based on the characteristics of CTG, such as baseline, variation, deceleration and uterine contraction. There are two existing evaluation methods for antenatal CTG, namely "scoring methods" and "ranking methods".

As for the scoring methods, there exits NST, Krebs, Fischer, and modified Fischer [18–20], but these scoring methods have some shortcomings. Firstly, the scoring systems are not uniform, ranging from 10 to 12. Secondly, the scoring items are inconsistent [19, 20]. Moreover, these methods cannot directly define whether the status of fetus is normal.

In the ranking methods for antenatal CTG, differences exist in different countries. The mainstream antenatal fetal monitoring guidelines include Canadian SOGC [21], American ACOG, British NICE, International Federation of Obstetrics and Gynecology FIGO [23, 24] and Chinese expert consensus [22]. Among them, SOGC, ACOG, NICE and FIGO all adopt three-level evaluation. But in Chinese experts' consensus, the conditions of fetuses are only divided into two levels, namely as "reactive" and "non-response" [25]. Besides, in Chinese "Obstetrics and Gynecology", SOGC is adapted in antenatal fetal monitoring [21]. In general, although the existing grading methods can define the specific conditions of the fetus, they have high sensitivity and low specificity in practical clinical applications [2, 3, 18, 25]. Especially when the CTG case is less than 40 min, it is prone to false positives, which will lead to overdiagnosis of fetal distress and unnecessary cesarean section for pregnant women [26].

2.2 The Machine-Learning-Based Models for Antenatal Fetal Monitoring

With the outbreak of big data and artificial intelligence, the progress of the intelligent fetal evaluation methods is dramatically driven by computer science and engineering. Many scholars have researched on the intelligent fetal monitoring models based on machine learning. One of the most contributing researches is an antenatal standard uterine contraction dataset published by the University of Porto in the Machine Learning Repository (UCI) [13]. Most antenatal fetal monitoring models based on machine learning, such as neural network, SVM, decision tree, fuzzy algorithm and hybrid algorithms, have achieved more than 90% total accuracy on this antenatal CTG data. But they mostly suffered from the imbalanced cardiotocography multi-classification [4–13]. The accuracy in suspicious and abnormal categories are mostly only 45%–84% and 66%–97%, respectively [6–13]. Many researchers have not realized that this is due to imbalanced multi-classification problem. And the imbalanced CTG data problem is very serious in clinical practice, especially in remote big data.

3   Materials and Methods

3.1   Dataset Description

The experimental dataset came from UCI repository [15]. This dataset contains 2126 Portuguese pregnant women CTG records from 29 to 42 gestational weeks. Each CTG record has 21 features, which were obtained through the CTG analysis program, named SisPorto 2.0 [16]. Three professional obstetricians evaluated fetal status from common classification features according to the FIGO guidelines. The records in the dataset were the ones consistently interpreted. Among the 2126 CTG records, 1655, 176 and 295 cases belonged to normal, suspicious or abnormal state, respectively.

From Fig. 1, it was obvious that the proportion of the fetal status was not uniform, the sample in the normal state accounted for 78%, and the total of suspicious and abnormal samples only accounted for 22%. It could be seen that there was a serious classification imbalance in the CTG dataset.

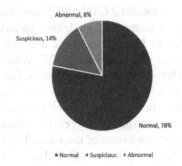

Fig. 1. CTG data distribution

3.2 Data Exploration and Preprocessing

By exploring the CTG data, the characteristics and the important features were found out for evaluating fetal health. The Pivot table was used to discover the important features of CTG and the correlation between fetal status and features (Figs. 2 and 3). Figure 2 showed that the UC range had a significant impact on fetal status assessment and 0.6% of uterine contractions per second was a watershed. In addition, Fig. 3 showed that the percentage of time spend with abnormal long-term variability (ALTV) played an important role in fetal status assessment. With the increase of ALTV value, the possibility of fetus being assessed as pathological and suspicious category increased.

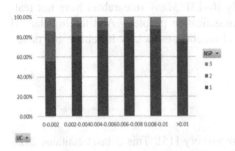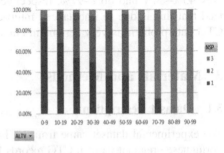

Fig. 2. Distribution of UC and fetal status   Fig. 3. Distribution of ALTV and fetal status

According to the results of the data exploration, AC, FM, DP, ASTV, ALTV, MLTV, Mode, Mean and Median features had a great role in evaluating fetal status. These features can be served as referenced input features of WRF model.

3.3 Weighted Random Forest for Intelligent Evaluation of Fetal Health Status

In the proposed weighted random forest model, the normal, suspicious and abnormal labels of CTG was defined as y = 0, 1 and 2, respectively, n is total number of CTG cases. Then, let m, l and n–m–l denoted the number of samples with labels 0, 1 and 2 respectively; and w_0, w_1 and w_2 were the weights of categories 0, 1, and 2, respectively.

$$w_0 = \frac{n}{3 \cdot m}, w_1 = \frac{n}{3 \cdot l}, w_2 = \frac{n}{3 \cdot (n - m - l)} \tag{1}$$

According to this, it can be seen that the penalty items of CTG categories were inversely proportional to the number of input samples. The larger the penalty items of a certain category, the higher the cost of misclassification would be considered. Hence, the WRF model was more sensitive to suspicious and abnormal categories.

$$H(x) = argmax \sum_{t=1}^{T} \prod (h_t(x) = y) \tag{2}$$

After that, the WRF model randomly chose K CTG features to obtain a subset xi. Then, it would construct decision tree $h_i(D_i)$, and made up random forest $\{h_1(D_1), h_2(D_2), h_3(D_3) \ldots\ldots h_{i-1}(D_{i-1}), h_i(D_i)\}$ Finally, the output prediction result was $\{H_1(x), H_2(x), H_3(x) \ldots\ldots H_{i-1}(x), H_i(x)\}$ (Fig. 4).

4 Results and Discussions

4.1 The Important CTG Feature for Antenatal Fetal Monitoring

As the experimental result, the number of CTG random features was determined to be 10, and the feature importance using WRF for antenatal fetal monitoring was shown in Fig. 5. It could be found that ALTV, ASTV, Median, Mean, AC, MLTV and Mode greatly contributed to fetal status discrimination. Moreover, these important features were consistent with the results of CTG data exploration.

4.2 Performance on Imbalanced Cardiotocography Multi-classification

Comparison with the Conventional Machine Learning Methods
In order to testify the performance on imbalanced CTG data of the proposed WRF model, the sensitivity, specificity, F1 score and ROC curve area of the six models were shown in the Table 1. Compared with traditional machine learning methods, the WRF model greatly improved the sensitivity (0.99 and 0.98) and specificity (0.96 and 0.95)

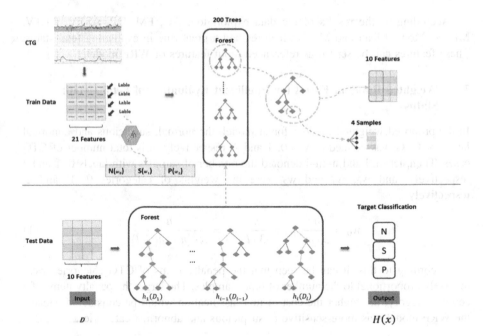

Fig. 4. Distribution of WRF and fetal status

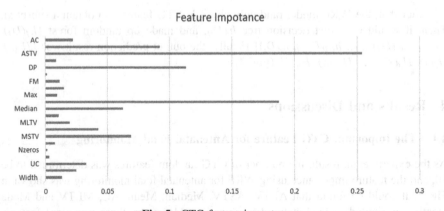

Fig. 5. CTG feature importance

in the categories of suspicious and abnormal. Meanwhile, according to the ROC curve area comparison chart (Fig. 6), it was demonstrated that the WRF model outperformed traditional machine learning models in reducing the probability of misdiagnosis. Furthermore, the WRF model had the highest accuracy and the shortest running time. The above results indicated that WRF model proposed could effectively solve the imbalance problem of multiple classifications CTG data.

Table 1. Comparison of overall classification evaluation and efficiency between WRF and other models

Evaluating indicator		Sensitivity	Specificity	F1	Auc	Running time (s)	Prediction error
WRF	**Normal**	**0.9981**	**0.9905**	**0.9975**	**0.9976**		
	Suspicious	**0.9923**	**0.9621**	**0.9768**	**0.9886**	**5.48**	**0.0438**
	Abnormal	**0.9834**	**0.9524**	**0.9524**	**0.9848**		
BP	Normal	0.9494	0.9785	0.9432	0.8884		
	Suspicious	0.8302	0.7586	0.7928	0.8083	35.82	0.0493
	Abnormal	0.9459	0.8333	0.8861	0.7782		
RF	Normal	0.9760	0.9442	0.9598	0.9538		
	Suspicious	0.9622	0.8750	0.8539	0.9504	26.51	0.0677
	Abnormal	0.9762	0.8913	0.9318	0.9475		
DT	Normal	0.9375	0.9443	0.9409	0.9376		
	Suspicious	0.7297	0.9923	0.7105	0.9236	23.38	0.0959
	Abnormal	0.8810	0.9024	0.8916	0.9105		
SVM	Normal	0.9495	0.8998	0.9240	0.7984		
	Suspicious	0.9595	0.8862	0.5152	0.7234	42.53	0.1274
	Abnormal	0.8905	0.8788	0.7734	0.6428		
KNN	Normal	0.9395	0.8758	0.9112	0.8343		
	Suspicious	0.8676	0.8846	0.6150	0.7568	38.34	0.1307
	Abnormal	0.8571	0.6207	0.7180	0.7523		

Note: The CPU configuration of the machine is Intel(R) Core (TM) i5-6200 CPU, 2.4 GHz, 8 GB of memory, and the system is 64 bits in the Chinese version of Win10.

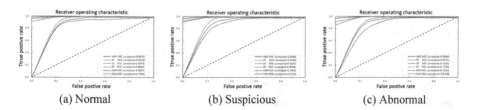

(a) Normal   (b) Suspicious   (c) Abnormal

Fig. 6. CTG Multi-classification ROC curve

In clinical practice, antenatal fetal monitoring often has serious multi-classification imbalance problem. To illustrate the WRF's adaptability to solve the imbalance problem of CTG data classification, the error classification spider-wed of seven classifiers, namely WRF, DT, RF, BP, SVM, KNN and opportunity, were plotted in Fig. 7. Among the six types of misclassification, the most dangerous one was to classify abnormal or suspicious errors as normal, because it will lead to missed optimal treatment time and even endanger fetal health. In addition, it was also dangerous to assess normal status as abnormal status, as it may lead to over-treatment, over-intervention and unnecessary cesarean section. The results showed that WRF model

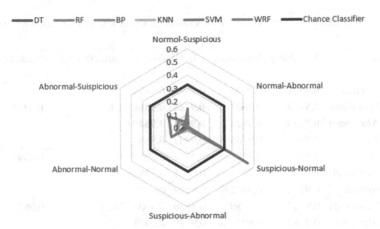

Fig. 7. Misclassification cobweb for seven classifiers.

had the lowest error classification rate among the three most harmful error classifications. Compared with other models, the WRF model greatly reduced the error classification rate of suspicious categories, and significantly improved the recognition ability of abnormal categories.

Comparison with the Existing Antenatal Fetal Monitoring Models
Compared with the existing antenatal CTG classification model (Table 2), the proposed WRF model had best classification performance in imbalanced fetal monitoring data. Table 2 showed that the F1 scores and accuracy of the proposed WRF model were higher than those of the existing antenatal fetal monitoring models. This further

Table 2. Comparison of overall accuracy and classification performance of existing CTG discriminant models

Model	Feature	Normal	Suspicious	Abnormal	F1	Accuracy
BP [9]	22	97.84%	45.14%	97.24%	80.07%	91.31%
GRNN [7]	21	95.70%	73.92%	84.88%	84.83%	91.86%
PNN [7]	21	95.91%	73.81%	85.45%	85.06%	92.14%
MLPNN [7]	21	95.00%	68.43%	80.50%	81.31%	90.36%
RF [11]	21	96.40%	79.60%	91.20%	89.07%	93.60%
IAGA [14] [1]	6	96.83%	79.15%	89.41%	88.46%	93.89%
DT-AdaBoost [10]	21	97.15%	83.69%	92.84%	91.23%	95.01%
DA [8]	10	89.69%	58.50%	65.58%	71.26%	82.03%
LS-SVM-PSO-BDT [12]	21	96.02%	72.98%	79.18%	82.73%	91.58%
DT [8]	10	93.31%	60.09%	66.43%	73.28%	86.31%
RF (this article)	10	96.53%	77.36%	89.16%	87.68%	93.43%
WRF (this article)	**10**	**99.75%**	**97.68%**	**95.24%**	**97.85%**	**99.71%**

demonstrated that the proposed WRF model had advantages in CTG data multi-classification. In general, the model had a good application prospect in the intelligent evaluation of antenatal fetal health using severely imbalanced CTG data (Fig. 8).

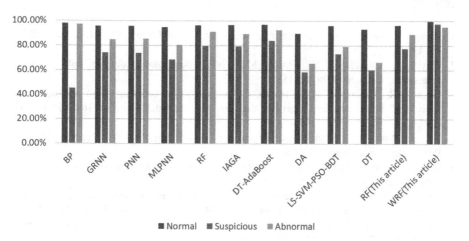

Fig. 8. Comparison of classification performance of existing CTG discriminant models

5 Conclusions

Diagnosis of fetal health is an essential task of antenatal fetal monitoring. Existing researches have implemented various machine learning algorithms to improve the accuracy for evaluation of antenatal fetal health status. However, they usually ignore that the fact that numbers of cases of abnormal and suspicious categories are very small in clinic. This will tent to result in the misdiagnosis the abnormal and suspicious cases as normal ones, and bring high risks to both fetuses and pregnant women. In this paper, we proposed a WRF model for antenatal fetal monitoring, which can intelligently and accurately evaluate the health status of the fetus using imbalanced cardiotocography data. Based on the mechanism of random forest algorithm, cost-sensitive learning was carried out by adjusting the class weights to solve the classification errors caused by imbalanced CTG data and reduced the miss-judgement of suspicious and abnormal classes. The experimental results showed that comparing with the existing 10 discriminant models of fetal monitoring, the proposed WRF model achieved the best performance, with an average F1 score of 97.85%. This verified the superiority of the WRF model in imbalanced multi-CTG data classification.

In the proposed WRF model, the CTG features were extracted from fetal heart rate and uterine contraction signals. There existed some calculating errors. Hence, improvement of CTG feature extraction should be studied further. Besides, the robustness of WRF should be optimized to the imbalance multi-classification problems in antenatal fetal monitoring.

Acknowledgement. This work is supported by The Medical Scientific Research Foundation of Guangdong Province under Grant No. A2019428, and the Natural Science Foundation of Guangdong Province under Grant No. 2015A030310312.

References

1. Haran, S., Everett, T.R.: Antenatal fetal wellbeing. Obstet. Gynaecol. Reprod. Med. **27**(2), 44–49 (2017)
2. Grivell, R.M., Alfirevic, Z., Gyte, G.M.L., et al.: Antenatal cardiotocography for fetal assessment. Cochrane Libr. (2015)
3. Gagnon, R., Campbell, M.K., Hunse, C.A.: comparison between visual and computer analysis of antepartum fetal heart rate tracings. Am. J. Obstet. Gynecol. **168**(3 Pt 1), 842 (1993)
4. Xie, X., Yan, W.: Obstetrics and Gynecology, 8 edn, pp. 118–120. People's Medical Publishing House, Beijing (2013)
5. Ocak, H., Ertunc, H.M.: Prediction of fetal state from the cardiotocogram recordings using adaptive neuro-fuzzy inference systems. Neural Comput. Appl. **23**(6), 1583–1589 (2013)
6. Ocak, H.: A medical decision support system based on support vector machines and the genetic algorithm for the evaluation of fetal well-being. J. Med. Syst. **37**(2), 9913 (2013)
7. Yılmaz, E.: Fetal state assessment from cardiotocogram data using artificial neural networks. J. Med. Biol. Eng. **36**(6), 820–832 (2016)
8. Huang, M.L., Hsu, Y.Y.: Fetal distress prediction using discriminant analysis, decision tree, and artificial neural network. J. Biomed. Sci. Eng. **05**(9), 526 (2012)
9. Sundar, C.M., Chitradevi, M.C., Geetharamani, G.: Classification of cardiotocogram data using neural network based machine learning technique. Int. J. Comput. Appl. **47**(14), 19–25 (2013)
10. Karabulut, E.M., Ibrikci, T.: Analysis of cardiotocogram data for fetal distress determination by decision tree based adaptive boosting approach. J. Comput. Commun. **02**(9), 32–37 (2014)
11. Arif, M.: Classification of cardiotocograms using random forest classifier and selection of important features from cardiotocogram signal. Biomater. Biomech. Bioeng. **2**(3), 173–183 (2015)
12. Yilmaz, E., Kilikçier, Ç.: Determination of fetal state from cardiotocogram using LS-SVM with particle swarm optimization and binary decision tree. Comput. Math. Methods Med. **2013**(2), 487179 (2013)
13. State Statistical Bureau. Statistical Yearbook of China. China Statistics Press, Beijing (2017)
14. Ravindran, S., Jambek, A.B., Muthusamy, H., et al.: A novel clinical decision support system using improved adaptive genetic algorithm for the assessment of fetal well-being. Comput. Math. Methods Med. **2015**, 11 (2015)
15. Asuncion, A., Newman, D.: UCI machine learning repository (2007)
16. Ayresde, C.D., Bernardes, J., Garrido, A., et al.: SisPorto 2.0: a program for automated analysis of cardiotocograms. J. Matern.-Fetal Med. **9**(5), 311–318 (2000)
17. Alfirevic, Z., Devane, D., Gyte, G.M.: Continuous cardiotocography (CTG) as a form of electronic fetal monitoring (EFM) for fetal assessment during labour. Cochrane Libr. **19**(3), CD006066 (2006)
18. Cheng, Z., Song, S.: Fetal electronic monitoring, 81–92 (2001)
19. Lyons, E.R., Bylsma-Howell, M., Shamsi, S., et al.: A scoring system for nonstressed antepartum fetal heart rate monitoring. Am. J. Obstet. Gynecol. **133**(3), 242–246 (1979)

20. Tian, C.: NST score and modified fischer scoring method to evaluate the correlation between fetal test results and newborn birth. CJ **16**(22), 28–29 (2009)
21. Society of obstetricians and gynaecologists of Canada. SOGC clinical practice guidelines. Guidelines for vaginal birth after previous caesarean birth. Number 155 (Replaces guideline Number 147), February 2005. Int. J. Gynaecol. Obstet. **89**(3), 319 (2005)
22. Santo, S., Ayres-de-Campos, D., Costa-Santos, C., et al.: Agreement and accuracy using the FIGO, ACOG and NICE cardiotocography interpretation guidelines. Acta Obstet. Gynecol. Scand. **96**(2), 166–175 (2017)
23. Ayres-de-Campos, D., Spong, C.Y., Chandraharan, E.: FIGO consensus guidelines on intrapartum fetal monitoring: cardiotocography. Int. J. Gynecol. Obstet. **131**(1), 13–24 (2015)
24. Chinese society of perinatal medicine. expert consensus on the application of electronic fetal heart rate monitoring. Chin. J. Perinat. Med. **2015**(7), 486–490 (2015)
25. Xie, X., Kong, B., Duan, T.: Gynecology and Obstetrics, 9th Edn, pp. 54–56. People's Health Publishing House, Beijing (2018)
26. Zhang, H.: Graphic analysis and management of 368 cases of abnormal non-stress test in fetal monitoring. Gen. Nurs. **14**(36), 3837–3838 (2016)

A Framework Design of National Healthy Diet Monitoring System

Lei Chen[1], Xiao-Qian Ma[1], and Wei Shang[2(✉)]

[1] Beijing Wuzi University, No. 321 FuHe Street, TongZhou District,
Beijing 101149, China
[2] Academy of Mathematics and Systems Science, Chinese Academy of
Sciences, No. 55 Zhongguancun East Rd, Beijing 100190, China
shangwei@amss.ac.cn

Abstract. Proper diet is one of the most important prerequisites for people's health. Resident nutrition and diet building are crucial to the success of national health program of China in its new stage of development. Although there has been numerous research on dietary and its relation of health, there is a lack of overall vision of the current dietary situations in China. In this paper, a national health diet monitoring system is proposed based on the national nutrition survey and the Internet nutrition diet related data, using the text knowledge discovery method. The purpose of the proposed framework is to find out the current situation of diet and nutrition of national residents, monitor the dietary purchase, dietary habits and changes of residents, and provide decision-making support for the formulation of relevant policies and the dietary guidance and improvement of residents.

Keywords: Nutrition and health · Decision support · System design

1 Introduction

The national nutrition plan (2017–2030), which was issued and implemented by the general office of the state council on June 30, 2017, is formulated to implement the outline of the "healthy China 2030" and improve national nutrition and health. Since the 19th CPC national congress, the main social contradictions in China have been the contradiction between the people's growing need for a better life and the unbalanced and inadequate development. With the development of social economy and the continuous improvement of people's living standard, the national demand for nutrition and health is higher and higher both in the premise of ensuring food safety, and in the pursuit of nutrition and health.

Nowadays, data quantity increases sharply [1], which is also a challenge to the formulation of policies. The rapid change of these demands means that the formulation of policies also needs to be followed up in time to solve the livelihood problems more efficiently. The major media pays more and more attention on the nutrition and health of the nation in different ways. However, in the era of big data, these reports are scattered all over the Internet. On the one hand, media information records the history; on the other hand, it also continuously provides users with new information, guiding

© Springer Nature Switzerland AG 2019
H. Chen et al. (Eds.): ICSH 2019, LNCS 11924, pp. 86–95, 2019.
https://doi.org/10.1007/978-3-030-34482-5_8

the public opinion in virtual world [2]. The theme of "healthy diet" is very close to People's Daily life. Public opinion monitoring and appropriate intervention on the national diet help to improve the national health level and reduce the risk of disease [3], and thereby improve the national happiness level [4]. However, it may also be exploited by illegal businesses, who make profits by spreading panic information. At present, the national nutrition and health detection system is still in the early stage of development, and the application of big data technology is not proficient [5]. Therefore, we hope to make use of computer technology, media data, text knowledge discovery model and other methods to design a national health diet monitoring system that can adapt to the characteristics of the times.

2 System Design

2.1 The Framework

Mission of the National Healthy Diet Monitoring System is to provide a real time inspection and analysis of residents' diet and related news reports. For the residents' diet and monitoring task, regular residents' diet survey data are collected and analyzed according to different monitoring tasks. The dietary survey of residents here comes from a nationwide regular dietary survey project. Internet news crawler gathered web pages with dietary and health topics. And these web-page texts are processed according to different themes and sentiments. Meaningful sentiment index is accordingly extracted from events detection and related policy. The framework is as shown in the following figure (see Fig. 1).

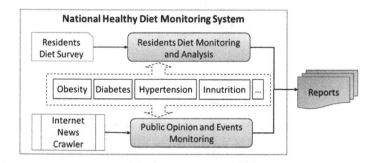

Fig. 1. System framework

2.2 Diet Survey

Diet survey in this research is a part of a national grain safety program. Respondents of the survey came from 31 provinces of China. The survey is regularly conducted four times a year to cover different season diet. Each survey covers about 3000 residents. The demographic features of our sample are statistically coincided with the whole nations using hieratical sampling methods. Respondents are required to take records of their daily meals, snacks and drinks for three continuous days including two weekdays and one weekend day. 927 interviewers are divided into 139 groups. Each group has a leader who is responsible for coaching the interviewers and checking the collected questionnaires. So far, 9382 questionnaires are collected and 251385 diet items are extracted for diet monitoring and analysis.

2.3   Web Page Text Mining

As an excellent background framework based on the python language, Django has efficient processing logic in URL accesses [6]. Its excellent performance in fluency has been tested [7]. And Scrapy is an excellent customizable framework [8].

Figure 2 is the system flow chart designed according to the requirements.

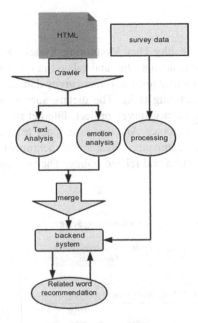

Fig. 2. Monitoring system path diagram

This paper uses Scrapy and Django framework to build background management system. Therefore, the whole system is composed of four major parts: text emotion analysis module, topic related word recommendation module, theme word frequency statistics module and related recommendation module.

Text emotion analysis module uses the emotional Thesaurus of Dalian University of Technology [9]. In this dictionary, each emotion word uses a seven-dimensional vector to represent seven emotions, so the word can be represented as $v_i(m_{i1}, m_{i2}, ..., m_{i7})$ where m_{ik} stands for the k emotion of the i word. After statistical calculation and transformation of all words, the emotion vector of the whole text can be represented by V_t, as shown in formula 1:

$$V_t = \left(\sum\nolimits_{i=0}^{n} m_{i1}, \sum\nolimits_{i=0}^{n} m_{i2}, \ldots, \sum\nolimits_{i=0}^{n} m_{i7} \right) \qquad (1)$$

Recommendation module of subject related words uses the word2vec model, which is evolved from the neural probabilistic language model. And word2vec model is an improved neural probabilistic language model, which is an extension of the n-gram statistical language model [10]. The original n-gram model is an efficient statistical language model [11], which assumes that a sentence W is composed of these words of a fixed order, then the probability of the occurrence of this sentence is $p(W)$, which can be regarded as joint probability of occurrence of k words (w_1, w_2, ..., w_k):

$$p(w_k | w_1, w_2, \cdots, w_{k-1}) = \frac{p(w_1, w_2, \cdots, w_{k-1}, w_k)}{p(w_1, w_2, \cdots, w_{k-1})} \qquad (2)$$

The neural probabilistic language model uses n-gram as a reference to express each word with a random word vector [12]. With the help of the neural network model, the final word vector is obtained through the iterative training of the corpus. According to the application needs, the system chooses CBOW as the training model [13], and we will analyze Chinese according to the word2vec model [14].

Text transformation into vector and text vector processing is a commonly used text analysis idea [15, 16]. TF-IDF is employed as a key method to judge the importance of a keyword vector in text in the subject word frequency statistics module of our system. The formula of TF-IDF is:

$$w_d = \frac{t_d}{t_a} \times \lg\left(1 + \frac{N}{n}\right) \qquad (3)$$

In formula (3), the td denotes the frequency of the word d appearing in t in this paper, ta represents the number of texts in the full text, N refers to the number of documents in the corpus, and n refers to the number of documents containing the word d.

In this system, We used TF-IDF to extract 7 theme words of each piece of information, and then counted the word frequency of these theme words, and selected the top 10 words to display in the "theme word frequency statistics model".

Meanwhile, in order to grasp the trend of public opinion in a more comprehensive way, we have trained the word2vec model using Wikipedia word base. When users monitor a keyword, we list some other keywords related to this keyword in "topic related word recommendation model", and recommend users to add these words at the same time.

3 Proof of Concepts

3.1 Diet and Obesity

In the diet survey, subjects' dietary information as well as their height, age, weight and other data are collected. As a proof of concept, we design a module to explore the relation between people's daily diet and obesity. Dietary items are classified according to the instruction from reports of the Chinese Dietary Guidelines and the obesity is calculated by BMI (Body Mass Index).

In this paper, the original data were filtered by using the Standard Score (z-score) based on the Median absolute deviation [17]. After removing the outliers in weight, height and BMI, a total of 8,230 valid data were obtained. Figure 3 shows the distribution of BMI of the respondents. The abscissa represents value of BMI, and the ordinate represents the proportion of current BMI in all BMI data:

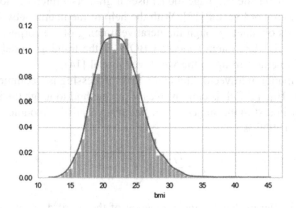

Fig. 3. BMI distribution of respondents

Table 1 describes the data distribution of height, weight and BMI of respondents:

Table 1. Statistical table of height, weight and BMI of respondents

	Height (m)	Weight (kg)	Age	BMI
Count	7706	7706	7706	7706
Mean	1.6	60.6	41.1	22.2
Std	0.1	11.9	20	3.3
Min	1.4	31	6	13.5
25%	1.6	52	24	19.7
50%	1.6	60	43	22
75%	1.7	69	56	24.3
Max	1.9	103	79	34.3

By comparing the diet structure of obese people (BMI higher than 24.9) and normal people (BMI between 18.5 and 24.9), we can compare the differences in dietary structure and dietary quantity between normal BMI and high BMI people.

Table 2 describes the diets that people with normal BMI and high BMI often eat, and then calculates the average number of times they eat these dishes per day.

Table 2. The top 5 frequently eaten food and average eaten times by people with high and normal BMI

No.	Food	Normal BMI	High BMI
1	Rice	0.72	3.32
2	Steamed bread	0.32	1.58
3	Noodles	0.15	0.70
4	Boiled egg	0.14	0.68
5	Millet gruel	0.13	0.66

As can be seen from Table 3, the diet structure of people with high BMI value is basically the same as that of people with normal BMI value.

Table 3. Comparison between high BMI diet and normal BMI diet

Diet	High BMI diet percentage	Normal BMI diet percentage
Total food	39.03%	38.78%
Eggs and products	7.38%	7.40%
Vegetables and products	30.58%	30.32%
Aquatic products	3.64%	3.70%
Meat and products	14.89%	15.25%
Milk and milk products	1.78%	1.84%
Beverage	1.13%	1.12%
Fruits and products	1.37%	1.37%
Nuts and seeds	0.14%	0.13%
Other or uncertain	0.06%	0.07%

Table 4 compares the average daily food intake of people with high BMI and those with low BMI.

According to the data in Tables 3 and 4, the main reason for the high BMI of nationals is that people with high BMI eat too much.

In the system, we added a "relevant Suggestions" module to provide some effective suggestions for certain search results. For example, according to this survey data, we can provide some suggestions such as "Eat less cook rice cakes and chicken hotpot" when users search for keywords such as "obesity" and "high BMI".

Of course, if you only want advice on dietary health, but do not need to know the information about national nutrition and health, you can also enter the keywords

Table 4. Average daily diet between high and low BMI people

Diet	High BMI average(g)	Normal average(g)
Total food	2261.25	470.05
Eggs and products	275.32	57.89
Vegetables and products	2027.08	417.94
Aquatic products	272.29	58.12
Meat and products	922.76	197.95
Milk and milk products	156.68	34.14
Beverage	126.09	26.43
Fruits and products	81.22	16.89
Nuts and seeds	3.13	0.65
Other or uncertain	2.18	0.49

directly to view this information. Because they will be stored into the database in advance and can be retrieved at any time.

3.2 Obesity Topic Monitoring

Here, as a proof of concept, we explored the Internet public and media opinions related to "obesity" from April 1 to 20, 2019. Using the proposed system to capture the "obesity" data for 20 consecutive days on the website of "Baidu news" from April 1, 2019, a total of 882 pieces of news data were obtained. Of these, 457 were successfully extracted by the system.

The visual data analysis results displayed in the system is shown in Fig. 4. It can be seen that during this period, the national attitude to healthy diet tends to be stable on the whole. At the same time, the "recommended addition" module provides key words related to obesity, such as "fat" and "dietary habit". The key words and their frequency in the 20-day news are shown in the "theme-related words". The order illustrates the link between "fat" and "healthy" and "weight loss" in people's minds. The "Suggestions" module prompts users to eat more healthy foods and eat less oily, fatty, greasy foods. For some users, useful opinions will also increase the user experience.

Through the system data export function, we can also enrich the research content and make full use of data to meet the needs of relatively professional data analysts. After exporting data in CSV format from the system, 457 news data generated in these 20 days, keywords corresponding to each news, and multidimensional emotional data corresponding to news content can be obtained.

3.3 Response to Hot Events

We can make further analysis with the help of the original data and five keywords extracted by TF-IDF. We assume that the subject words of n articles contain the word, then we can use formula (4) to express the emotion represented by each word with the current data:

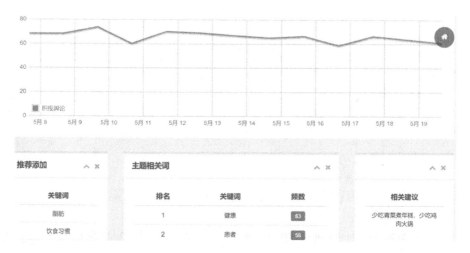

Fig. 4. "Obesity" news.baidu.com data between April 1 and 20, 2019.

$$word_{vk} = \frac{\sum\limits_{i=1}^{n} motion_{vi}}{n} \tag{4}$$

Where, emotion vector $motion_{vi}$ represents the emotion vector for article I that contains the word. And then we do this for every word that appears, and finally we get the emotional distribution of the word in the current situation. It can be seen from the results that the expressions of disgust, namely "parent", "education", "heart", "gut", "slimming" and "sleep" are the most frequent words in the heat text, which is also valuable information for some data analysis teams. In certain cases, it may identify bad businesses that use the Internet to spread false information and rumors for profit. The original data crawled by the system provide the basis for policy making and scientific research.

When trying to verify an emergency event or a hot news headline with the system, we hope the system can highlight emergencies according to the analysis of public opinion. However, most headline events are related to food safety, so we try to analyze the latest food safety emergencies with a systematic analysis method. These data is based on solstice's information on the topic of "food safety" from September 15, 2016 to October 31, 2016 (see Fig. 5).

In mid-September 2016, the "Cao Lin rice noodle case" in Shanghai was one of the headlines that attracted more attention in China. In the middle of September 2016, "Cao Lin rice noodles" was suspected of forcibly adding poppies into food, and forcibly distributing condiment bags packaged with poppies to more than 100 branches, causing a bad impact. On October 12, 2016, The owner of "Cao Lin rice noodles" and the other persons involved were sentenced according to law. In order to compare with the previous case, we verified the effectiveness of the system by using 1,048 pieces of news data that can extract emotions on September 16, 2016 and October 31, 2016. The

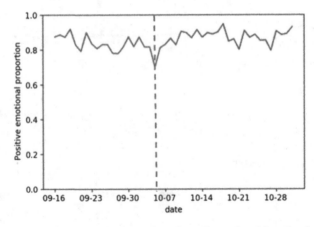

Fig. 5. Percentage of positive emotions from September 16 to October 31

analysis results verified that we can detect some emergencies related to the current topic through this system, so as to provide support for the timely response of relevant institutions.

4 Conclusions

In this paper, a framework of national healthy diet monitoring system is designed. The system provides two main functions to improve national health by promoting better diet suggestions. One is residents' diet monitoring and analysis of a national wide residents' diet survey project. The other is public opinion and events monitoring based on Internet documents. The system is designed as a general decision support system targeted at resident nutrition and diet related topics, such as obesity, diabetes, hypertension and nutrition, etc. Obesity monitoring, for example, provides useful information of the relationship between obesity and diet and public opinion on obesity-related topics. In the future, research will focus on other issues related to national healthy diet and relevant decision-making tasks.

Acknowledgement. This project is supported by the Key Project of Chinese Academy of Sciences (No. KJZD-EW-G20), Projects of Social Science Program of Beijing Education Commission (No. SM201810037001 and SM201910037004) and Social Beijing Social Science Foundation (No. 18GLB022)

References

1. Lynch, C.: Big data: how do your data grow? Nature **455**(7209), 28 (2008)
2. Zhu, H., Bin, H.: Impact of information on public opinion reversal – an agent based model. Phys. A **512**, 578–587 (2018)

3. Young, C., et al.: Supporting engagement, adherence, and behavior change in online dietary interventions. J. Nutr. Educ. Behav. **51**(6), 719–739 (2019)
4. Koronakos, G., et al.: Assessment of the OECD's better life index by incorporating the public opinion. Soc. Econ. Plann. Sci. (2019, in press). https://doi.org/10.1016/j.seps.2019.03.005
5. Guo, Q.Y., et al.: Comparative analysis of 1959, 1982, 1992, 2002 and 2010–2013 Chinese residents' nutrition and health status survey/monitoring. Health Res. **45**(4), 542–547 (2016). (in Chinese)
6. Holovaty, A., kaplin-moss, J.: The definitive guide to Django: Web development done right. Apress (2009)
7. Pu, W., Cao, L., Xia, B.: Design of keyword ranking monitoring system based on Django framework. Microcomput. Appl. **20**(2017), 97–100. (in Chinese)
8. Feng, C., Yang, B.: Design and implementation of JD data analysis system based on scrapy framework. Value Eng. **28**, 111 (2018). (in Chinese)
9. Xu, L., et al.: Construction of affective lexical ontology. Acta Intell. **27**(2), 180–185 (2008)
10. Rong, X.: Word2vec parameter learning explained. arXiv preprint arXiv:1411.2738 (2014)
11. Pauls, A., Klein, D.: Faster and smaller n-gram language models. In: Proceedings of the 49th Annual Meeting of the Association for Computational Linguistics: Human Language Technologies-Volume 1. Association for Computational Linguistics (2011)
12. Bengio, Y., et al.: A neural probabilistic language model. J. Mach. Learn. Res. **3**, 1137–1155 (2003)
13. Ma, L., Zhang, Y.: Using Word2Vec to process big text data. In: 2015 IEEE International Conference on Big Data (Big Data). IEEE (2015)
14. Zhang, D., et al.: Chinese comments sentiment classification based on word2vec and SVMperf. Expert Syst. Appl. **42**(4), 1857–1863 (2015)
15. Trstenjak, B., Mikac, S., Donko, D.: KNN with TF-IDF based framework for text categorization. Procedia Eng. **69**, 1356–1364 (2014)
16. Huang, C.-H., Yin, J., Hou, F.: A text similarity measurement combining word semantic information with TF-IDF method. Jisuanji Xuebao (Chin. J. Comput.) **34**(5), 856–864 (2011)
17. Leys, C., et al.: Detecting outliers: do not use standard deviation around the mean, use absolute deviation around the median. J. Exp. Soc. Psychol. **49**(4), 764–766 (2013)

The Research on Spatial Accessibility to Healthcare Services Resources in Tianhe, Guangzhou

Juhua Wu[1], Zhenyi Zhao[1(✉)], Shunjun Jiang[2], and Lei Tao[1]

[1] School of Management, Guangdong University of Technology,
Guangzhou 510520, China
zhaozhenyi1994@outlook.com
[2] The First Affiliated Hospital of Guangzhou Medical University,
Guangzhou 510120, China

Abstract. The rational allocation of medical service resources can affect the convenience of residents to obtain health care services. Therefore, the uneven distribution of medical resources is currently a prominent problem in the process of building medical and health services in China. The spatial accessibility analysis can assess areas of lack of medical resources and serve as a scientific measure for assessing the rationality of spatial allocation of medical services. This study uses the route planning module based on the online map API to calculate the distance of residents arriving at medical institutions, through the spatial accessibility analysis method based on the gravity model, and use Arc-GIS to geographically visualize the results. The spatial accessibility in the northeastern part of Tianhe was much lower than that in the southwestern part, indicating that there is still a large spatial accessibility difference in medical facilities in Tianhe District, and the layout of medical facilities lacks certain rationality. Where healthcare service resources are concentrated but medical care is crowded, hospital pressure should be minimized and some patients should be referred to the surrounding areas. At the same time more medical services should be offered to improve the allocation of local medical resources where medical resources are scarce.

Keywords: Healthcare services resources · Spatial accessibility · Gravity model · Geographic visualization

1 Introduction

With the aging of the social population structure, the aggravation of urbanization, and the improvement of people's health awareness, the demand for basic public service facilities such as health care and medical service is growing rapidly. One of the major contradictions in China's healthcare service industry is the serious imbalance between the supply and the demand of medical resources, which is manifested in the unequal distribution of medical resources in the region. Even in the same urban area, there is a problem of uneven distribution of supply. The rational allocation of medical service

© Springer Nature Switzerland AG 2019
H. Chen et al. (Eds.): ICSH 2019, LNCS 11924, pp. 96–105, 2019.
https://doi.org/10.1007/978-3-030-34482-5_9

resources has become a problem that cannot be ignored in the development and construction of medical and health services in China.

In the context of the policy of equalization of basic public services, an important goal of basic medical resource allocation and optimization of hospital layout planning is to achieve a fair allocation of medical service resources [1] to achieve safety, effectiveness, fairness, and Basic public health services and basic healthcare services. The spatial accessibility assessment method can identify scarce areas of healthcare service resources and is an effective way to measure the fairness of healthcare service facilities layout [2].

With the development of cities in first front, the distribution of large general hospitals is excessively concentrated in economically developed areas, while the undeveloped areas far from the central areas of cities, including urban-rural integration, are relatively lack of healthcare services resources, which make the uneven of healthcare service resources very serious.

The accessibility of medical services is a multidimensional and comprehensive concept [3], which is not limited to objective geographic distance measurements, but also includes subjective measurements [4]. In addition, accessibility creates unmet health care needs, not only because of barriers to distance, but also because of the unavailability of health care services and the acceptability of individual medical services to patients [5, 6].

Considering the convenience and accuracy of measuring, spatial accessibility is often used as a key indicator of accessibility measurement. Spatial accessibility is also the combination of two-dimensions which mean "accessibility" and "availability" [7]; therefore, travel time and appointment time can be considered as a unit of measure for interpreting "spatial accessibility." This study also uses this indicator as the main target of the measurement. Among that, accessibility is the geographical spatial relationship between patients and health care institutions [8], which refers to the separation between population and health care services [9], e.g., the travel time from a location of the population to the location of the health care service. And availability generally refers to the number of health care services a patient can choose, that is, the relationship between what provided by the supplier and the patient's needs [8], but other indicators such as waiting time may also be considered, like the waiting time [10]. We can find that among many spatial accessibility evaluation methods, 2SFCA and potential model method are the most widely used [11–13]. The 2SFCA method and gravity model both consider the factors comprehensively, which also share a similar theoretical basis of the model [14].

This study takes Tianhe District as an example to evaluate the rationality and equality of regional healthcare service resources distribution by analyzing the spatial accessibility distribution of them.

2 Material and Method

2.1 Study Area

As shown in Fig. 1, Tianhe, the study area, is located in Guangzhou, Guangdong province. It is the main district of Guangzhou, which also is one of the most developed regions. Since the establishment officially in the 1980s, Tianhe has experienced miraculous rapid growth for more than 30 years. Tianhe has grown into a district with 1.6979 million permanent residents and an administrative area of 137.38 km². There are 21 subdistrict units (called Jiedao in Chinese) in Tianhe, including Wushan, Yuancun, Shahe, Chepi, Shipai, Tianhenan, Linhe, Shadong, Xinghua, Tangxia, Tianyuan, Xiancun, Liede, Yuangang, Huangcun, Longdong, Changxing, Fenghuang, Qianjin, Zhuji, Xintang. Tianhenan and Shipai are the developed sub-district with the densest population in Tianhe. This study takes the subdistrict as the minimum spatial unit in following calculation.

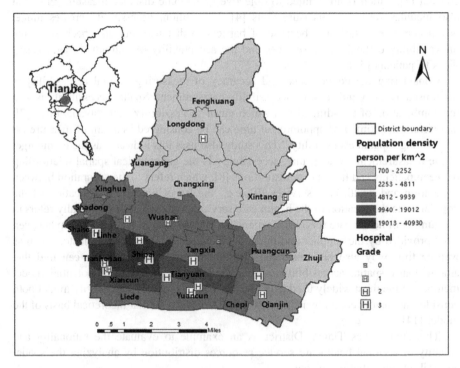

Fig. 1. Population density distribution in Tianhe District

2.2 Data

The population data at the sub-district level used in this study comes from the national economic statistics of Tianhe District (2017), which is the latest official population census data at the sub-district level. Due to the lack of population data at a finer scale, the geometry centroids of sub-districts are used to denote the demand nodes.

List and addresses of healthcare facilities in Tianhe are obtained from the official website of Guangzhou Government Data Unified Open Platform (http://data.gz.gov.cn). The latest time of visiting the website was April 4, 2019. Our analysis only includes the hospitals listed on the above website.

Since the community healthcare centers are usually small-scaled and dispersed in the space, and their service capacities are unknown, they are not considered in this study. In addition, the specialized hospitals for certain types or a few types of diseases have also been excluded, this study focuses on the general hospitals that provide general healthcare and medical services for residents. As shown in Fig. 1, there are 23 hospitals which can supply general medical services for citizens in Tianhe. The number of hospital beds is used to denote the service capacity of each hospital in this paper.

APIs of online map developers such as Google Map or Baidu Map are usually used to estimate travel time [15–17]. Researchers can make use of the dynamically updated transport network data and the routing rules maintained by map developers to obtain a reliable estimation of travel time [16]. In this study, Datamap, which developed based on the Amap API, is utilized to estimate the travel time from the residential area to hospital under the driving-mode, and the analysis and calculation is performed by Excel to construct the O-D cost matrix.

2.3 Method

The gravity model is one of the classic models for studying the interaction between social and economic space. It is widely used to compare the size of urban attraction or the advantages and disadvantages of comparative development. This study uses a gravity model to measure the attractiveness of hospitals in the region to residential areas as a measure of the spatial accessibility of healthcare service resources. A population size impact factor is added to the gravitational model, which measures the cumulative value of the attractiveness of medical institutions (resources) in all populations by simulating the formula of the law of universal gravitation. It considers the service capabilities of the facility, the distance to the facility, the spatial attenuation, and the distribution of population around the facility [18, 19, 22]. As follows, the spatial accessibility can be expressed as a function:

$$A_i = \sum_{j=1}^{n} \frac{S_j}{D_{ij}^{\beta} V_j} \tag{1}$$

The function of Vj can be used an exponential form to express and considering a time measure instead of a distance measure, we can formulate the following equation:

$$V_j = \sum_{k=1}^{m} \frac{P_k}{D_{kj}^{\beta}} \tag{2}$$

For our study, Ai represents a spatial accessibility measure, and Sj represents a measure of the healthcare service supply, that is the service supply capacity of services (the number of hospital beds); Pk is the population living in the administrative area (in this study, a street district); Finally, D_{ij}^{β} represents the time that an healthcare user have taken to travel to the healthcare service; β is the distance attenuation coefficient, the effect of spatial impedance increases as β gets larger, and vice versa, when β is less than 1.0, the distance attenuation effect is not obvious. The study found that the actual value of β is mostly concentrated between [1, 2, 18], so we experimentally select 1, 2 as the value of β, and the space obtained by the two is reachable.

By the functions of "join", "Summarize" and "Fieldcalculator" of ArcGIS, the spatial accessibility is calculated with the attribute table. Then, using the Kriging method (In statistics, originally in geostatistics, kriging is a method of interpolation for which the interpolated values are modeled by a Gaussian process governed by prior covariances) to interpolate the entire Tianhe District with calculated results, and rasterizing the GA (geostatistical analyst) layer that obtained from Kriging method, and extracting it by mask according to the district-level administrative map, to obtain the visualization results of the accessibility distribution of medical service resources in Tianhe District.

3   Results

Table 1 shows the descriptive statistics of the spatial accessibility under different β. The results are shown in Table 1 below. When β = 2, the spatial accessibility of each point in the region fluctuates more and the degree of dispersion is larger; when β = 1, the data is relatively concentrated. Therefore, when β = 2, the spatial accessibility of medical resources in each street has better performance in showing the difference in the distribution of healthcare service resources.

Table 1. Descriptive statistics of Ai under different β

	Min	Max	Mean	SD
β = 1	1.6321	3.0437	2.1129	0.31379
β = 2	0.83069	3.6415	1.8818	0.61773

Figure 2 shows a spatial representation of spatial accessibility in the survey zones when β is different, respectively. Compare β = 1, the spatial accessibility of healthcare service resources in the eastern and the southwestern of Tianhe District have a better performance when β = 2. In addition, the trend of spatial distribution of healthcare service resources in Tianhe District do not change significantly under different values of β. Overall, the area is greener means a higher accessibility for residents, while the red area indicates the lack of accessibility. As Fig. 2 shows, the study find that the spatial accessibility reaches the highest value in the southern part of Tianhe District, and gradually decreases outwards.

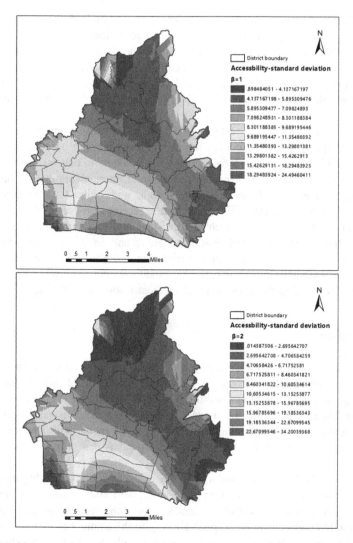

Fig. 2. Healthcare service resources spatial accessibility-standard deviation in survey zones

As shown in Fig. 2, the distribution of healthcare accessibility by gravity model shows significant spatial disparity. Specifically, the accessibility in the southern edge region is higher than the others part of Tianhe. Sub-districts with the highest healthcare accessibility are mainly located in Yancun, followed by Tianyuan, Tangxia and Shipai. These sub-districts have advantages in access to healthcare services because of their economic central locations. Longdong and Fenghuang, the most northern sub-district in Tianhe District with sparely population, which are the most peripheral sub-districts in Tianhe, have the lowest accessibility. The other peripheral region such as Zhuji located in east of Tianhe, and Liede located in southwest of Tianhe lack of accessibility as well.

Overall, with the spatial accessibility index, areas located in the southern of the city are areas that have high predictive values of spatial accessibility. And we also observed that accessibility varies more in the southern of the district than in other areas of Tianhe. The area with the lowest spatial accessibility index value (less than 2.696) is located in the northern of Tianhe. The red color in this zone shows that there are similarly low values of healthcare accessibility in the extremely south-west and south-east of Tianhe.

As Fig. 2 shows, the south-west part of Tianhe is a densely populated area. And as a result, excessive population reduces the convenience brought by concentrated hospitals in the region and increases the pressure on residents to pay for hospitals in the southwestern part of Tianhe District. The over-concentrated population has led to overloading of hospital admissions in this area, and reduces the availability of healthcare services. The accessibility of healthcare service resources in the northeastern part of Tianhe District is low, which is consistent with the characteristics of sparse population distribution, scattered residential areas and relatively small number of general hospitals. As a result, although Tianhe Nan and Shipai is the most developed area in Tianhe District with intensively distributed hospitals, the dense population in this area has diminished the advantages of medical resources in the region.

4   Conclusion

The general healthcare service is one type of public resources provided to residents. Spatial equality accessibility is very essential to the general healthcare service. How to eliminate spatial disparities of accessibility to general healthcare services for residents is an urgent issue for government. In order to detect the spatial disparity of healthcare service centers for local people, this study utilize gravity model with ArcGIS to obtain the characteristic of geographical distribution of hospitals that supply general medical service.

The study finds the medium and low values of the spatial accessibility index are in the northern areas, as well as in the extreme south-west and north-east of the district. The north Tianhe is an industrial–residential zone, inhabited by people with lower socio-economic conditions than the people living in the south. The extreme north-east of the district is also characterized by socio-economically deprived neighborhoods. The values of the spatial accessibility index had high variations in the southern of the city. This situation could be related to the presence of an important number of healthcare services in this zone. Indeed, the south Tianhe is the zone which has the highest concentration of public healthcare services in the district as the Fig. 1 shows, the road network is also more developed in these sub-districts which is helpful to get healthcare service.

According to the spatial accessibility distribution of healthcare service resources in Tianhe District, the supply of hospital services should be increased in the areas with insufficient accessibility, such as increasing hospital beds, introducing medical technicians, and promoting the transfer of high-quality medical resources from central urban areas to rural areas. Optimizing the layout of medical resources and promoting the establishment of a graded diagnosis and treatment system are good options for improving the efficiency of medical and health services. And promoting medical cooperation between universities and research institutions and small and medium-sized medical institutions is helpful to the rational allocation of medical resources in the region. The results in this study lead to a better understanding of healthcare disparities or inequalities, and can thus be considered as important tools for decision makers towards more efficient decisions regarding the health system in the study area.

There are still limitations in this paper: Firstly, the units selected for analysis are small. In fact, the radiation coverage of medical services in some large general hospitals may exceed the boundary of district-level administrative units. Residents in other adjacent districts and residents in Tianhe District will across the district for higher level of medical experience. Secondly, considering the influence of the friction coefficient β on the reachability results, in the future research, it may be considered to collect real data to determine the friction coefficient. Thirdly, this paper uses the administrative center of the neighborhood as the residential area to analyst. If the OD cost matrix can be constructed with a more realistic location of the residential area, the accuracy of the research results can be further improved.

Future research related to the medical spatial accessibility could include the incorporation of more detailed information regarding the population age composition regional. People of different ages have varying degrees of demand for medical services. For example, an area with large number of older adults require a high level of medical spatial accessibility. It will also be important to relate the travel behavior of residents since the spatial accessibility is an integrated result of vehicle, traffic congestion, public parking facilities and so on. In fact, the accessibility is also influenced by residents' behavior. Bertakis [19] found that the racial, social hierarchy, gender, age and income of residents also have an impact on their possibility of receiving medical services; and Wang et al. [20] divided these non-spatial factors that affect accessibility into four categories: social demographic structure, socio-economic factors, living environment and education service. Finally, there could be another potential role of the index for the explanation of the health inequalities in relation to specific health problems, such as chronic diseases or epidemics.

Acknowledgments. The authors would like to acknowledge the reviewers and editor for their insightful and constructive comments. The presented work has been funded by the National Natural Science Foundation of China (PM. Juhua Wu, NO. 71771059), the Philosophy and Social Science Foundation of Guangzhou (PM. Juhua Wu, NO. 502170111), and the Key Laboratory of Guangdong Science and Technology Finance and Big Data Analysis (NO. 2017B030301010).

References

1. Tao, Z., Cheng, Y.: Research progress of the two-step floating catchment area method and extensions. Prog. Geogr. **35**, 5 (2016)
2. Song, Z., Chen, W., Yuan, F., Wand, L.: Formulation of public facility location theory framework and literature review. Prog. Geogr. **29**(12), 1499–1508 (2010)

3. Andersen, R.M.: Revisiting the behavioral model and access to medical care: does it matter? J. Health Soc. Behav. 1–10 (1995). https://doi.org/10.2307/2137284

4. Comber, A.J., Brunsdon, C., Radburn, R.: A spatial analysis of variations in health access: linking geography, socio-economic status and access perceptions. Int. J. Health Geogr. **10**(1), 44 (2011). https://doi.org/10.1186/1476-072x-10-44

5. Aday, L.A., Andersen, R.: A framework for the study of access to medical care. Health Serv. Res. **9**(3), 208 (1974)

6. Chen, J., Hou, F.: Unmet needs for health care. Health Rep. **13**(2), 23–34 (2002)

7. Guagliardo, M.F.: Spatial accessibility of primary care: concepts, methods and challenges. Int. J. Health Geogr. **3**(1), 3 (2004)

8. Penchansky, R., Thomas, J.W.: The concept of access: definition and relationship to consumer satisfaction. Med. Care, 127–140 (1981). https://doi.org/10.1097/00005650-198102000-00001

9. Delamater, P.L.: Spatial accessibility in suboptimally configured health care systems: a modified two-step floating catchment area (M2SFCA) metric. Health Place **24**, 30–43 (2013). https://doi.org/10.1016/j.healthplace.2013.07.012

10. Cavalieri, M.: Geographical variation of unmet medical needs in Italy: a multivariate logistic regression analysis. Int. J. Health Geogr. **12**(1), 27 (2013). https://doi.org/10.1186/1476-072x-12-27

11. Apparicio, P., Abdelmajid, M., Riva, M., Shearmur, R.: Comparing alternative approaches to measuring the geographical accessibility of urban health services: distance types and aggregation-error issues. Int. J. Health Geogr. **7**(1), 7 (2008). https://doi.org/10.1186/1476-072x-12-27

12. Hu, R., Dong, S., Zhao, Y., Hu, H., Li, Z.: Assessing potential spatial accessibility of health services in rural China: a case study of Donghai County. Int. J. Equity Health **12**(1), 35 (2013). https://doi.org/10.1186/1475-9276-12-35

13. Fransen, K., Neutens, T., De Maeyer, P., Deruyter, G.: A commuter-based two-step floating catchment area method for measuring spatial accessibility of daycare centers. Health Place **32**, 65–73 (2015). https://doi.org/10.1016/j.healthplace.2015.01.002

14. Cabrera-Barona, P., Blaschke, T., Kienberger, S.: Explaining accessibility and satisfaction related to healthcare: a mixed-methods approach. Soc. Ind. Res. **133**(2), 719–739 (2017). https://doi.org/10.1007/s11205-016-1371-9

15. Cheng, G., et al.: Spatial difference analysis for accessibility to high level hospitals based on travel time in Shenzhen, China. Habitat Int. **53**, 485–494 (2016). https://doi.org/10.1016/j.habitatint.2015.12.023

16. Wang, F., Xu, Y.: Estimating O-D travel time matrix by Google maps API: implementation, advantages, and implications. Ann. GIS **17**(4), 199–209 (2011). https://doi.org/10.1080/19475683.2011.625977

17. Gu, W., Wang, X., McGregor, S.E.: Optimization of preventive health care facility locations. Int. J. Health Geogr. **9**(1), 17 (2010). https://doi.org/10.1186/1476-072x-9-17

18. Hansen, W.G.: How accessibility shapes land use. J. Am. Inst. Planners **25**(2), 73–76 (1959). https://doi.org/10.1080/01944365908978307

19. Joseph, A.E., Bantock, P.R.: Measuring potential physical accessibility to general practitioners in rural areas: a method and case study. Soc. Sci. Med. **16**(1), 85–90 (1982). https://doi.org/10.1016/0277-9536(82)90428-2

20. 宋正娜, 陈雯. 基于潜能模型的医疗设施空间可达性评价方法. 地理科学进展 **28**(6), 848–854 (2009)

21. Bertakis, K.D., Azari, R., Helms, L.J., Callahan, E.J., Robbins, J.A.: Gender differences in the utilization of health care services. J. Fam. Pract. **49**(2), 147 (2000)
22. Wang, F., Luo, W.: Assessing spatial and nonspatial factors for healthcare access: towards an integrated approach to defining health professional shortage areas. Health Place **11**(2), 131–146 (2005). https://doi.org/10.1016/j.healthplace.2004.02.003

A Comprehensive Database Based on Multiple Data Sources to Facilitate Diagnosis of ASD

Tao Chen[1,2(✉)]

[1] School of Information Management, Wuhan University, Wuhan, China
chentao1979@126.com
[2] Suzhou Zealikon Healthcare Co., Ltd., Suzhou, China

Abstract. Autism spectrum disorder (ASD) is a neurodevelopmental disorder which has an increasing prevalence in children. ASD is clinically highly heterogeneous and lacks objective diagnostic criteria. In recent years, magnetic resonance imaging and genomics have been widely used in the diagnosis of ASD, and some valuable biomarkers have been found, which has improved people's understanding of the neural and molecular development mechanism of ASD. However, most studies focus on limited data sources with lack of integration research, thus leading to inconsistent or biased results. In this paper, we design a compute-aided diagnosis framework based on multiple ASD-relevant data sources for purpose of distinguishing the ASD patients more accurately. We first establish a multiple data collection procedure from initial diagnosis to regular follow-up visits. Various medical big data including structured and unstructured forms are collected from different devices or protocols and then they are deposited and accessed based on Hadoop platform. Furthermore, we design a classification framework to identify ASD patients by integrating the complementary information from multiple data sources. Deep learning is used to extract features from each data source automatically, and then all extracted features are integrated by the multiple kernel learning method for improving the diagnostic accuracy of ASD.

Keywords: Autism Spectrum Disorder · Multiple data sources · Database · Big data · Classification · Multiple kernel learning · Deep learning

1 Introduction

Autism Spectrum Disorder (ASD) is a neurodevelopmental disorder characterized by social and communication difficulties, repetitive and restricted behaviors [1]. ASD is now diagnosed mainly based on Diagnostic and Statistical Manual of Mental Disorders, Fifth Edition (DSM-5) [2] criteria and various behavior scales such as Autism Diagnostic Observation Schedule (ADOS) [3], Autism Diagnostic Interview, Revised (ADI-R) [4]. However, the clinical symptoms of ASD patients may vary greatly among individuals and the diagnosis accuracy mainly depends on the physician's experience. With the development of artificial intelligence research in medical image analysis, computer aided diagnostic techniques based on magnetic resonance imaging have emerged, and many studies have found meaningful imaging biomarkers, providing

H. Chen et al. (Eds.): ICSH 2019, LNCS 11924, pp. 106–113, 2019.
https://doi.org/10.1007/978-3-030-34482-5_10

some guidance for the early discovery of ASD. However, the biomarkers obtained in these imaging studies are not always consistent, making it impossible to achieve clinical reliability by relying only on medical imaging [5, 6]. The reason for this inconsistence lies in that ASD is a highly heterogeneous and complex disease with unknown etiology but associated with neurological, genetic, environmental and other factors. At present, there are studies explaining the imaging heterogeneity of ASD patients from molecular perspective. For example, Qureshi et al. found that 16p11.2 chromosome deletion leads to an increase in brain volume, while its duplication leads to a decrease in brain volume [7]. Some studies also revealed how ASD risk genes (such as CNTNAP2, MET) affect brain structure and function networks [8, 9]. These studies have emphasized the important role of inheritability in ASD disease. And combining genes and imaging can facilitate the discovery of more accurate ASD imaging biomarkers. In 2009, the National Institute of Mental Health (NIMH) conducted a research project called Research Domain Criteria (RDoC) [10], which aims to transcend the limits of traditional classification method, combining genetics, neuroscience, behavioral science and other methods to clarify the neural basis and biomarkers of mental illness. This project implies that integration of multiple data sources such as genetic, neuroimaging, behavioral assessment, and patient clinical history can facilitate to improve ASD classification performance and investigate specific subtypes for better personalized healthcare.

In the last decade, many large-scale ASD data repositories have emerged for open access such as the National Database for Autism Research (NDAR) [11], the Simons Simplex Collection (SSC) [12], the Autism Genetic Resource Exchange (AGRE) [13], the Autism Brain Imaging Data Exchange (ABIDE) [14]. Among these data repositories, only NDAR contains a wide range of data sources such as clinical assessments of symptoms and functioning, genetic and genomic findings, imaging modalities, utilization of health and education resources, and quantitative behavioral assessments such as eye movement tracking, while SSC and AGRE include clinical and genetic data, and ABIDE includes clinical and imaging data. These open-access data repositories offer great opportunities to explore and advance scientific discoveries in the research of ASD. Although these large databases have promoted the identification of many new ASD susceptibility genes, as well as neurophysiological and neurobehavioral characteristics associated with ASD, they still have some limitations such as absence of longitudinal follow-up data that may reveal long-term genetic or neurological impact to ASD phenotypic manifestation, and narrow coverage of ethnic populations that may differ in the genetic background and environmental exposures. Furthermore, the number of samples including the complete set of data sources from the same individual is relatively small.

To address these issues, we propose to establish a large-scale ASD database including participants of some main Chinese ethnic populations such as Han, Hui, etc. And this dataset intends to contain longitudinal follow-up data for understanding the evolution of different pathological factors over the course of ASD development. The integration of various medical data from the same participant is beneficial to characterize the full manifestation of one specific ASD subtype and to identify its etiology and corresponding treatment plans. In order to effectively manage and analyze the multiple medical data sources, we design a storage scheme based on the big data technology. Considering the low cost and good scalability, we choose the Apache Hadoop platform to construct the architecture for data access and analysis. In addition, we also propose a classification framework based on multiple data sources to distinguish ASD patients from healthy controls.

2 Multiple Data Collection and Storage

Due to the heterogeneity of ASD etiology, we should collect data from different sources and deposit them in high-performance database system for a better integration analysis. Similar to NDAR database, the following ASD-relevant data will be collected such as clinical assessment including ADOS and ADI-R scores, neuroimaging, genetics, eye movement tracking, electroencephalography (EEG) recording, electronic health records (EHR). Participants will be diagnosed as ASD based on the DSM-5 criteria, and then be followed up every six months for three years. Figure 1 shows the data collection procedure and different data sources.

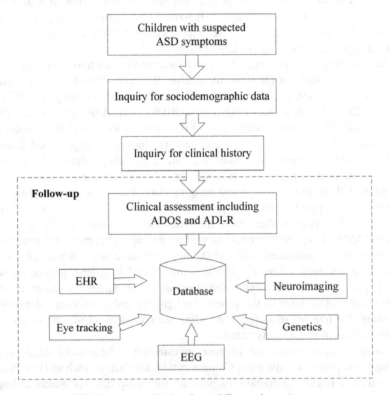

Fig. 1. Data collection from different data sources

The data collection protocols and data structures vary greatly for different data sources. The clinical assessment data are based on standard diagnosing scales such as

ADOS and ADI-R. Eye movement tracking and EEG recording data are generated from digital-based medical devices. The sociodemographic data is usually derived from the Hospital Information System (HIS) that is built on a Relational Database Management System (RDBMS). The above are all structured data that can be assembled into the RDBMS or directly into HDFS that is the core storage part of Hadoop. As for the unstructured data such as neuroimaging, genetics and EHR, they are preprocessed with ETL tools and then are deposited into HDFS. Except for HDFS, there are two high-level storage abstractions: Hive and HBase. The Hive tool is built on top of Hadoop for providing large-scale data query and analysis. It can map the structured data into a database table and use SQL-like query syntax to maximize compatibility with SQL standards. Hive is suitable for statistical analysis of large datasets without demanding high speed of data load and query. However, some clinical diagnosis may need to be determined with the real-time requirement. Such kind of data can be deposited into the distributed HBase data store, and by integrating with other components like Apache Spark, HBase can achieve fast, random reads and writes to those data that require real-time analysis. The overall storage scheme based on Hadoop components are shown in Fig. 2.

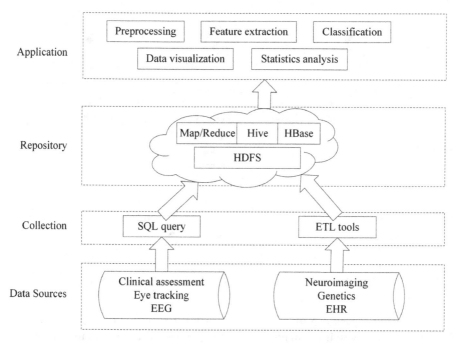

Fig. 2. Data storage scheme based on Hadoop platform

3   Integrated Classification Model for Identify ASD Patients

Most studies are focusing on ASD computer-aided diagnosis based on one or some few data sources. Each data source is assumed to convey distinct information or contain a different perspective from other data source, and the integration of multiple data sources provides more comprehensive characterization of ASD, leading to better classification performance and disease assessment than the single data source based method. Because the raw data collected from most sources are high-dimensional, it is not suitable to feed them directly to the classification model. Deep learning methods can effectively extract more discriminative features from high-dimensional and complex data [15]. To utilize fully the features extracted from various data sources and boost the overall classification performance, some feature integration methods should be used instead of simply concatenating the feature matrix of each data source. The integrated ASD classification framework is shown in Fig. 3.

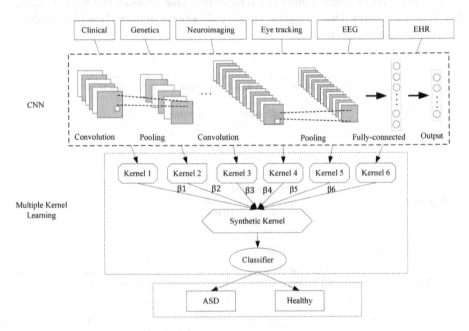

Fig. 3. Integrated classification framework to identify ASD

Convolutional Neural Network (CNN) is a feedforward neural network derived from biological nerves. It is a multi-layer perceptron model designed to recognize two-dimensional images and has certain invariance to image transformation. CNN is composed of three components including the convolutional layer, the pooling layer, and the fully connected layer, and it has some advantages such as network weight sharing and direct input of the original image. Although CNN is mainly used in the field of computer vision, its powerful feature analysis capabilities can also be used for the processing of genetics data [16]. There are many CNN models, e.g., LeNet-5,

Inception v3, that can be utilized to automatically extract the high-level features. This automated extraction method can learn features from raw medical data without prior knowledge, which can avoid the poor model performance cause by strong assumption in handcrafted feature design.

Support Vector Machine (SVM) [17] is a supervised learning method and commonly used in classification problems, which separates the classes with largest gap. For non-linearly separable data problems, SVM uses kernels which can transform the data from input space to a new high dimensional feature space where data can be separated with a linear surface. The optimal performance of SVMs is highly dependent on the kernel function used. Cross-validation is the standard approach to select the best kernel function among a set of candidates such as linear kernel, polynomial kernel and gaussian kernel. However, SVM is not suitable for analyzing multiple data sources using a single kernel function. We can use Multiple Kernel Learning (MKL) method to combine kernels calculated on different data source to obtain better predictive performance [18, 19]. There are many MKL toolboxes that are publicly available such as SimpleMKL [20] and Group Lasso [21].

4 Discussion

Medical big data have emerged and grew rapidly in the past decade, and it continues to bring opportunities to the compute-aided diagnosis development, which is especially important to those complex diseases like ASD. Benefiting from current popular open-access data repositories like NDAR, we introduce a data collection procedure and the possible data sources that may help to characterize ASD from perspectives of behavioral, cognitive, neurological, physiological, and genetic. These data are different in acquisition protocols and their data structures also vary greatly. Most of them show the characteristics of big data. From the long term, it is necessary to build a comprehensive database to deposit and manage these big data using relevant technologies such as Hadoop, or to take advantage of existing big data platform if the medical institution already has one for sake of saving costs. Of note, it will make more sense to collect these data from the same individuals at each time of data collection. A variety of studies have revealed the association with ASD of each data source. If they are integrated effectively, the complementary power of various features is assumed to improve the classification accuracy of ASD prediction model. Furthermore, integration of multiple data sources may be beneficial to the early detection and diagnosis of ASD since some sources may embody the early symptoms of ASD while others may not.

In order to combine the potentially complementary information, we propose an ASD classification framework to integrate these different data sources. Multiple CNN networks are used to extract discriminative features from different data sources. In order to differentiate the contributions or weights to the classification of each data source, we intend to leverage the MKL technique to learn the optimal combination coefficients of different kernel functions, which is expected to improve the classification accuracy than simply using the concatenation of different features. Furthermore, by collecting longitudinal follow-up data for each individual the early neurological or genetic biomarkers are expected to be found, which may improve identification and prognosis of ASD. More importantly, we believe that such data integration may improve our ability to classify ASD into more homogeneous subtypes that holds the promise of better personalized healthcare and precision medicine for ASD patients with specific manifestations.

Acknowledgments. This research was supported by a grant from National Natural Science Foundation of China (No: 61772375) and Independent Research Project of School of Information Management Wuhan University (No: 413100032).

References

1. Simonoff, E., et al.: Psychiatric disorders in children with autism spectrum disorders: prevalence, comorbidity, and associated factors in a population-derived sample. J. Am. Acad. Child Adolesc. Psychiatry **47**(8), 921–929 (2008)
2. Hu, R.J.: Diagnostic and Statistical Manual of Mental Disorders (DSM-IV). Academic Press, New York (2003)
3. Gotham, K., Pickles, A., Lord, C.: Standardizing ADOS scores for a measure of severity in autism spectrum disorders. J. Autism Dev. Disord. **39**(5), 693–705 (2009)
4. Cox, A., et al.: Autism spectrum disorders at 20 and 42 months of age: stability of clinical and ADI-R diagnosis. J. Child Psychol. Psychiatry **40**(5), 719–732 (1999)
5. Just, M.A., Cherkassky, V.L., Keller, T.A., Minshew, N.J.: Cortical activation and synchronization during sentence comprehension in high-functioning autism: evidence of underconnectivity. Brain J. Neurol. **127**(Pt 8), 1811–1821 (2004)
6. McFadden, K., Minshew, N.J.: Evidence for dysregulation of axonal growth and guidance in the etiology of ASD. Front. Hum. Neurosci. **7**, 671 (2013)
7. Qureshi, A.Y., et al.: Opposing brain differences in 16p11.2 deletion and duplication carriers. J. Neurosci. Off. J. Soc. Neurosci. **34**(34), 11199–11211 (2014)
8. Dennis, E.L., et al.: Altered structural brain connectivity in healthy carriers of the autism risk gene, CNTNAP2. Brain Connect. **1**(6), 447–459 (2011)
9. Rudie, J.D., et al.: Autism-associated promoter variant in MET impacts functional and structural brain networks. Neuron **75**(5), 904–915 (2012)
10. Insel, T., et al.: Research domain criteria (RDoC): toward a new classification framework for research on mental disorders. Am. J. Psychiatry **167**(7), 748–751 (2010)
11. Payakachat, N., Tilford, J.M., Ungar, W.J.: National Database for Autism Research (NDAR): big data opportunities for health services research and health technology assessment. Pharm. Econ. **34**(2), 127–138 (2016)
12. Buxbaum, J.D., et al.: The autism simplex collection: an international, expertly phenotyped autism sample for genetic and phenotypic analyses. Molecular autism 534 (2014)
13. Geschwind, D.H., et al.: The autism genetic resource exchange: a resource for the study of autism and related neuropsychiatric conditions. Am. J. Hum. Genet. **69**(2), 463–466 (2001)
14. Di Martino, A., et al.: The autism brain imaging data exchange: towards a large-scale evaluation of the intrinsic brain architecture in autism. Mol. Psychiatry **19**(6), 659–667 (2014)
15. Najafabadi, M.M., Villanustre, F., Khoshgoftaar, T.M., Seliya, N., Wald, R., Muharemagic, E.: Deep learning applications and challenges in big data analytics. J. Big Data **2**(1), 1 (2015)
16. Yu, H., Samuels, D.C., Zhao, Y.Y., Guo, Y.: Architectures and accuracy of artificial neural network for disease classification from omics data. BMC Genom. **20**(1), 167 (2019)
17. Cortes, C., Vapnik, V.: Support-vector networks. Mach. Learn. **20**(3), 273–297 (1995)

18. Rahimi, A., Gonen, M.: Discriminating early- and late-stage cancers using multiple kernel learning on gene sets. Bioinformatics **34**(13), i412–i421 (2018)
19. Tao, M., et al.: Classifying breast cancer subtypes using multiple kernel learning based on omics data. Genes **10**(3) (2019)
20. Rakotomamonjy, A., Bach, F., Canu, S., Grandvalet, Y.: SimpleMKL. J. Mach. Learn. Res. **9**(11) (2008)
21. Bach, F.: Consistency of the group Lasso and multiple kernel learning. Comput. Sci. (2007)

Social, Psychosocial and Behavioral Determinants of Health

An Empirical Study on the Influencing Factors of the Continued Usage of Fitness Apps

Yu Yu[✉] and Qing Chen

Commercial College, Central South University, Changsha 410083, Hunan, China
2221401862@qq.com

Abstract. In order to improve users' fitness frequency and to promote the sustainable development of fitness apps, it is necessary to study factors that influence the continued usage of fitness apps to provide some suggestions for providers. Based on the task-technology fit theory, a research model of the continued usage behavior of fitness apps was constructed. Through a questionnaire survey, 331 valid samples were collected, and then an empirical test was carried out on the model. The results showed that the task characteristics and technology characteristics significantly and positively influenced the task-technology fit; the task-technology fit positively affected the performance impacts, continued usage attitude and continued usage behavior; performance impacts was positively related to continued usage attitude and continued usage behavior; continued usage attitude had a significantly positive impact on continued usage behavior; the mediating roles of continued usage attitude with respect to the relationship between the task-technology fit and performance impacts, as well as continued usage behavior, were supported by empirical results; and the performance impacts played a significant intermediary role between task-technology fit and continued usage behavior. Therefore, according to the research results, providers can improve the matching degree between fitness apps' functions and the users' needs, enhance users' perception of fitness apps' using effects and prompt users to maintain a positive attitude during the continuous use process to promote the continued usage of apps and to improve users' fitness frequency.

Keywords: Fitness apps · Task-technology fit theory · Fitness frequency · Continued usage behavior

1 Introduction

With the rapid development of the economy, people's material and spiritual lives are becoming more and more abundant, but at the same time, the health condition is worrying. Economic development has provided people with adequate food, but it has also increased the health risks due to excessive calorie intake. In addition, with the advancement of science and technology, the mode of production has developed from manual labor to mental labor, and the number of calories burnt has greatly decreased. At the same time, a series of problems such as the rapid development of computers and mobile applications, the lack of sports facilities, and the accelerated pace of life have also resulted in people being less engaged in exercise. Therefore, the outlook for the

© Springer Nature Switzerland AG 2019
H. Chen et al. (Eds.): ICSH 2019, LNCS 11924, pp. 117–133, 2019.
https://doi.org/10.1007/978-3-030-34482-5_11

health level is not optimistic. In 2014, the Chinese government issued the "Several Opinions of the State Council on Accelerating the Sports Industry to Promote Sports Consumption." The opinion pointed out that national fitness should be promoted to a national strategy, and the strengthening of people's physical fitness level and the improvement of their health level should be the fundamental goals of the development of the sports industry.

As a kind of physical exercise ancillary tool based on the Internet, mobile devices and wearable technology, fitness apps can effectively promote physical exercise and formation of exercise habits [1]. Fitness apps represent the application of information systems in exercise. These types of applications can provide users with a variety of services [2], including allowing users to set fitness goals, track activities, collect workout ideas, obtain fitness coaching, and share progress on social media and so on [3]. The organic integration of apps and fitness provides a new solution to promote people's fitness.

Although fitness apps can effectively improve the fitness level, according to statistics, the current users' fitness frequency is still at a low level. Bida Consulting's "3rd Quarter 2017 China Sports Fitness App Product Market Research Report" pointed out that 56.7% of users exercise two times or less per week, 28.5% of users exercise three to four times a week, and only 14.8% of users exercise five to seven times a week [4]. The Speedway Institute's report also provided similar statistical results: 61.7% of users exercised two times or less per week, 24.5% of users exercised three to four times a week, and only 13.8% of users exercised five to seven times per week [5]. In addition, Han Zhang et al. [6] conducted a questionnaire survey on 1904 people who used fitness apps, and the statistical results also provided similar data.

In the online health situation, users' fitness and app use are integrated. Therefore, the users' fitness frequency can be improved by promoting the users' use of fitness apps, that is, promoting continued usage behavior. Continued usage behavior refers to post-adoption behavior, which is the repetitive use behavior of users after accepting a system [7], often measured by the frequency of use [8]. Continued usage is important to both users and providers. For the users, in the context of online health, strengthening the continued usage behavior is related to the improvement of the fitness frequency and the improvement of the fitness level. For providers, the initial adoption by users is only the first step toward achieving a system's overall success, and post-adoption behavior is at least as important. Bhattacherjee [7] even said that "the long-term viability of the system and its ultimate success depend on its continued use rather than its first use. Therefore, it is necessary to study the factors that influence the continued usage of fitness apps in order to provide some suggestions for providers about how to improve the products and services, promote the continued usage of users and users' fitness frequency, and then realize the success of apps.

In the field of information systems, considering the importance of continued usage, many scholars have conducted a series of studies on the continued usage of users, and the relevant literature is rich, but the research on the continued usage intention accounts for the majority, with few studies on continued usage behavior [9, 10]. The models and theories widely applied in the continued usage studies mainly include the expectation confirmation model of information system continuance (ECM-ISC) [7], technology acceptance model (TAM) [11, 12], diffusion of innovations theory (DOI) [13], uses and gratification theory (U&G) [14] and so on. At present, scholars study the continued usage of information systems mainly by expanding, integrating or modifying these theories or models to build continued usage models for different situations [15–19]. As a kind of emerging application in recent years, there have been insufficient researches on fitness apps, and there are fewer studies on their continued usage. Moreover, the only researches on the continued usage of fitness apps are mainly on continued usage intention, lacking further exploration of continued usage behavior. In addition, in these studies, there have been very few studies involving fitness apps' system characteristics and task characteristics [20–26]. The fitness app is an organic combination of fitness and app technology. It has different system characteristics from other systems, and the tasks that need to be completed by it also have different characteristics from other tasks. These factors both have impacts on the users' usage. Alter [27] pointed out that in order to adequately understand the use of information systems, it is necessary to simultaneously consider the roles of the systems and the actual working factors. Although the above-mentioned widely used information systems continued usage theory in information systems field can effectively explain the continued usage of users, they don't comprehensively consider the impacts of factors related to tasks and systems very well. Therefore, in order to better understand the continued usage of fitness apps and build a continued usage model that is more suitable for fitness apps, this paper used a theory that better considers factors of these two aspects to study the continued usage of fitness apps.

2 Theoretical Basis

In Alter's series of articles, he strongly recommends that information systems research should focus on the relationship between technology and work [27–30]. He points out that in order to adequately understand the use of information systems, we should not only focus on the system itself but also take into account the actual work [27]. Task-technology fit theory is a theory that explicitly explores the relationship between technology and work-related factors and helps people understand the use of information systems effectively [31]. Although the task-technology fit theory is originally used to explain the user's adoption behavior, scholars believe that task-technology fit also has an important impact on continued usage [32]. Larsen et al. [33] pointed out in his article that the task-technology fit model has considerable potential for explaining the users' continuance. Subsequent studies confirmed this view empirically, illustrating the feasibility of using task-technology fit theory to explain the continued usage in the field of information systems [34–38]. Therefore, in order to properly understand the use of fitness apps, this article applied the task-technology fit theory to this research. Of course, in addition to the factors related to tasks and systems, the users' behaviors can also be affected by personal psychological factors. Attitude is such an important psychological variable that affects the continued usage of users [39, 40], therefore, in order to build a more overall continued usage model, this paper added attitude into the model.

The task-technology fit theory (TTF) was first proposed by Goodhue and Thompson in 1995 [31]. They pointed out that if information technology needs to achieve a good performance, then the technology must be used, and it must have a good match with the task. Goodhue used the "technology-to-performance chain" to describe the basic framework of task-technology theory: task characteristics, technology characteristics, and personal characteristics have direct or interactive effects on task-technology fit, and task-technology fit has a direct effect on performance impacts. Performance impacts can be influenced by the expected results of use and the behavior of use. Individuals receive feedback after performance. If performance does not match their expected results, then individuals will adjust their expectations. Because the complete model is difficult to measure, the author and subsequent researchers often use a simplified ask-technology fit model for measurement purposes. The specific relationships of each variable are shown in Fig. 1.

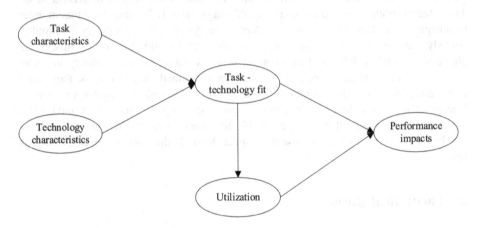

Fig. 1. Task-technology fit model

The task-technology fit theory originated in the field of information systems and has since been applied by scholars in various fields. In the field of information systems, it is mainly used to study the initial adoption of systems, but Larsen et al. [33] pointed out that the task-technology fit theory has great potential for explaining the users' continuance of information systems. Therefore, in their research, the task-technology fit model was integrated with the expected confirmation model, and a comprehensive theoretical model was constructed to explain the users' continuance of information systems. Subsequent empirical testing of the model confirmed the important predictive power of the task-technology fit theory for continued usage. In order to study the determinants of the continued usage intention of users of virtual learning systems, Lin et al. [34] used the task-technology fit theory to construct the continued usage model in online learning situation, and then empirically tested the model. The results showed that task-technology fit can significantly positively affect users' satisfaction, and satisfaction can positively affect the users' continued usage intention. In addition, task-technology fit can directly affect the continued usage intention. To study the relationship between environmental factors and the continued usage of mobile services, Liang et al. [41] established an integrated continued usage model based on task-technology fit theory and planned behavior theory and tested it empirically. The results showed that the task-technology fit can significantly affect the users' attitude of use, thus affect the users' continued usage intention. In the research of continued usage of online learning services, Cheng et al. [42] used the task-technology fit theory and the expectation confirmation theory to determine the influencing factors of the users' continued usage intention and made assumptions about their mechanisms of action. Then they verified the assumptions through empirical evidence. The results showed that task-technology fit can influence the users' continued usage intention through perceived usefulness and satisfaction and can also directly affect the continued usage intention. Later, many scholars also applied the task-technology fit theory to their continued usage researches, and empirically confirmed the applicability of using task-technology fit theory to study the users' continued usage [43–45]. Therefore, this paper used the task-technology fit theory as a framework to study the continued usage of fitness apps.

3   Research Hypotheses and Model

3.1   Task-Technology Fit Model

Task characteristics are factors that encourage users to rely more strongly on one aspect of technology [46]. Wagner et al. [47] used demand characteristics to replace task characteristics in their blog on social computing research because they believe that task execution is driven by demand, so using demand characteristics measurements will be more realistic. Since then, many scholars have used the users' demands to measure the characteristics of the task [48, 49]. Therefore, this study also used the demands of fitness apps' users to measure task characteristics. Wang et al. [50] pointed out that display and interaction, follow learning and improvement, intuitive feedback and goal management, as part of the intrinsic motivations are related to the users' task. The users' reports from Bida consulting data center and iResearch both counted the demands of fitness apps' users [51, 52]. The statistical results were in line with the above four demands. Therefore, this paper used the four demands to measure characteristics of fitness apps' users.

Technology characteristics refer to the characteristics of the tools that users use to carry out a task [46]. In related researches about task-technology fit theory, technology characteristics are often defined as the functional characteristics of the research objects and are embodied as actionable questions during measurement [53, 54]. Because the technological characteristics are closely related to the characteristics of the specific research objects, different technology characteristics should be extracted according to the specific research objects when conducting different studies. Wu and Wang [55] summarized the characteristics of fitness apps, pointing out that fitness apps have anytime and immediate characteristics, scientific and instructional characteristics, and private and social characteristics. Therefore, this paper used these characteristics to measure technology characteristics.

Goodue and Thompson [31] proposed the task-technology fit model and explained the relationships between the variables in the model. The task characteristics and technology characteristics positively affect the task-technology fit; the task-technology fit positively affects the performance impacts and users' utilization; and the users' utilization positively affects the performance impacts. After the task-technology fit theory was proposed, scholars applied it to many different information system backgrounds and proved the relationships between variables with empirical results [54, 56, 57]. Therefore, this paper proposed the following hypotheses:

H1: The task characteristics positively affect the task-technology fit.
H2: Technology characteristics positively affect the task-technology fit.
H3: Task-technology fit positively affects the performance impacts.

3.2 Task-Technology Fit and Continued Usage Behavior

The task-technology fit is the degree to which a technology assists an individual in completing a series of tasks [31]. Although the task-technology fit theory was first used to study the initial use, it is later applied by scholars to continued usage researches, and the relationship between task-technology fit and continued usage is discussed. In the research of online learning systems, Larsen et al. [33] pointed out that task-technology fit can affect the continued usage intention through perceived usefulness. Wen et al. [35] proved that task-technology fit can positively influence the continued usage intention by using empirical results. In addition, Yang [58] also found a significant positive effect of the task-technology fit on the continued usage intention of college students' online teaching platforms. Yuan et al. [44] also obtained results consistent with these studies. According to the theory of planned behavior, intention is positively related to behavior [59]. Therefore, this article proposed the following hypothesis:

H4: Task-technology fit positively affects the continued usage behavior.

3.3 Performance Impacts and Continued Usage Behavior

Performance refers to the completion of a series of tasks [31]. The performance impacts here refer to the performance perceived by the users, that is, the degree to which the users believe the apps help them complete fitness tasks. Regarding the relationship between performance impacts and continued usage, Westbrook [60] pointed out in his research that perceived performance is an important antecedent factor of consumers' continued usage. In the ECM-ISC model proposed by Bhattaeherjee, the perceived usefulness as an important part of perceived performance positively affects the users' continued usage intention through satisfaction and also directly affects the users' continued usage intention [7]. Zhang [61] conducted an empirical test on the positive correlation between consumer perceived performance and continued usage intention and proved this relationship. Gan [62] confirmed this relationship in her study of mobile books. In addition, the theory of planned behavior states that intention is significantly related to behavior [59]. Therefore, this paper inferred that performance impacts can positively affect the users' continued usage behavior. In addition, based on the positive correlation between task-technology fit and performance impacts, this article inferred that task-technology fit can affect the continued usage behavior of users through the intermediate variable—the performance impacts. Therefore, the following hypotheses were proposed:

H5: Performance impacts positively affect the continued usage behavior.

H6: Task-technology fit positively influences the users' continued usage behavior through the intermediary role of the performance impacts.

3.4   Task-Technology Fit and Continued Usage Attitude

Regarding the relationship between task-technology fit and attitude, McGill [63] pointed out that task-technology fit affects users' attitude, and attitude further affects the users' use of a system. Yu et al. [64] demonstrated that the task-technology fit can positively affect the attitude of use in their e-learning system research. Staples et al. [65] also found a significant relationship between task-technology fit and attitude. The studies of Gan and Harrati et al. confirmed this relationship [62, 66]. Therefore, the higher the degree of task-technology fit is, the more willing users are to use the fitness apps, and the more positive the attitude towards continued usage of the apps is. And according to the theory of planned behavior, behavioral attitude can significantly affect behavior [59]. Therefore, this paper inferred that task-technology fit can affect the continued usage behavior of users through the intermediate variable—continued usage attitude. Therefore, this paper proposed the following hypotheses:

H7: Task-technology fit positively affects the continued usage attitude.

H8: Task-technology fit positively influences the users' continued usage behavior through the intermediary role of the continued usage attitude.

3.5   Performance Impacts and Continued Usage Attitude

The technology acceptance model considers that attitude is affected by perceived usefulness [67]. Hwang et al. [68] pointed out that perceived usefulness positively affects attitude. Wu et al. [45] confirmed this view in their research of continued usage. Perceived usefulness is an important part of perceived performance. Therefore, it can be inferred that the perceived performance can also positively influence attitude. Xin [69] confirmed this inference in his research. The higher the level of performance impacts perceived by the users are, the more the benefits of fitness apps perceived by the users are. Then, the attitude towards continuing the use of the fitness apps to support their fitness will be more positive. In addition, because behavioral attitude can significantly affect behavior [59], this paper inferred that the performance impacts can indirectly affect users' continued usage behavior through the continued usage attitude. Therefore, this paper proposed the following hypotheses:

H9: Performance impacts positively affect the continued usage attitude.

H10: Performance impacts positively influence the users' continued usage behavior through the intermediary role of the continued usage attitude.

3.6   Continued Usage Attitude and the Continued Usage Behavior

Ajzen [59, 70] proposed the theory of planned behavior and explained the relationships between variables. Attitude positively influences behavioral intention, and intention positively affects behavior. Attitude refers to the positive or negative feelings that individuals hold about behavior. After the theory of planned behavior was proposed, scholars applied it to various fields and tested the relationships between variables with empirical evidence [71–75]. Thus, according to the theory of planned behavior, this paper inferred that the continued usage attitude can positively influence the continued usage behavior. Therefore, the following hypothesis was proposed:

H11: Continued usage attitude positively affects the continued usage behavior.

Based on the above hypotheses, this paper proposed the integrated continued usage research model of fitness apps (see Fig. 2):

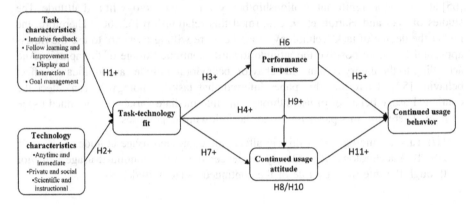

Fig. 2. Theoretical model

4 Research Methods

4.1 Variable Measurement

This paper used a questionnaire survey to verify the research model. In order to ensure the content validity of the questionnaire, the measurement items in this study were adapted from the mature scales in the existing literature. The measurement scale of task characteristics was adapted from the studies of Zhou et al. and Wang et al. [49, 50]. The measurement scale of technology characteristics was adapted from the studies of Zhou et al. and Wu et al. [49, 55]. The measurement scale of task-technology fit was adapted from the study of Lu et al. [76]. The measurement scale of performance impacts was adapted from the study of Goodhue et al. [31]. The measurement scale of continued usage attitude was adapted from the study of Cheng et al. [77]. The measurement scale of continued usage behavior was adapted from the study of Limayem et al. [8] (see Table 1).

4.2 Data Collection

This questionnaire survey distributed questionnaires to various kinds of fitness apps' users who had used fitness apps for a period of time through online platforms. A total

Table 1. List of measures.

Constructs	Measures
Task characteristics (TAC)	TAC1: I need to obtain intuitive feedback on my fitness level (e.g., exercise data, exercise history, self-monitoring data, etc.)
	TAC2: I need to conduct the followed learning to improve my fitness level (e.g., increasing fitness knowledge, obtaining fitness guidance, paying attention to exercise examples, etc.)
	TAC3: I need to display my fitness status and interact with others (e.g., record exercise experience, share photos of myself, interact with others, accept and send exercise messages or videos, etc.)
	TAC4: I need to manage my fitness goals (e.g., formulate fitness goals, set exercise reminders and ensure supervision of completing preset goals, etc.)
Technology characteristics (TEC)	TEC1: The fitness apps provide anytime and immediate services
	TEC2: The fitness apps provide private and social services
	TEC3: The fitness apps provide scientific and instructional services
Task-technology fit (TTF)	TTF1: In helping me to exercise, the functions of fitness apps are appropriate
	TTF2: In helping me to exercise, the functions of fitness apps are sufficient
	TTF3: In general, the functions of fitness apps fully meet my exercise needs
Performance impacts (PI)	PI1: The fitness apps have a strong positive impact on the efficiency and outcome of my fitness
	PI2: The fitness apps provide important and valuable help for enhancing my fitness effect
Continued usage attitude (CUA)	CUA1: I think that continuously using fitness apps is a good idea
	CUA2: I think that continuously using fitness apps for exercise would be a wise idea
	CUA3: I think that continuously using fitness apps is pleasant
	CUA4: In my opinion, it is desirable to continuously use fitness apps
Continued usage behavior (CUB)	CUB1: How often did you use fitness apps during the last 4 weeks? (never/always)
	CUB2: How often did you use fitness apps during the last 4 weeks? (once a month/once a day)

of 528 questionnaires were collected, and then invalid samples were removed, resulting in a total of 331 valid questionnaires. The basic information of the samples is shown in Table 2.

Table 2. Sample profile of survey (N = 331).

Items	Demographics	Number	Percentage %
Gender	Male	166	50
	Female	165	50
Age	<18 years old	3	0.9
	18–25 years old	59	17.8
	26–35 years old	189	57.1
	36–45 years old	66	19.9
	46–55 years old	12	3.7
	56–65 years old	2	0.6
Education level	High school/high school or below	4	1.2
	Secondary school	9	2.7
	College	84	25.4
	Bachelor	210	63.4
	Master's degree	24	7.3
	PhD and above	0	0
Career	Student	28	8.4
	Corporate staff	230	69.5
	Institution staff	36	10.9
	Administrative staff	5	1.5
	Other occupation	32	9.7
Mobile application experience	Never used	0	0
	Less than 1 year	4	1.2
	1 to 3 years	53	16
	3 to 5 years	134	40.5
	5 to 10 years	120	36.3
	More than 10 years	20	6

5   Empirical Analysis

5.1   Measurement Model Analysis

The average variance extracted (AVE) and outer loadings almost reached levels of 0.5 and 0.7, respectively, indicating that the measurement model of this study had good convergence validity (see Table 3). The square roots of the AVE of each construct were greater than their correlations with other constructs, which shows that the model had good discriminant validity. Next, the composite reliability (CR) and Cronbach's alpha coefficient were used to measure the reliability of the questionnaire. All of the CR values and Cronbach's alpha values of the model are higher than 0.8 and 0.7, respectively, indicating that the measurement model of this study had good internal consistency (see Table 3). Overall, our findings provided satisfactory empirical supports for measuring the reliability, convergence and discriminant validity of this model (Table 4).

Table 3. AVE, CR and Cronbach's Alpha values of the measurement model.

Constructs	AVE	CR	Cronbach's Alpha
Continued usage attitude (CUA)	0.655	0.883	0.824
Continued usage behavior (CUB)	0.809	0.895	0.766
Performance impacts (PI)	0.788	0.881	0.731
Task characteristics (TAC)	0.563	0.836	0.737
Technology characteristics (TEC)	0.635	0.839	0.714
Task-technology fit (TTF)	0.632	0.837	0.708

Table 4. AVE square roots and correlation coefficients of the latent variables.

	CUA	CUB	PI	TAC	TEC	TTF
CUA	0.809					
CUB	0.660	0.900				
PI	0.685	0.576	0.888			
TAC	0.650	0.614	0.615	0.750		
TEC	0.640	0.540	0.591	0.643	0.797	
TTF	0.703	0.617	0.679	0.640	0.624	0.795

5.2 Structural Model Analysis

The data were analyzed using SmartPLS3.0. The path coefficients and significances between each variables are shown in Fig. 3.

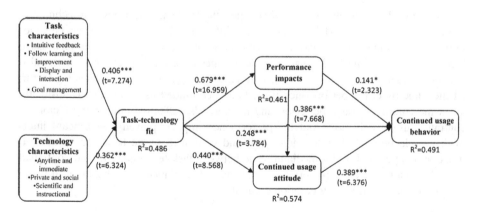

Fig. 3. Research model results

Note: *$p < 0.05$, **$p < 0.01$, *** $p < 0.001$.

According to Fig. 3, all results of the hypothetical paths were significant. That is to say, hypotheses H1 (task characteristics → task-technology fit), H2 (technology characteristics → task-technology fit), H3 (task-technology fit → performance impacts), H4 (task-technology fit → continued usage behavior), H5 (performance impacts → continued usage behavior), H7 (task-technology fit → continued usage attitude), H9 (performance impacts → continued usage attitude), H11 (continued usage attitude → continued usage behavior) were supported.

In order to test the mediation effects, this paper performed a Sobel test on the hypotheses. The results showed that performance impacts had a significant mediating effect between task-technology fit and continued usage behavior (Sobel test $z = 4.87 > 1.96$); hypothesis H6 was supported. In addition, task-technology fit had a significant impact on continued usage behavior, so performance impacts played a partial intermediary role. Furthermore, continued usage attitude had a significant mediating effect between task-technology fit and continued usage behavior (Sobel test $z = 6.07 > 1.96$); hypothesis H8 was supported. In addition, task-technology fit had a significant effect on continued usage behavior, so continued usage attitude played a partial intermediary role. Finally, continued usage attitude also had a significant mediating effect between performance impacts and continued usage behavior (Sobel test $z = 4.95 > 1.96$); hypothesis H10 was supported. The effect of performance impacts on continued usage behavior was significant, so continued usage attitude played a partial intermediary role.

6 Conclusion

6.1 Main Conclusions

According to the research results in this paper, the task characteristics and technology characteristics in this model can positively influence the continued usage behavior through task-technology fit, and the task-technology fit can affect the continued usage behavior through continued usage attitude and performance impacts. And it can also affect continued usage behavior directly. It's a very important direct influencing factor. At the same time, the performance impacts and continued usage attitude can directly affect the continued usage behavior, and they are also effective influencing factors of continued usage behavior. And the performance impacts played a significant intermediary role between task-technology fit and continued usage behavior. Continued usage attitude also played a mediating role between task-technology fit and continued usage behavior, as well as performance impacts and continued usage behavior. It was a very important intermediary emotional variable.

6.2 Theoretical Contributions

Based on the task-technology fit theory, this paper constructed an integrated model of continued usage behavior of fitness apps and tested it through empirical evidences. The conclusions had certain theoretical significance. First of all, this paper studied the continued usage behavior and enriched the literature on the continued usage behavior in the field of information systems. Secondly, this paper applied the task-technology fit framework to the online health situation and verified the applicability and effectiveness of the theory in studying the users' continued usage behavior in this situation. Finally, this study comprehensively considered the characteristics of fitness apps, the special needs of fitness apps' users and personal psychological factor and built an integrated continued usage model that is more suitable for online health situation, which deepened the understanding of influencing factors of the continued usage of fitness apps and their mechanisms of action.

6.3   Practice Implications

The conclusions of this research can be used to guide strategies for promoting users' continued usage behavior and improving fitness frequency. Fitness apps' providers can promote continued usage of the apps through the applications of the following information:

(1) Because the task-technology fit can effectively affect the users' continued usage, fitness apps' providers should fully understand the users' needs according to the market and user surveys. Then they need to design and improve the apps' various functions to ensure that the apps can effectively meet the needs of users. For example, if users need intuitive feedback about their fitness, then the providers should improve the apps' feedback system, such as offering more detailed and professional exercise data, explaining the data more vividly and so on. Moreover, functional modules customization services can be provided according to the different needs of users, so that the apps can be more suitable for the users' needs.

(2) Because the perceived performance impacts can promote the continued usage of fitness apps, the providers of fitness apps should strive to enhance the users' perceptions of the fitness apps' degree of help for improving fitness performance. For example, in fitness apps, providers could set up various psychological hints for displaying the effectiveness of the fitness apps, provide phased feedback on fitness results, and propagate various successful cases of users who achieved good fitness results after using the fitness apps.

(3) Since the users' continued usage attitude is related to the continued usage of the apps, the providers should try to keep the users' attitude positive throughout the use process. For example, highlighting the meeting of fitness needs supported by the apps, enhancing the feedback of the users' effect after usage, improving the users' perceptions of the usefulness of the apps, and setting up various sports-related entertainment or prize-winning activities to enhance the users' pleasure when using.

References

1. Chuan-hai, L., Qing-mei, W., Jun-wei, Q.: The influence of sports apps on the promotion of physical exercise behavior and the formation of exercise habits. J. Nanjing Sport Inst. (Soc. Sci. Edition) **29**(03), 109–115 (2015)

2. Litman, L., et al.: Mobile exercise apps and increased leisure time exercise activity: a moderated mediation analysis of the role of self-efficacy and barriers. J. Med. Internet Res. **17**(8), 15 (2015)
3. Sama, P.R., et al.: An evaluation of mobile health application tools. Jmir Mhealth Uhealth **2**(2), 6 (2014)
4. Bida consultancy: 3rd quarter 2017 sports fitness apps product market research report in China. in Beijing: Bida consultancy (2017)
5. Institute: Fitness app market report for the first half of 2017. Internet World **09**, 32–34 (2017)
6. Zhang, H., Liu, X.: Resources and use of fitness instruction APP. J. Wuhan Inst. Phys. Educ. **51**(10), 37–42 (2017)
7. Bhattacherjee, A.: Understanding information systems continuance: an expectation-confirmation model. MIS Q. **25**(3), 351–370 (2001)
8. Limayem, M., Cheung, C.M.K.: Understanding information systems continuance: the case of Internet-based learning technologies. Inf. Manag. **45**(4), 227–232 (2008)
9. Yang, H., Yuan, W., Wang, W.: A review of domestic and foreign researches on users continuance of social apps. Inf. Sci. **35**(03), 164–170 + 176 (2017)
10. Hui-ping, C., Ling, J.: Analysis on the research status of domestic IT/IS user continuance usage. Inf. Sci. **36**(04), 171–176 (2018)
11. Davis, F.D.: A technology acceptance model for empirically testing new end-user information systems: theory and results. Sloan School of Management, Massachusetts Institute of Technology (1986)
12. Davis, F.D.: Perceived usefulness, perceived ease of use, and user acceptance of information technology. MIS Q. **13**(3), 319–340 (1989)
13. Rogers, E.M.: Diffusion of Innovations, 4th edn., pp. 1–20. Clarendon Press, New York (1995)
14. Blumler, J.G., Katz, E.: The uses of mass communications: current perspectives on gratifications research. Am. J. Sociol. **3**(6), 318 (1974)
15. Hong, S.J., et al.: Understanding the behavior of mobile data services consumers. Inf. Syst. Front. **10**(4), 431–445 (2008)
16. Kim, M.J., et al.: Dual-route of persuasive communications in mobile tourism shopping. Telematics Inform. **33**(2), 293–308 (2016)
17. Gan, C.M., Li, H.X.: Understanding the effects of gratifications on the continuance intention to use WeChat in China: a perspective on uses and gratifications. Comput. Hum. Behav. **78**, 306–315 (2018)
18. Lu, Y., Papagiannidis, S., Alamanos, E.: Exploring the emotional antecedents and outcomes of technology acceptance. Comput. Hum. Behav. **90**, 153–169 (2019)
19. Joo, Y.J., Park, S., Shin, E.K.: Students' expectation, satisfaction, and continuance intention to use digital textbooks. Comput. Hum. Behav. **69**, 83–90 (2017)
20. Yuan, S.P., et al.: Keep using my health apps: discover users' perception of health and fitness apps with the UTAUT2 model. Telemed. E-Health **21**(9), 735–774 (2015)
21. Gowin, M., et al.: Health and fitness app use in college students: a qualitative study. Am. J. Health Educ. **46**(4), 223–230 (2015)
22. Lee, H.E., Cho, J.: What motivates users to continue using diet and fitness apps? application of the uses and gratifications approach. Health Commun. **32**(12), 1 (2016)
23. Lee, S., Kim, S., Wang, S.: Motivation factors influencing intention of mobile sports apps use by applying the unified theory of acceptance and use of technology (UTAUT). IJASS (Int. J. Appl. Sport. Sci.) **29**(2), 115–127 (2017)

24. Beldad, A.D., Hegner, S.M.: Expanding the technology acceptance model with the inclusion of trust, social influence, and health valuation to determine the predictors of German users' willingness to continue using a fitness app: a structural equation modeling approach. Int. J. Hum.-Comput. Interact. **34**(9), 882–893 (2018)

25. Park, M., et al.: Why do young people use fitness apps? cognitive characteristics and app quality. Electron. Commer. Res. **6**, 1–7 (2018)

26. Li, J., et al.: Users' intention to continue using social fitness-tracking apps: expectation confirmation theory and social comparison theory perspective. Inform. Health Soc. Care, 1–15 (2018)

27. Alter, S.: 18 Reasons why IT-reliant work systems should replace the IT artifact as the core subject matter of the IS field. Commun. Assoc. Inform. Syst. **12**(23), 365–394 (2003)

28. Alter, S.: Are the fundamental concepts of information systems mostly about work systems? Equine Vet. J. **44**(5), 621–625 (2001)

29. Alter, S.: Which life cycle–work system, information system, or software? Commun. Assoc. Inf. Syst. **7** (2001)

30. Alter, S.: Architecture of Sysperanto: a model-based ontology of the IS field (2005)

31. Goodhue, D.L., Thompson, R.L.: Task-technology fit and individual performance. MIS Q. **19**(2), 213–236 (1995)

32. Ferratt, T.W., Vlahos, G.E.: An investigation of task-technology fit for managers in Greece and the US. Eur. J. Inf. Syst. **7**(2), 123–136 (1998)

33. Larsen, T.J., Sorebo, A.M., Sorebo, O.: The role of task-technology fit as users' motivation to continue information system use. Comput. Hum. Behav. **25**(3), 778–784 (2009)

34. Lin, W.S.: Perceived fit and satisfaction on web learning performance: IS continuance intention and task-technology fit perspectives. Int. J. Hum Comput Stud. **70**(7), 498–507 (2012)

35. Lin, W.S., Wang, C.H.: Antecedences to continued intentions of adopting e-learning system in blended learning instruction: a contingency framework based on models of information system success and task-technology fit. Comput. Educ. **58**(1), 88–99 (2012)

36. Yang, S.Q., et al.: Understanding consumers' mobile channel continuance: an empirical investigation of two fitness mechanisms. Behav. Inf. Technol. **34**(12), 1135–1146 (2015)

37. Ajayi, I.H., et al.: A conceptual model for flipped classroom: Influence on continuance use intention. In: 2017 5th International Conference on Research and Innovation in Information Systems (2017)

38. Lin, K.Y.: User communication behavior in mobile communication software. Online Inf. Rev. **40**(7), 1071–1089 (2016)

39. Lin, K.M., Chen, N.S., Fang, K.T.: Understanding e-learning continuance intention: a negative critical incidents perspective. Behav. Inf. Technol. **30**(1), 77–89 (2011)

40. Hong, S., Kim, J., Lee, H.: Antecedents of use-continuance in information systems: toward an inegrative view. J. Comput. Inf. Syst. **48**(3), 61–73 (2008)

41. Liang, T.P., et al.: Contextual factors and continuance intention of mobile services. Int. J. Mobile Commun. **11**(4), 313–329 (2013)

42. Cheng, Y.M.: What drives nurses' blended e-learning continuance intention? J. Educ. Technol. Soc. **17**(4), 203–215 (2014)

43. Chang, I.C., et al.: Assessing the performance of long-term care information systems and the continued use intention of users. Telematics Inform. **32**(2), 273–281 (2015)

44. Yuan, S.B., et al.: An investigation of users' continuance intention towards mobile banking in China. Inf. Dev. **32**(1), 20–34 (2016)

45. Wu, B., Chen, X.H.: Continuance intention to use MOOCs: Integrating the technology acceptance model (TAM) and task technology fit (TTF) model. Comput. Hum. Behav. **67**, 221–232 (2017)

46. Hong, T., Xu, F.: Research review of task-technology fit model. R&D Manage. **24**(04), 24–31 (2012)
47. Ip, R.K.F., Wagner, C.: Weblogging: a study of social computing and its impact on organizations. Decis. Support Syst. **45**(2), 242–250 (2008)
48. Lu, H.P., Yang, Y.W.: Toward an understanding of the behavioral intention to use a social networking site: an extension of task-technology fit to social-technology fit. Comput. Hum. Behav. **34**(5), 323–332 (2014)
49. Zhou, T., Lu, Y.B., Wang, B.: Integrating TTF and UTAUT to explain mobile banking user adoption. Comput. Hum. Behav. **26**(4), 760–767 (2010)
50. Wang, S., Zhang, J., Liu, Y.: The effective factor study of sports app promote public exercise adherence. J. Fujian Norm. Univ. (Philos. Soc. Sci. Ed.) (06), 88–99 + 170–171 (2018)
51. Bida consultancy: July 2016 sports fitness apps users monitoring report. in Beijing: Bida consultancy (2016)
52. iResearch consultancy: Case studies: user insights and case studies on the big data sports apps, in iResearch consultancy (2018)
53. Wells, J.D., et al.: Studying customer evaluations of electronic commerce applications: a review and adaptation of the task-technology fit perspective. In: Hawaii International Conference on System Sciences (2003)
54. Gebauer, J., Shaw, M.J.: Success factors and impacts of mobile business applications: results from a mobile e-procurement study. Int. J. Electron. Commer. **8**(3), 19–41 (2004)
55. Ruoxi, W., Qingjun, W.: Fitness app: development status, problems and countermeasures. J. Shandong Sport. Univ. **31**(04), 18–22 (2015)
56. D'Ambra, J., Wilson, C.S.: Use of the world wide web for international travel: integrating the construct of uncertainty in information seeking and the task-technology fit (TTF) model. J. Am. Soc. Inform. Sci. Technol. **55**(8), 731–742 (2004)
57. Yen, D.C., et al.: Determinants of users' intention to adopt wireless technology: an empirical study by integrating TTF with TAM. Comput. Hum. Behav. **26**(5), 906–915 (2010)
58. Yang, G.: Research on continuous use and performance influencing factors of network teaching platform under mixed learning mode. E-Educ. Res. **36**(07), 42–48 (2015)
59. Ajzen, I.: The theory of planned behavior. Organ. Behav. Hum. Decis. Process. **50**(2), 179–211 (1991)
60. Westbrook, R.A.: Product/Consumption-based affective responses and post purchase processes. J. Mark. Res. **24**(3), 258–270 (1987)
61. Zhang, X.: The model construction and empirical research of consumer's continuance intention on using e-commerce web sites. Zhejiang Gongshang University (2013)
62. Chunmei, G.A.N.: Empirical analysis on continuance intention to use mobile library services. Libr. Trib. **36**(01), 79–84 (2016)
63. McGill, T.J., Klobas, J.E.: A task-technology fit view of learning management system impact. Comput. Educ. **52**(2), 496–508 (2009)
64. Yu, T.K., Yu, T.Y.: Modelling the factors that affect individuals' utilisation of online learning systems: an empirical study combining the task technology fit model with the theory of planned behaviour. Br. J. Edu. Technol. **41**(6), 1003–1017 (2010)
65. Staples, D.S., Seddon, P.B.: Testing the technology-to-performance chain model. J. Organ. End User Comput. **16**(4), 17–36 (2004)
66. Harrati, N., Bouchrika, I., Mahfouf, Z.: Investigating the uptake of educational systems by academics using the technology to performance chain model. Libr. Hi Tech **35**(4), 629–648 (2017)
67. Davis, F.D., Bagozzi, R.P., Warshaw, P.R.: User acceptance of computer technology: a comparison of two theoretical models. Manage. Sci. **35**(8), 982–1003 (1989)

68. Hwang, C., Chung, T.L., Sanders, E.A.: Attitudes and purchase intentions for smart clothing: examining U.S. consumers' functional, expressive, and aesthetic needs for solar-powered clothing. Cloth. Text. Res. J. **34**(3) (2016)
69. Xin, G.: The model construction and empirical research of user's continuance intention towards LBS applications. Wuhan University of Technology (2015)
70. Ajzen, I.: From Intentions to Actions: A Theory of Planned Behavior. Springer, Heidelberg (1985)
71. Rai, A., Lang, S.S., Welker, R.B.: Assessing the validity of IS success models: an empirical test and theoretical analysis. Inf. Syst. Res. **13**(1), 50–69 (2002)
72. Pavlou, P.A., Fygenson, M.: Understanding and predicting electronic commerce adoption: an extension of the theory of planned behavior. MIS Q. **30**(1), 115–143 (2006)
73. Luarn, P., Lin, H.H.: Toward an understanding of the behavioral intention to use mobile banking. Comput. Hum. Behav. **21**(6), 873–891 (2005)
74. Jian, L., Ning, Z.: A study on intention of taking high-speed rail based on theory of planned behavior. Chin. J. Manag. **11**(09), 1403–1410 (2014)
75. Wang, D., Yao, F., Zheng, Y.: A study on credit cards usage intention and its marketing strategies based on theory of planned behavior. Chin. J. Manag. **8**(11), 1682–1689 + 1713 (2011)
76. Lu, H.P., Yang, Y.W.: Toward an understanding of the behavioral intention to use a social networking site: an extension of task-technology fit to social-technology fit. Comput. Hum. Behav. **34**, 323–332 (2014)
77. Cheng, T.C.E., Lam, D.Y.C., Yeung, A.C.L.: Adoption of internet banking: an empirical study in Hong Kong. Decis. Support Syst. **42**(3), 1558–1572 (2006)

Understanding Opioid Addiction
with Similarity Network-Based Deep Learning

Jiaheng Xie[1]([✉]), Zhu Zhang[2], Xiao Liu[3], and Daniel Zeng[1]

[1] University of Arizona, Tucson, USA
xiej@email.arizona.edu
[2] Chinese Academy of Sciences, Beijing, China
[3] University of Utah, Salt Lake City, USA

Abstract. Opioid use disorder (OUD) refers to the physical and psychological reliance on opioids. OUD costs the US healthcare systems $504 billion annually and poses significant mortality risk for patients. Understanding and mitigating the barriers to OUD treatment is a high-priority area for healthcare and IS researchers, practitioners, and policymakers. Current OUD treatment studies largely rely on surveys and reviews. However, the response rate of these surveys is low because patients are reluctant to share their OUD experience for fear of stigma in society. In this paper, we explore social media as a new source of data to study OUD treatments. Drug users increasingly participate in social media to share their experience anonymously. Yet their voice in social media has not been utilized in past studies. We develop the SImilarity Network-based DEep Learning (SINDEL) to discover barriers to OUD treatment from the patient narratives and address the challenge of morphs. SINDEL significantly outperforms state-of-the-art baseline models, reaching an F1 score of 76.79%. Thirteen types of OUD treatment barriers were identified and verified by domain experts. This study contributes to IS literature by proposing a novel deep-learning-based analytical approach with impactful implications for health practitioners.

Keywords: Deep learning · Health analytics · Text mining · Computational data science

1 Introduction

The misuse of and addiction to opioids, involving nonmedical use, misuse, or abuse of opioid medications (e.g., pain relievers), and use of illicit opioids (e.g., heroin), are epidemic and have become a serious public health crisis in the United States. It was estimated that in 2016, 11.8 million Americans misused prescription opioids or used illicit opioids (SAMHSA 2017). Among them, 2.1 million suffered from opioid addiction.

This growing crisis devastates millions of Americans with opioid use disorder (OUD). OUD causes serious medical and financial consequences for patients and healthcare systems. In 2017, the number of overdose deaths involving opioids was six times higher than that in 1999 (CDC 2018). The Council of Economic Advisors at the

H. Chen et al. (Eds.): ICSH 2019, LNCS 11924, pp. 134–141, 2019.
https://doi.org/10.1007/978-3-030-34482-5_12

White House estimated that in 2015, the cost of OUD was $504 billion, or 2.8% of the GDP that year (White House 2017).

In response to the growing burden of OUD, society needs to work together to improve the access to treatment. Although many medical studies show that OUD treatments are effective and could prevent further ramifications, only 17.5% of patients with OUD receive treatment (NIDA 2018). In 2018, the US Surgeon General stressed the urgency of understanding and removing the barriers to OUD treatment. Understanding these barriers forms the premise to decrease overdose mortality, reduce the transmission of infectious diseases, and lower healthcare expenditure. In this study, we aim to propose and evaluate an innovative computational approach to understand the barriers to OUD treatment.

Existing studies employed surveys to understand the barriers to OUD treatment. These survey studies are challenged by the narrow patient population, as individuals struggling with OUD often are difficult to reach if they are not actively under treatment. Social media can bridge this gap. In drug forums, in particular, patients share their experiences of taking prescription and illicit opioids. Due to the anonymous nature of these forums, patients are willing to elaborate on their real decision-making on OUD treatments. To our best knowledge, no social media analytical approach has been taken in OUD treatment research.

Significant challenges still exist to understand patient perspectives in drug forums despite their enormous potential. Patients prefer to use a wide variety of morphs (fake alternative names) to describe drugs and treatment options in order to avoid censorship and surveillance, entertain readers, or use personal writing styles. The literal meanings of the morphs are distant from their contextual meanings. To understand OUD treatment barriers in drug forums and address the challenge of morphs, we propose a novel computational method: SImilarity Network-based DEep Learning (SINDEL).

Our study makes the following contributions to information systems literature, data analytical methodology, and healthcare practice. First, we develop a deep learning framework (SINDEL) to extract OUD treatment barriers from drug forums. SINDEL can be generalized to extract information from many other text genres containing specialized morphs, such as hacker forums, health social media, and product reviews. Second, our study falls into the category of computational design science research that aims to design analytical solutions to problems with social impact (Rai 2017). Third, our empirical findings complement current behavioral health science research on OUD treatments with comprehensive patient experience data. We discover 13 types of OUD treatment barriers. Many of the OUD treatment barriers that we discover have not been noted by prior survey studies.

2 Literature Review

Surveys and interviews are commonly used to investigate the barriers to OUD treatment. The barriers to OUD treatment identified in these studies can be categorized into three categories: (1) System-related: the factors related to healthcare systems and regulations, such as government and insurance policies and funding barriers (Knudsen et al. 2011); (2) Provider-related: the factors related to health providers, such as lack of

DEA waiver, lack of institutional support, and lack of resources (Wolfe et al. 2010); (3) Patient-related: patient-specific factors, such as the fear of pain and lack of information on treatments (Hassamal et al. 2017).

The surveys only capture a snapshot of barriers. In reality, many patient-level barriers are complicated by patient characteristics and policy changes, causing them to vary over time. Furthermore, patients are reluctant to disclose their issues with OUD treatments, especially illicit drug users. Innovative approaches are needed to understand barriers to OUD treatments, patient behaviors, and potential measures that can deliver the care to patients in need. Health big data from social media not only provide real-time and dynamic information but also cover an unprecedent scale of the patient population with heterogeneous characteristics. Yet, no social media analytical approach has been taken in OUD treatment studies.

To understand OUD treatment barriers in health social media, significant challenges need to be addressed, because users invent new slang and idiomatic expressions to describe their experience. Related work in morphology addresses the challenges of understanding slang, synonyms, and other types of word variations in unstructured text. The main body of literature in morphology utilizes distributed representation and deep learning methods, such as word embedding and BLSTM, to interpret the semantics of morphs. We, therefore, devise a deep learning-based method to extract OUD treatment barriers from drug forums while tackling the morphs.

3   Research Method

We propose an OUD treatment barrier mining approach. This approach receives a sentence from drug forums as the input. Two parallel representation models represent the sentence with two vectors. Branch 1 utilizes word embedding to generate semantic vectors for each word. Branch 2 creates a similarity network of words and generates a network representation for each word. The two representations are concatenated in the hidden layers which further recognize the OUD treatment barriers in the sentence. A clustering model is utilized to cluster the extracted barriers into meaningful categories of OUD treatment barriers. This approach is called SImilarity Network-based DEep Learning (SINDEL).

The proposed similarity network-based representation contains two parallel representations. The first representation is a word embedding representation to capture the semantic meaning of words, so that morphs can be interpreted as their intended meaning. Let S be a training sequence $[w_1, w_2, \ldots, w_T]$. Variable w_i denotes word i in the sequence. The training objective is to maximize the objective function in Eq. 1. Parameter c is the window size (the words that appear within a distance of c words). Variables w_{t+j} are the words surrounding w_t.

$$L = \frac{1}{T} \sum_{t=1}^{T} \sum_{-c \leq j \leq c, j \neq 0} \log p(w_{t+j}|w_t). \tag{1}$$

The second representation aims to construct a network of words in order to capture the interconnected relationships among morphs. In this network $G = (V, E)$, each node V is a word, and the edge E is the semantic similarity between words. As such, each word is linked to a set of words that are closely related. For instance, oxy will be linked with O.C. and Oxycet, because they are the most similar morphs. This word similarity network is capable of addressing the limitation of word embedding by considering the semantic relationships among entities of interests. Instead of using the representation of the focal word, we use similar words that are connected to the focal word as the second representation for the focal word. Figure 1 shows an example.

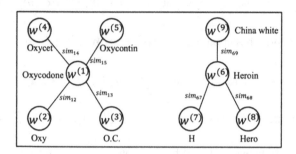

Fig. 1. An example of a word similarity network

In the simple example in Fig. 1, Oxycodone ($w^{(1)}$) is linked to oxy, O.C., Oxycet, and Oxycontin, because they belong to the same drug class. We use $w^{(2)}$, $w^{(3)}$, $w^{(4)}$, and $w^{(5)}$ to represent $w^{(1)}$. Likewise, China white, H, and hero are linked to heroin. We use $w^{(7)}$, $w^{(8)}$, and $w^{(9)}$ to represent $w^{(6)}$. In our corpus, we construct a similarity network for all words and compute the similarity between each pair of words. We select a set of most similar words for each word and link them together. Word similarity is computed using the cosine similarity of word embedding as shown in Eq. 2.

$$sim_{ij} = \frac{x^{(i)} \cdot x^{(j)}}{\| x^{(i)} \| \| x^{(j)} \|}. \tag{2}$$

Variables $x^{(i)}$ and $x^{(j)}$ are the word embedding of word $w^{(i)}$ and $w^{(j)}$. Given word w, let $w^{(1)}, w^{(2)}, \ldots, w^{(10)}$ be the top ten words that are the most similar to word w. Let $sim^{(1)}, sim^{(2)}, \ldots, sim^{(10)}$ be the similarity between word w and the other ten words. Let $x^{(1)}, x^{(2)}, \ldots, x^{(10)}$ be the word embedding for $w^{(1)}, w^{(2)}, \ldots, w^{(10)}$. The similarity network representation of word w is defined in Eq. 3.

$$x_s = \sum_{i=1}^{10} sim^{(i)} x^{(i)}. \tag{3}$$

To effectively extract the barriers to OUD treatment, we utilize a bidirectional long short-term memory (BLSTM) architecture. We devise a multi-view BLSTM model that processes the word embedding representation and the similarity network representation in parallel. The multi-view BSLTM model contains two branches. Each branch has independent BLSTM layers that contain LSTM units. The computational process for branch two is shown in Eqs. 4–9. The computational process in the first branch is the same, except that the input at each time step is word embedding $x^{(t)}$ instead of similarity network representation $x_s^{(t)}$.

$$\text{Similarity network–based input gate} : i_s^{(t)} = \sigma\left(W_{si}x_s^{(t)} + U_{si}h_s^{(t-1)} + b_{si}\right); \quad (4)$$

$$\text{Similarity network–based forget gate} : f_s^{(t)} = \sigma\left(W_{sf}x_s^{(t)} + U_{sf}h_s^{(t-1)} + b_{sf}\right); \quad (5)$$

$$\text{Similarity network–based output gate} : o_s^{(t)} = \sigma\left(W_{so}x_s^{(t)} + U_{so}h_s^{(t-1)} + b_{so}\right); \quad (6)$$

$$\text{Similarity network–based cell state} : u_s^{(t)} = \sigma\left(W_{su}x_s^{(t)} + U_{su}h_s^{(t-1)} + b_{su}\right); \quad (7)$$

$$\text{Similarity network–based memory cell} : c_s^{(t)} = i_s^{(t)} \circ u_s^{(t)} + f_s^{(t)} \circ c_s^{(t-1)}; \quad (8)$$

$$\text{Similarity network–based hidden state} : h_s^{(t)} = o_s^{(t)} \circ \tanh\left(c_s^{(t)}\right). \quad (9)$$

Variable $x_s^{(t)}$ is the current input, and $h_s^{(t-1)}$ is the previous hidden state. Parameters W, U, and b are weight parameters with values between 0 and 1. Each forward or backward hidden state has 128 dimensions. We condense useful information from the 300-dimensional $x^{(t)}$ to 128 dimensions in the LSTM cell. The learning rate in gradient descent is 0.1. The dropout rate is 0.2. Each branch obtains a hidden state in the last time step. The final hidden states of branch one and two are further concatenated as an integrated model. Finally, a Softmax layer (Eq. 10) is stacked on the top to predict the word type (OUD treatment barrier or not). Variable y is the predicted word type. Variable x is the input to the Softmax layer. Parameter w is the weight parameter.

$$p(y = j|x) = \frac{e^{x^T w_j}}{\sum_{k=1}^{K} e^{x^T w_k}}. \quad (10)$$

4 Empirical Analyses

The research testbed comes from a leading health IT platform Drugs-Forum.com. We collected the posts from Drugs-Forum related to drug use from the start of Drugs-Forum to September 1, 2018. The raw dataset encompasses 27,154 posts. We randomly sampled 3,000 posts related to OUD treatment. Four expert annotators read the posts and annotated the OUD treatment barriers for model training purposes. The IOB labeling scheme is adapted to assign tags for each word in a sentence. To test inter-annotator reliability, we leverage Cohen's Kappa. The Kappa value for the OUD treatment barrier annotation is 0.92, indicating excellent reliability.

We evaluate our model on the annotated dataset, with 70% for training, 10% for validation, and 20% for testing. We repeat the training procedure for each model 20 times and report the average performance in Table 1. Our SINDEL model outperforms all baseline models by a very large margin in F1 score and precision.

Table 1. Evaluation of SINDEL against baseline methods

Method	Precision	Recall	F1 score
SVM	58.10%	40.09%	47.40%
LR	45.25%	61.15%	50.01%
NB	22.54%	**95.50%**	36.47%
CRF	78.46%	36.59%	49.90%
RNN	75.19%	48.49%	58.80%
LSTM	71.90%	54.48%	61.77%
BLSTM	81.91%	62.65%	70.98%
SINDEL (Ours)	**85.31%**	70.14%	**76.97%**

The SINDEL model could extract the OUD treatment barriers from the research data. These barriers are the actual expressions that patients used in the drug forums. Many expressions may indicate the same type of treatment barrier. We, therefore, cluster the extracted treatment barriers to identify the general types. We use k-means as the clustering method. Thirteen clusters are identified. Table 2 shows the types of OUD treatment barriers.

Table 2. Types of OUD treatment barriers

Type	Description	Percentage
Lack of motivation	The patient does not have motivation to quit opioids	24.67%
Lack of medical literacy	The patient lacks knowledge of consequences of addiction	21.88%
Concerns about social stigma and job opportunities	The patient is concerned about social stigma or afraid of losing jobs	12.67%
Afraid of withdraw reactions	The patient is afraid of the withdrawals after quitting	12.35%
Side effects of treatment	The patient is concerned about the side effects of treatment	9.13%
Reliance because of chronic pain/fatigue	The patient cannot stop opioids because of chronic pain	5.64%

(*continued*)

Table 2. (*continued*)

Type	Description	Percentage
Concerns about buprenorphine/methadone addiction	The patient is concerned about buprenorphine or methadone addiction	3.85%
High cost of treatment	The patient cannot afford the treatment or insurance does not cover	2.91%
Poor patient-physician relationship	The patient does not have good relationship with the providers	2.19%
Enjoy euphoric feeling of drugs	The patient enjoys the euphoric feeling of opioids and does not want to quit	1.70%
Depressed mental status	The patient is depressed and does not want to receive treatment	1.57%
Lack of accessibility	Treatment is not accessible to patients	0.63%
Others	Others	0.82%

The results shed valuable insights to understand patient's decisions about receiving OUD treatment. Lack of motivation is the most common barrier to receiving OUD treatments (24.67%). To motivate these patients, social support and family encouragement are essential to help them receive treatment. In addition to the barriers that confirm prior literature, we also identified new barriers that have not been noted in prior survey studies, such as side effects of treatment, concerns about buprenorphine or methadone addiction, poor patient-physician relationships, and depressed mental status. These barriers have not been identified by survey studies because these barriers are sensitive and involve personal behavior. The patients are willing to share these undisclosed opinions in drug forums because of the anonymity.

5   Conclusion

We designed a novel deep-learning-based approach to collect relevant patient discussions from drug forums, extract the OUD treatment barriers, and analyze the types of barriers. In line with the design science research methodology, we rigorously evaluated our model which outperforms all the baseline models, attributed to the similarity network-based component. The SINDEL model can be generalized in many other information retrieval tasks involving morphs. The OUD treatment barriers detected in this study allow stakeholders to gain rich insights from the patient perspective and understand the real barriers faced by the patients. Being aware of these barriers allows proactive intervention and early preventions to avoid harmful outcomes caused by OUD.

References

CDC. Multiple Cause of Death Data on CDC WONDER (2018). https://wonder.cdc.gov/mcd. html. Accessed 22 Dec 2018

Hassamal, S., Goldenberg, M., Ishak, W., Haglund, M., Miotto, K., Danovitch, I.: Overcoming barriers to initiating medication-assisted treatment for heroin use disorder in a general medical hospital. J. Psychiatr. Pract. **23**(3), 221–229 (2017). https://doi.org/10.1097/PRA. 0000000000000231

Knudsen, H.K., Abraham, A.J., Oser, C.B.: Barriers to the implementation of medication-assisted treatment for substance use disorders: the importance of funding policies and medical infrastructure. Eval. Prog. Plann. **34**(4), 375–381 (2011). https://doi.org/10.1016/j. evalprogplan.2011.02.004

NIDA. Overview | National Institute on Drug Abuse (NIDA) (2018). https://www.drugabuse. gov/publications/research-reports/medications-to-treat-opioid-addiction/overview. Accessed 22 Dec 2018

Rai, A.: Editor's comments: diversity of design science research. MIS Q. **41**(1), iii–xviii (2017)

SAMHSA. Results from the 2016 National Survey on Drug Use and Health: Detailed Tables | CBHSQ (2017). https://www.samhsa.gov/data/report/results-2016-national-survey-drug-use-and-health-detailed-tables

White House. The Underestimated Cost of the Opioid Crisis (2017). https://www.whitehouse. gov/sites/whitehouse.gov/files/images/TheUnderestimatedCostoftheOpioidCrisis.pdf

Wolfe, D., Carrieri, M.P., Shepard, D.: Treatment and care for injecting drug users with HIV infection: a review of barriers and ways forward. The Lancet. **376**(9738), 355–366 (2010)

Analysis of Smart Health Research Context and Development Trend Driven by Big Data

Ying Qu, Moran Fan, Xiaowei Zhang, and Weige Ji[✉]

School of Economics and Management, Hebei University
of Science and Technology, Shijiazhuang 050000, Hebei, China
1065085918@qq.com

Abstract. In the context of new healthcare reform in China, smart health has gradually developed into a necessary link for health service. To comb the research context of smart health based on academic achievements and to explore the development priority of the leading research will help to perfect the theoretical studies and practical applications of smart health. Through Python crawler technology, accessed 922 documents as a data source from CNKI; Using word segmentation, statistical techniques, visualization analysis research context; CiteSpace V software is used to analyze the research profile and development priority from the literature sources, cooperation teams and key words. Through the qualitative analysis of research context and the quantitative analysis of the number of different types of literature, it reveals the process of the development of smart health from the theoretical start, idea formation, practical application, technological progress, cross-border cooperation to the final relatively stable. But found some problems such as underutilization of data, lack of informationization of critical illness, low recognition of family health systems, and problems between government and patients. Therefore, we should strengthen the government's promotion, application stability, hospital data information processing ability, etc. in the development priority. These foreseeability trend and development context will provide new ideas for theoretical research and make up for the deficiencies in practical application.

Keywords: Smart health · Research focus · Bibliometrics · Word cloud visualization · Cooccurrence network

1 Introduction

Smart health is the use of Internet of Things technology to realize the interaction between patients, medical personnel, medical institutions and medical equipment, and gradually achieve informationization. The smart health service system is widely used in humanistic theory, software application, data analysis, high-tech innovation, remote decision-making and other related fields because of its integration of technology development, social needs, and healthcare research. China, as the large country in population, faces the shortage of medical resources. The development of smart health undoubtedly alleviates the uneven distribution of resources, difficult medical treatment and expensive medical treatment. At the same time, with the improvement of the Chinese people's living standard, the demand for health diagnosis and disease

© Springer Nature Switzerland AG 2019
H. Chen et al. (Eds.): ICSH 2019, LNCS 11924, pp. 142–154, 2019.
https://doi.org/10.1007/978-3-030-34482-5_13

treatment has gradually increased. Taking advantage of the huge number of seek medical advice in China, this is useful for the intelligent medical decision-making, regional remote guidance and accurately carry out the smart health. At the same time, it provides a new platform for big data decision-making, Internet technology and remote sensing technology. This paper combed the research context of smart health in China, refined the research development process, found out the shortcomings in this research, and provides inspiration for similar research.

- Through analysis of the general situation of China's smart health research teams, this paper divided the research field of smart health and found the focus of discipline distribution, and research direction is explored from the discipline perspective.
- Research on document theme in time sequence. This paper qualitatively combed the theme direction of the annual smart health research. Through the evolution of time, it showed the insufficiency of research and the development of technology, and provided the basis for forecasting the frontier development of intelligent medical research from the perspective of textual analysis.
- By dividing the smart health service system, we can get the number of documents in the relevant systems and find the shortcomings in the research from the quantitative point of view, and then combine the qualitative analysis of the above points to get the reasons for the research defects, and finally provide strategies for the next step of the smart health research.

Through this study, there are some problems in China's "Smart Health":

- According to the research category and team analysis of smart health, it was found that most of the breakthroughs in smart health research started from the medical point of view, and the research of related technologies was out of touch with the development of medicine.
- According to the analysis of the research process, with the implementation of "smart health", there are too many deficiencies in government propaganda, policy formulation and supervision methods, which lead to obvious differences between urban and rural areas, and the gap of people's telemedicine consciousness. How to take into account the overall situation, balanced development and eliminate local differences is the focus of future research.
- Analysis based on leading research. The development of smart health has matured in some fields, however, the research on doctor workstations, smart prescriptions and epidemic situation release has not been in-depth, which leads to the narrow research on smart health in China and needs breakthroughs.

2 Literature Review

Around the problem of smart health service system, scholars have explored and analyzed from such dimensions as humanities study, software application, data analysis, high-tech innovation and telemedicine. **(1) Humanities study in smart health.** Surk et al. analyzed the trend of the elderly in smart health, and validated the effectiveness of intelligent health care technology on the health of the elderly [1]; Yang solves the problem of providing for the aged by creating an integrative medical service model of medical care and maintenance [2]; Rui conducted an applied research on the prevention and treatment of chronic diseases with high morbidity rate through smart health big data [3]. (**2**) **Software application in smart health.** Wang implemented iOS-based smart health system by using iOS client + background server + database three-tier architecture model, which provided technical support for the implementation of mobile medicine [4]. (**3**) **Data analysis in smart health.** Koutkias et al. proposed that electronic health records, clinical records and biological data all reflect the high performance of large data, which provides possibilities for smart health strategy [5]; Lou built a smart health data analysis platform based on cloud platform and Hadoop to prevent disease and reduce costs [6]; Gu qin studied the function of data mining system for children's rehabilitation information through medical big data processing [7]. (**4**) **High-tech innovation in smart health.** Karthi et al. use Android mobile devices to perform intelligent health monitoring on automated databases [8]; Jia realizes the deep integration with the medical industry from the key technologies of artificial intelligence such as image recognition and deep learning [9]; He et al. elaborated the role of cloud computing in smart health management model, including server and storage center, desktop terminal, regional smart health platform architecture and other aspects [10]. (**5**) **Telemedicine in smart health.** Sung-hee et al. proposed to use a special key encryption system to ensure the collection of personal health information in telemedicine and ensure its privacy [11]; Jun receives Zigbee wireless module data through RS232 serial port of PC terminal monitoring system, and stores, calculates, filters, analyzes and draws 12-channel real-time dynamic ecg waveform to achieve remote health monitoring [12].

Although such studies are common, there is still room for improvement. For example, Current research focuses on technology application, few scholars focused on the analysis of management mode and the construction of service system, while the technical support of smart health will become stronger and stronger, and the problems of service and management will become more and more prominent. In addition, the current research content of smart health research is widely distributed. In order to clarify the development context and research trends of China's smart health, based on the perspective of smart health service system, this study combines the latest research literature, adopts text metrological analysis technology, and makes a comparative study, review and summary of existing academic achievements in China, It is concluded that: ① The research and construction of rural smart health institutions will be the research focus of China's smart health in regional development; ② Patients' awareness and the government's efforts to promote the development of smart medicine are obstacles. Therefore, strengthening the analysis and research on the management mode and service system, and qualitative analysis on the necessity of the development of smart health in China are new driving forces for the development of smart health; ③ The research of artificial intelligence technology will be a new idea for the development of smart health, which will make up for the problem of unreal simulation of conscious thinking in telemedicine technology; ④ The formation of the ecosystem of medical enterprises provides support for smart health in economy, technology, policy and other aspects.

3   Data Acquisition and Preprocessing

Based on the data of academic journals, doctoral dissertations, master's dissertations and conference papers in China Knowledge Network (China Knowledge Infrastructure Database), received 992 academic articles on the topic of "smart health". Firstly, the structure and content of the article are preliminarily understood and the data items needed are determined. In this paper, five data items including "title", "abstract", "author introduction", "author" and "publication date" are selected in the process of climbing; Secondly, using Python "crawler" technology, the resource locator 1 (URL) of the network where the data is located and the HTML identifier number of the page where the data item is located are determined. Through Python technology, the get function requests.get (URL) in the requests package is invoked to open the required web address, and the BeautifulSoup package is used to locate the "crawling" data in the web page, according to the above identified URL and data item ID, the "crawl" article content is stored in ECXEL (the description of the data source acquisition section is shown in Table 1.

Table 1. Data source acquisition description (partial)

Data source acquisition description section			
		Article title	Abstract
Web page HTML identifier		<h1 class="xx_title">	<div class="xx_font">
Python get statement		soup. find_all (HTML identification)	
Data source example	Example 1	The development of 'smart health' in China under the— background of digital divide	[abstract]: With the use of information technology in the field of medical and health services...
	Example 2	Introduction to the normative construction of key links in the smart health chain	[abstract]: Explain the service tenet and composition of the smart health chain...
	Example n	...	...

The data of "title", "abstract", "author introduction" and "author" are text types, there is a similar data, a null value, the code, etc., therefore, the data sources acquired need to be pre-processed such as de-duplication and deletion of redundant characters. For example, the obtained article will appear the abstract and date is not standard, space and carriage return character redundant and other conditions, the consequences of text segmentation and word frequency statistics errors, leading to the research context is not clear, refining the topic and other issues.

4 Smart Health Research Context Analysis

4.1 Disciplinary Distribution and Teamwork Analysis

Research Category Distribution

Chinese academic achievements are mainly divided into two categories: journals and master PhD thesis. Through the professional screening of the author's briefing and the statistics of journal publishing categories, the proportion of research categories related to smart health was obtained. As shown in Table 2, among the academic achievements published by Journal of smart health, the medical and health science and technology category accounted for 47.39%. There are significant differences between the master PhD thesis and the journal articles, and telecom technology, computer software and computer applications account for 54.38%. Smart health supports only 4 medical schools in the master PhD thesis, which shows that the research direction of "smart health" in universities are more focused on the process of "smart". Most of the publishing units of journals are hospitals and related research institutes. Therefore, the development of medical practice in smart health relies on medical workers and medical researchers. In summary, in the research on the theme of "smart health", universities focus on the technical issues related to "wisdom", while hospitals and research institutes focus on the medical and practical issues related to "Medical Treatment".

Table 2. Smart health research category

Master PhD thesis distribution	Ratio (%)	Journal category distribution	Ratio (%)
Telecommunications technology	29.82	Medical and health technology	47.39
Computer software and computer application	24.56	Information Technology	10.53
Information Economy and Postal Economy	8.77	Medical and Health Policy and Regulations	10.53
Instrumentation industry	7.10	Electronic information science synthesis	5.26
Medical and Health Policy and Regulations	7.01	Computer software and computer application	5.26
Business economy	7.00	Economics and management science	5.26
Internet technology	7.00	Social science	5.26
Automation technology	5.26	Information Economy and Postal Economy	5.26
Radio electronics	3.50	Medical Education and Medical Marginal Studies	5.26

Teamwork Analysis

An article with two or more authors is called a research team, referring to CiteSpace V Statistical Tool, co-occurrence analysis of authors was carried out, as shown in Fig. 1.

① Li Rui Team: The main research on the application of big data to diabetes prevention in the context of smart health. The team is mainly based on clinical medicine and explains the research of smart health from a medical perspective. ② Qian Hui Team: Research on policy and development strategies for smart health and medical care. ③ Sun Xiaohe team, through the contribution of mobile terminals and mobile Internet to smart health, including: the application of mobile terminals in the golden time rescue process, the application of wireless rounds, the application of mobile phone appointment registration, etc. ④ Lu Weiliang team used technological innovation as the research background to provide research ideas for the innovation and research and development of new technologies for smart health.

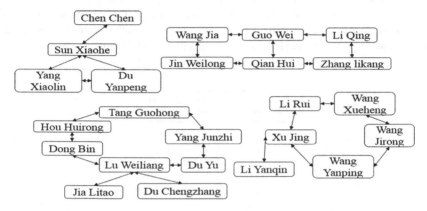

Fig. 1. Author co-occurrence network

4.2   Qualitative Analysis of Hot Issues in Research Process

Using the Jieba package of Python, this paper makes a qualitative analysis of the word segmentation and word frequency of the abstract part of academic achievements, obtains the keywords and word frequency of each year, and forms a visual word cloud (as shown in Fig. 2). From the research context chart, we can see that the process of smart health research in China is from landing, starting, development and application, the research themes at different stages are obviously different.

Landing. Since the promulgation of the new medical reform document in April 2009, the vision of "basic medical and health services for all" has become the goal of unremitting efforts of health departments and medical institutions throughout the country. In the same month, IBM Medical Industry Solutions Laboratory was established, which means that IBM smart health solutions series has landed in China.

Starting. The new type of health informationization construction is to provide a business and technology platform for collecting, transmitting, storing and processing data of the health industry in a digital form within a certain area. Since 2010, the emergence of Internet of Things technology has added a booster to the construction of new health information technology, and promoted the new development of health informationization. At the same time, the people pay more attention to their own health and enhance their health awareness.

Consensus. In 2011, different entities expanded the experience of smart medical care and expanded the application requirements of smart medical care. ① for the patients, the use of archived past inspection data to provide personalized inspection resource allocation schemes reduced patient diagnosis time and cost, improve the satisfaction of medical treatment [13]. ② for doctors, smart health can realize the needs of cross-regional diagnosis and treatment through image and data transmission at the same time, doctors can use the patient's past data to identify the patient's physical condition and family genetic history to achieve effective and effective treatment [14]. ③ for some diseases, 'smart health' can be combined with the professional procedures set by various medical experts for a common disease, such as the prevention, first aid, diagnosis, treatment and rehabilitation of patients with cerebral hemorrhage, it can provide multi-level solutions [15] so that treatment can be found.

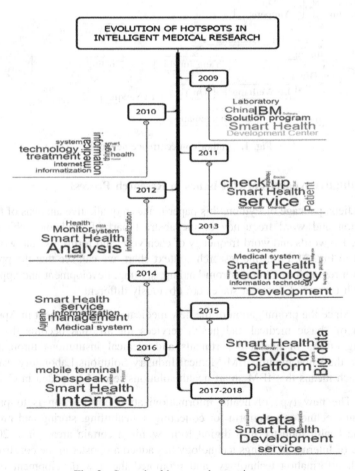

Fig. 2. Smart health research venation map

Medical Big Data Analysis Started. On December 15, 2012, Wu Hequan, academician of the Chinese Academy of Engineering, introduced the application of medical big data. In the process of medical digitalization, hospitals have become an important source of big data. The application of big data is the first to be smart health. The intelligent information processing technology used in 'smart health' includes information collection technology, information mining technology, etc. [16], and the rational use of data provides a possibility for medical deep research and patient self-examination.

Support Technology Diversification. Since 2013, many technologies supporting smart medicine have been put into practice, including personnel positioning and clinical medical system supported by RFID technology; medical management scheme supported by radio frequency identification technology, mobile communication technology and computer network technology; radio ward rounds, wireless nursing and wireless mobile communication supported by wireless communication technology have promoted the multi-level development of intelligent medicine.

Soft Environment Construction. In 2014, with the improvement of the hardware environment, the improvement of the soft environment is imminent. The main focus on ① the new development path of 'smart health', robotics and automatic sensor recognition technology to track hospital assets, optimize the hospital business optimization and reengineering and help to reduce the availability of medical resources. ② the problem of 'smart health' has gradually emerged. There is a phenomenon of 'one enterprise is an island' in China. In the process of the realization of smart health, there is also a shortcoming of low medical information sharing rate. Therefore, the key to the breakthrough of smart health lies in Interconnection of information. ③ 'Smart Health' service quality and management research, quality control in smart health, in the development of smart health technology, the efficiency of doctors and patients is improved, but the quality control of doctors and patients cannot be ignored. The quality of service cannot be weakened. Therefore, in 2014, 'Smart Health' also carried out innovation in the diagnosis and treatment service model [17]. Smart health combined with efficient medical treatment process has improved the quality of medical care and management in smart health. Therefore, in addition to an efficient information support system, a standardized information standard system and a normalized information security system, a scientific supervision system is also necessary for the development of smart health [18].

The Medical Big Data and Cross-Border Cooperation Network Market Has Developed in Parallel. Since 2015, the theory and application of smart health big data have gradually deepened and the cross-border cooperation in medical science has arisen. It mainly focuses on ① resident health card, information exchange platform, resident health file, two-way patient system, health monitoring sensor, medical image which are medical data provided by 'smart health'. The acquired different medical data has the characteristics of heterogeneity, so big data technology has become the basis of 'smart health' data research. Semantic networks, associated data networks [19], data transformation, data segmentation [20] and other data mining technologies have effectively applied medical data, providing new vitality for the development of smart medical care, and forming various medical storage databases, to make medical resources more shared. ② the network market of cross-border cooperation is applied in 'smart health', and the cooperation between smart health and geographic big data enables technology alliance, data sharing and scientific research cooperation. As a temporary barrier to entry for smart healthcare, science and technology will gradually disappear over time, and market pioneers with a vibrant ecological network will gain economies of scale and thus create sustainable barriers to entry [21].

Mobile 'Smart Health' Test. In 2016, the research on smart health was gradually graded, including: the continuous innovation of 'smart health' platform construction technology, the depth exploration of the storage and application of big data in 'smart health', and the advantages of 'smart health' comprehensive promotion and application. As the research progress of smart health continues to deepen, people pay more and more attention to self-inspection of their own health conditions, the popularity of mobile terminals and mobile Internet provides an effective way for patients to seek medical treatment and inquiry. WeChat, mobile medical APP reduce the time for patients to see a doctor in the hospital, and the use of mobile phones is also more convenient, which is another new breakthrough in the development of smart medical care.

The Emergence of Medical Enterprise Cooperative Ecosphere. Since 2017, Alibaba, private capital and hospitals have diversified and supported the technology, economy and information cooperation in the smart health industry. However, it is worth mentioning that patients' awareness and recognition of Internet medical use are not high, and the phenomenon of hospital queues still exists. It is difficult to blame for the lack of Internet medical platform construction and insufficient promotion. It fails to demonstrate the advantages of smart health.

Since 2009, the development of smart health in China is full of opportunities and challenges. ① from the perspective of technology development, Internet of Things technology provides the conditions for the development of smart health. The data mining of big data and cloud computing increases the accuracy of medical remote decision making. Internet + and AI technologies add infinite possibilities to smart health terminals and tele induction; ② from the perspective of themes, China's smart health expands the demand for smart health applications to the problems between hospitals, society and patients, thus using technology and policy-related means to solve problems, and finally forming a relatively stable; ③ at the regional level, the construction of medical informationization originated from medical institutions in large and medium-sized cities. With the increase of people's attention to health, community-based medical institutions gradually integrated into smart medicine. Eventually, due to the development of technology and the realization of telemedicine, it brought hope to remote rural professional medicine. Nevertheless, after 2017, there are still some problems, such as weak implementation of grass-roots government and serious supervision problems. It leads to the outdated primary medical facilities, the lack of medical and health personnel, the patients do not believe that the radiation capacity of primary medical care and health services is limited, and the construction of smart health is difficult.

5   Leading Development Theme Analysis

The comprehensive application and service system of smart health mainly consists of three parts: intelligent hospital system, regional health system and family health system. Through the keyword screening statistics of textual big data, the corresponding classification topics are obtained. For example, the family health system in smart health, through the classification of the topical word segmentation related to the family health system, the visual result is shown in Fig. 3. The results show that the attention of family health system is mainly caused by the increase of chronic diseases, demand for old-age care, people's attention to their own health and the maturity of related technologies. Secondly, the number of articles in the corresponding topic is filtered out (as shown in Fig. 4), and find the short board in smart health from a quantitative point of view. At the same time, combined with the qualitative analysis of the above research hotspots, it is concluded that the future development trend of each theme of the three smart medical service systems in China is mainly as follows:

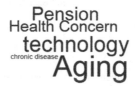

Fig. 3.   Family health system theme cloud

(1) The service system of doctor workstations and smart prescriptions needs to be improved. The doctor workstation is a service system established in the hospital for the storage, conversion, analysis and application of medical data for medical workers, smart prescription is to provide an effective medical decision-making service system through medical big data. It can be seen that although big data is prevalent in the medical field, there are some problems in the use of big data in the hospital system. On this basis, the hospital digests its own data reasonably, combines with relevant data analysis and decision-making technology, establishes a mature doctor's workstation, and the shape of the wisdom prescription becomes natural.

(2) The service system of scientific research institutions management and epidemic situation release and control system in the regional health system service system needs to be improved. Because people's general demand for community health care and community health care to a certain extent alleviate many advantages such as medical resources, research on community health services and health supervision system in regional health service system is more diversified. On the contrary, it is precisely because the needs of community health care are mostly reflected in the diagnosis and treatment of conventional diseases such as chronic diseases and geriatric diseases, which ignores the problem that epidemics are easy to spread in the region and that major diseases need timely diagnosis

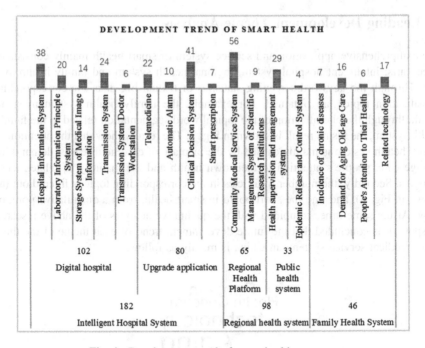

Fig. 4. Development trend of smart health category

and treatment. In the scientific research work of smart medical care, medical experience, effective data and regional basic conditions are used to construct epidemic distribution and control system, and establish a rapid medical treatment process for major diseases in the community. It is a new perspective for the research of community public health service system.

(3) The service system of family health system is the weakest compared with other fields; the main reason is that people have different health needs. Starting from China's national conditions, the problem of aging is serious, and patients with chronic diseases need timely monitoring. Therefore, China's family health service system is formed. However, most patients pay less attention to their own health. Patients with chronic diseases tend to visit hospitals or communities. How to promote the family health service system and reduce the cost of family health care has become the focus, and the government and society have become the dominant force. At the same time, in academic research, family health needs of fine investigation, remote and artificial intelligence technology development, the purpose is to improve the accuracy and timeliness of family medical treatment, enhance people's recognition of the family health system, from a scientific point of view to promote the system.

6 Conclusion

This study is based on the relevant data of CNKI online, and integrates the methods of quantitative analysis, visual display, qualitative and quantitative analysis, etc., to reveal the hot topic context and frontier development trend of Chinese smart health research. In the context of research, the regional development of smart health can be roughly divided into large and medium-sized urban medical institutions $\rightarrow$ community primary medical institutions $\rightarrow$ rural medical institutions; the development of smart health subjects has generally experienced the development of smart health in China $\rightarrow$ initial development $\rightarrow$ smart medical advantages $\rightarrow$ medical data Interconnections $\rightarrow$ technology development $\rightarrow$ problem highlighting $\rightarrow$ medical big data analysis and mining $\rightarrow$ cross-border cooperation $\rightarrow$ application of mobile terminals $\rightarrow$ patient cognition and government promotion; technology development is generally IoT technology $\rightarrow$ big data technology $\rightarrow$ cloud computing $\rightarrow$ Internet + $\rightarrow$ artificial intelligence. From the perspective of cutting-edge development trend, internal storage and analysis of hospital data need to be strengthened to support the convenience of intelligent decision-making process. In addition, the smart health of major diseases cannot be ignored, and timely prevention and control of major epidemics is a new challenge for smart health; The promotion of family service system is closely related to the awareness of the government and people. Only by increasing the support of the government can the popularization of family health service system be accelerated.

Acknowledgements. This paper is supported by the Scientific and Technological Research Projects of Colleges and Universities in Hebei Province 'Research on Risk Knowledge Management of Software Project Driven by Big Data' (Project No. ZD2017029).

References

1. Yi, E.S.: The physical activity and smart health care of trend for the elderly. J. Digit. Converg. **15**(8), 511–516 (2017)
2. Yang, X.: Creating intelligent medical service model of medical maintenance integration. Inf. Syst. Eng. **02**, 22 (2018)
3. Li, R.: Application of intelligent medicine in the old-age service industry based on the model of medical-nursing integration. World Latest Med. Inf. Dig. **18**(74), 190+192 (2018)
4. Wang, H.: Design and Development of Intelligent Medical Software Based on iOS. Beijing University of Posts and Telecommunications (2017)
5. Koutkias, V., Thiessard, F.: Big data - smart health strategies: findings from the yearbook 2014 special theme. Yearb. Med. Inform. **9**(1), 48–51 (2014)
6. Lou, X.: Design and Implementation of Intelligent Health Data Analysis Platform. China Ocean University (2015)
7. Gu, L.: Applied research on data mining of children's rehabilitation information for intelligent medical treatment. Shandong Ind. Technol. **2018**(09), 190+220 (2018)
8. Karthi, A., Rajendran, R., Mathiarasan, P., et al.: Smart health surveillance with automated database using android mobile device. Braz. Arch. Biol. Technol. **60** (2017)
9. Jia, L.: Artificial intelligence: prying intelligent medicine. China Informatiz. **05**, 85–87 (2018)

10. He, Y., Xiong, Y., Shangwu. Creating intelligent medical management model by cloud computing. J. Med. Inform. **37**(04), 39–42+62 (2016)
11. Bemont, C.: The development of robust structural health monitoring sensors utilizing TRIP steel. IEEE Sens. J. **9**(11), 1449–1455 (2009)
12. Jun, W.: Design and implementation of intelligent medical monitoring platform based on web and PC client. Beijing University of Posts and Telecommunications (2015)
13. Chi, W.: Design and implementation of ICH inspection and diagnosis service system based on trust. Harbin University of Technology (2011)
14. Jian, R.: Intelligent medicine. Technol. Entrep. **11**, 6 (2011)
15. Zhang, X.: Design and implementation of S3HC-ICH treatment and rehabilitation service system. Harbin University of Technology (2011)
16. Zhu, R., Zhao, L., Gong, X., Li, Y.: Research on key information technologies and their applications for "Intelligent Medicine". Comput. Knowl. Technol. **8**(05), 1137–1138 (2012)
17. Weilina: Research on Quality Control of Digital Intelligent Medical Ward. Southern Medical University (2014)
18. Yuan, F.: Exploration of intelligent medical application. J. Med. Inform. **35**(12), 2–7 (2014)
19. Tu, Z., Wu, D.: Investigation and research on open associated data sets in medical related domains. Libr. Inf. Work. **59**(18), 14–23+76 (2015)
20. Xiong, Y.: Study on liver CT image conversion and segmentation based on openEHR. Zhejiang University (2015)
21. Jiang, L.: Innovative map and ecological network of mobile health and intelligence medical business model. China Science and Technology Forum (06) (2015)

The Impact of Physician's Login Behavior on Patients' Search and Decision in OHCs

Qin Chen, Xiangbin Yan[(⊠)], and Tingting Zhang

Donlinks School of Economics and Management,
University of Science and Technology, Beijing Xueyuan Road 30,
Beijing 100083, China
xbyan@ustb.edu.cn

Abstract. With the dramatic development of Web2.0, the occurrence of online health communities (OHCs) appeals to increasing number of patients and physicians to involve in this type of healthcare platform. Extant literatures have primarily discussed the various influential factors of patients' choices in OHCs. However, scant studies have been conducted to explore the effect of physicians' login behavior on patients' choices, and the roles of physicians' online reputation and offline reputation. Drawing on the signaling theory, a two-equation model was proposed and tested using collected data from a Chinese OHC to examine the effects of physician's login behavior on patients' search and decision, and the moderation effects of physician's online reputation and offline reputation. The results indicate that physicians' login behavior has positive effects on patients' search and decision. Furthermore, physicians' online reputation and offline reputation moderate these positive relationships. Especially, the moderation effect of offline reputation is higher than online reputation in the search stage, and lower in the decision stage. This study not only enriches the literature on patient behavior, but also advances the understanding of physicians' login behavior in OHCs. The results have implications for the management of OHCs.

Keywords: Online health community · Login behavior · Search · Decision · Online reputation · Offline reputation

1 Introduction

With the support of Health 2.0 technology, more and more people use the Internet to satisfy their health-related needs [1]. Online health community (OHC) has gained popularity in recent years. OHC can be divided into online physicians communities, online physician-patient communities, and online patients communities according to user composition and communication model [2]. This study focuses on the online physician-patient community, and OHC in this paper refers to the online physician-patient community. OHC provides a platform on which physicians can provide serve and help patients. Compared with other types of online communities, OHC has several special characteristics: First, disease is unique for every patient [3]. Second, the stakes are life and death [4]. Third, information asymmetry is more serious between physicians and patients. Since the provision of healthcare services mainly relies on physicians [5], the information of physicians has significant effects on patients' choice [6]. All the above characteristics suggest that a comprehensive investigation of patients' online behavior and determinants of physicians' performance in OHCs is essential.

Patients need to go through two stages for choosing a physician to consult, which includes the process of search and decision in OHCs. Combining the information obtained in the two stages, patients decides whether to choose a physician [7]. Studies have shown that the roles of reviews [8], word of mouth (WOM) [9, 10], patient-generated and system-generated information [7] in patients' search and decision. However, many physician who provide healthcare consultation service online, and also have a job in clinics or hospitals [7]. These physicians must use their spare time to provide healthcare services online [11]. In addition, physicians' satisfaction with OHC causing differences in physicians' login behavior. To a certain extent, the physician's login behavior represents the timeliness of online healthcare services, may influence patients' search and decision. Therefore, there existing an impact of physician's login behavior on patients' search and decision in OHCs.

Reputation has been recognized as one of the most influential factors affecting the consumer's behavior and seller's performance, especially in online markets. Considering people live in a blended environment composed of both offline and online world [12]. Therefore, in OHCs, a physician's reputation also includes two aspects [13]: (1) offline reputation (medical title and academic title), influence patients' consultation behaviors [8, 14], appointment [9], satisfaction [15], online contribution level [16], social and economic returns [17]; (2) online reputation (patients' evaluation), influence patients' appointment [13], posting treatment experience [18]. Reputation in their empirical analyses has not formally integrated both offline and online reputations. This study attempts to narrow this research gap by exploring the impact of reputation, and examining the moderation effect of online reputation and offline reputation between physician's login behavior and patients' search and decision in OHCs.

This study' contribution is three-fold. First, it is one of the earliest attempts to consider physicians' login behavior in OHCs, offers important theoretical contributions. Second, our research adds to online healthcare literature by examining the effects of physicians' login behavior on patients' choices in different stage: search and decision stages. Third, our research provides a comprehensive and in-depth analysis of physicians' reputation, finds the difference between online reputation and offline reputation in the search and decision stages.

This paper is organized as follows: In Sect. 2, literature on OHCs, patient choice, online reputation are reviewed. Research model and hypotheses are presented in Sect. 3. A pilot study is presented in Sect. 4. In Sect. 5 concludes this paper.

2   Literature Review

2.1   Patients' Search and Decision

Due to the lack of medical knowledge, patients must depend on considerable information to select physicians. There are two stages in the process of selecting a physician online: search stage and decision stage. In the search stage, according to their needs, patients search for physicians' initial information (e.g. titles, workplace, services, and dynamic behavior) to select alternatives, and then determine whether to visit the homepage of a physician to get more information. In the decision stage, patients visit the physician's homepage and obtain more information (e.g. articles, patient number, evaluations). Finally, the patient makes a decision whether to consult the physician [7].

Researchers have investigated the impact of physicians' information and indicate that it affects patients' healthcare decisions [19]. Li et al. researched the impact of reviews of physicians on patients' telephone consultation [8]. Lu and Wu explored the impact of WOM about physicians' service quality on patients' appointment [9]. Cao et al. conducted an empirical study from elaboration likelihood perspective, revealed that service quality and WOM both had positive effects on patients' consulting intention [10]. Liu et al. found that overall satisfaction and review volume both have positive impacts on patients' online decisions [20]. Although there are many studies on patients' choices, limited attention has been given the influence of physician's login behavior on patients' choice (search and decision). This study uses the number of visits and patients representative patients' search and decision.

2.2   Physicians in OHCs

OHCs is changing the way that physicians provide services for patients [21]. Indeed, physicians are now enabled to provide services not just in clinics or hospitals, but also in OHCs. Moreover, physicians can also construct their own personal communities within OHCs to link to both their online and offline patients. Such dynamic behaviors of physicians within OHCs are becoming increasingly important for healthcare delivery [7]. However, physicians are also being overloaded with their usual work in hospitals (offline services), use their off-duty hours to help patients in the OHCs (online services), so that the time spent by physicians in OHCs is limited and not fixed [22]. Hence, physicians' login behavior within OHCs could also greatly affect healthcare delivery efficiency, which probably influences patients' perception towards them.

At present, many studies have explored the physician's knowledge sharing [23], online workload [24], services number [15], doctor-patient interaction [25, 26] and so on. To date, few studies have provided a formal understanding physician's login behavior in OHCs, especially its role in patients' decision-making process in OHCs.

2.3   Online Reputation

With the development of Web 2.0 technologies, social media provides a unique platform for product and services to be evaluated by their purchasers and users. A large number of online websites have already provided a reputation mechanism [9], allowing consumers to look for other consumers' experiences and ratings [27]. Therefore, consumers can make decisions based on public information such as reputation. In healthcare field, OHCs also shows physician's reputation (e.g. recommendation generated from system), by which patients can get information about the quality of physician services, helps patients to explore the relationship between physicians' healthcare quality and patients' online behaviors.

Most of the previous research is the direct influence of physicians' online reputation. Wu and Lu found that the reputation of physicians has a positive impact on the number of patients sharing treatment experience [18]. Liu found that the online reputation affected the consultation volume [28]. Liang et al. had studied that the efforts and reputations of physicians have a significant impact on the number of new patients [29]. Therefore, there is lack of research on the moderation of physician's online reputation in OHCs.

3 Research Model and Hypotheses

3.1 Signaling Theory

Signaling theory is used to explain behaviors when players have different information. Because the players hold different quantities and levels of information, there is significant information asymmetry between them [30], signaling theory seeks to define how information asymmetry between two players is minimized [31]. Hence, the information conveyed by the information superiority can help the information inferior to make better decisions.

In the healthcare field, the participants include physicians and patients in OHCs, Compared to the physician, the patient is in a disadvantage, must entrust the physician to help him/her make the right decision [32]. Hence, patients should fully consider all aspects of the physician (e.g. title, workplace, dynamic behavior, evaluation) when choosing their own agent, to serve themselves [28]. Therefore, the signaling theory can be used to explain the relationship of physician's login behavior and patients' search and decision.

3.2 Physician's Login Behavior and Patients' Search & Decision

Most physicians provide healthcare services not only in clinics or hospitals (offline services), but also in an OHC, even in multiple OHCs (online services). The time spent by physicians in OHCs is limited and not fixed [22]. Such dynamic behaviors of physicians within OHCs are becoming increasingly important for healthcare delivery [7]. Due to the special feature of healthcare services, patients are more willing to choose a physician who frequently login OHC to get a more timely response.

In the search stage, patients need to search physicians' information to select alternatives for consultation. However, only parts of the physician's information are available at initial stage of search, including the information about the physician's login behavior (e.g. last online time, reflecting whether the physician has logged recently), will affect the patient whether enters the physician's homepage to see more information about the physician.

When visiting a physician's homepage, patients can learn about more information and decide whether to choose this physician for online consultation by evaluating a physician's information [7, 10]. As an important signal reflecting the physician's online behavior, a physician's login behavior indicates that whether he/she can provide healthcare services in time. Therefore, it is hypothesized that:

H1: Physician's login behavior positively affects patients' search.

H2: Physician's login behavior positively affects patients' decision.

3.3 The Moderation of Physician's Online Reputation

There exists an online reputation mechanism in OHCs, which can be used as an effective signal to help patients distinguish between different online reputation levels. The higher the online reputation level is, the more the physician's service quality and service level are recognized by the majority of patients who consult online [33, 34]. According to the signaling theory, the physician transmits online reputation as a signal to patients, effectively helping patients to distinguish physicians [28].

Therefore, in the search stage, physicians' online reputation can transmit a signal of physicians' capabilities and service qualities, determine whether to visit the selected physician's homepage to obtain more information, especially for physicians who log in more frequently. In the decision stage, online reputation is more objective and credible than traditional information from acquaintances [35]. For patients, they rely on physician's online reputation(e.g. recommendation), to judge the service quality of a physician [10]. In addition, patients could find more information about physicians' online behavior to determine their service delivery process (e.g. physicians' login behavior), which is important in affecting patient's online decision-making. Therefore, it is hypothesized that:

H3a: Physician's online reputation positively moderates the relationship between login behavior and patients' search.

H3b: Physician's online reputation positively moderates the relationship between login behavior and patients' decision.

3.4 The Moderation of Physician's Offline Reputation

The physician's medical and academic title are considered to represent his/her offline reputation, with patients believing it to be involved with the physician's ability. Since the physician's title represents his/her status and treatment levels, can assist patients in evaluating medical ability, provide more objective information for patients [17]. According to the signaling theory, the effectiveness of signaling can be enhanced by repetitive signals [31]. Indeed, when several signals present consistent information, the strength of these signals is strong. Following the same logic, if a physician's offline reputation is positive, patients should regard the signals as more credible. Physicians with high offline reputation level are likely to attract more patients, people are willing to trust such physicians whose services offered are usually considered 'credence services'. Thus, physicians' offline reputation can be a signal to patients, make up for the effects of physicians' online behavior, influences patients' search and decision. So, it is hypothesized that:

H4a: Physician's offline reputation positively moderates the relationship between login behavior and patients' search.

H4b: Physician's offline reputation positively moderates the relationship between login behavior and patients' decision.

In China, physicians have four medical titles(resident physicians, chief physicians, deputy chief physicians, and attending physicians) [36] and three academic titles (professor, associate professor, and lecture). These titles refer to the physician's medical status as evaluated by the government according to the physician's comprehensive abilities [13]. The physician's medical and academic title are considered to represent his/her offline reputation, with patients believing it to be involved with the physician's ability. Since physician's title represents the physician's status and treatment levels, can assist patients in evaluating a physician's ability, provide more objective information for patients [36]. High offline reputation are likely to attract more patients, people are willing to choose physicians whom they think are able to offer better treatment. Physicians' offline reputation can be a signal to patients, make up for the effects of physicians' online behavior, influences patients' search and decision. So, it is hypothesized that:

H5a: Compared to the physician's offline reputation, online reputation has a greater effect on login behavior and patients' search.

H5b: Compared to the physician's offline reputation, online reputation has a greater effect on login behavior and patients' decision.

The research model is shown in Fig. 1.

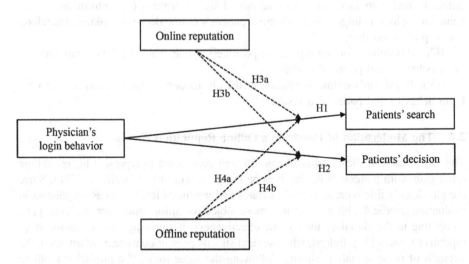

Fig. 1. Research model

4 A Pilot Study

4.1 Data and Description of Variables

This study used data from Haodf.com (http://www.haodf.com/), a leading OHC in China, and took physicians with coronary heart disease as an example. After deleting invalid data, 5758 physicians' data were obtained. This study used a two-equation model to examine the effects of physician's login behavior on patients' search and decision.

This study uses the number of visits and patients as proxies for patients' search and decision, respectively. To reduce reciprocal causality between dependent variables and independent variables, this study uses the difference between two periods of data as the dependent variable for this model. More specifically, this study collected the data twice in March and April, 2019, respectively.

The independent variable is the physician's login behavior. This study uses the physician's last online time as proxy for login behavior. If the physician's last online time is less than one month, it means that the physician has logged in this month, marked 1; else, marked 0. Data for measuring independent variables and moderators were collected in March, 2019, respectively. The control variables in this paper are physicians' sex and hospital level. Table 1 presents the description of variables. Tables 2 and 3 show the descriptive statics and correlations of variables, respectively. Since the dimensions of the two moderators are different, this study normalizes them by the following formula (1) and (2):

$$Online\ reputation = STD(Recommendation) \tag{1}$$

$$Offline\ reputation = STD[STD(Medical\ title) + STD(Academic\ title)] \tag{2}$$

Table 1. Variable description

Variable type	Variable	Description	Proxy
Independent variable	Login behavior	The last time the physician logged OHC, determine if he/she is logged in this month	Login
Dependent variable	Patients' search	Patients search for physicians' initial information to select alternatives and determine whether they should visit the homepage of a physician	Visits
	Patients' decision	Patients evaluate information and make a decision to consult a physician online	Patients
Moderator	Online reputation	The information reflecting physicians' service quality	Recommendation
	Offline reputation	The information representing physicians' ability	Medical title
			Academic title
Control variable	Gender	The physician's gender	Gender
	Hospital level	The level of the physical hospital where a physician work for	Hospital level

Table 2. Descriptive statistics (N = 5758)

Variable	Mean	Std. deviation	Min	Max
Gender	0.199	0.399	0	1
Hospital level	2.882	0.443	0	3
Login	0.323	0.468	0	1
Patients	5.450	25.949	0	678
Visits	3807.685	13579.460	53	461922
Recommendation	3.698	0.279	2.7	5
Medical title	3.132	0.908	0	4
Academic title	1.073	1.274	0	3

Table 3. Correlations of variables (N = 5758)

Variable	1	2	3	4	5	6	7	8
1 Gender	1							
2 Hospital level	0.066**	1						
3 Login	−0.081**	−0.002	1					
4 Visits	−0.057**	0.001	0.266**	1				
5 Patients	−0.036**	0.032*	0.294**	0.581**	1			
6 Recommendation	0.034*	0.200**	0.398**	0.321**	0.383**	1		
7 Medical title	0.201**	0.115**	−0.075**	0.055**	0.030*	0.262**	1	
8 Academic title	0.052**	0.093**	0.015	0.122**	0.072**	0.392**	0.499**	1

** Correlation is significant at the 0.01 level (2-tailed); * Correlation is significant at the 0.05 level (2-tailed)

4.2   Model Estimation

To test hypotheses, this study formulates Eqs. (3) and (4). While the former examines the effects of physician's login behavior on patients' search, the latter examines the effects of physician's login behavior on patients' decision. Since the distribution of dependent variables may not be normal, we use $\ln(X + 1)$ transformations for these variables. The search Eq. (3) and decision Eq. (4) are as follows:

$$\Delta \ln(Visists + 1) = \ln(Visits_t - Visits_{t-1} + 1)$$
$$= \alpha_1 + \alpha_2 Gender + \alpha_3 Hospital\ level_{t-1} + \alpha_4 Login_{t-1} +$$
$$\alpha_5 Online\ reputation_{t-1} + \alpha_6 Offline\ reputation_{t-1} + \alpha_7 Login_{t-1} *$$
$$Online\ reputation_{t-1} + \alpha_8 Login_{t-1} * Offline\ reputation_{t-1} + \varepsilon$$

$$(3)$$

$$\Delta \ln(Patients + 1) = \ln(Patients_t - Patients_{t-1} + 1)$$
$$= \beta_1 + \beta_2 Gender + \beta_3 Hospital\ level_{t-1} + \beta_4 Login_{t-1} +$$
$$\beta_5 Online\ reputation_{t-1} + \beta_6 Offline\ reputation_{t-1} + \beta_7 Login_{t-1}*$$
$$Online\ reputation_{t-1} + \beta_8 Login_{t-1} * Offline\ reputation_{t-1} + \varepsilon$$

$$(4)$$

For the search equation, α_1 to α_8 are the parameters to be estimated. $\Delta \ln(Visits + 1)$ denotes the number of patients visiting the physician's homepage in one month. For the decision equation, β_1 to β_8 are the parameters to be estimated. $\Delta \ln(Patients + 1)$ denotes the number of patients consulting the physician in one month.

4.3   Results

Table 4 presents the results of the search equation, shows the results with only control variables in Model 1, and then adds the independent variables and moderators in Model 2–5. The R^2, Adjust -R^2 and F are reasonable and significant. The results of the VIF statistics for the variable indicate no multicollinearity (the VIF statistic of every variable is not greater than 4.0). According to Model 2 of Table 4, the coefficient of login ($B = 1.742$, $T = 51.42$, $P < 0.01$) is positive and statistically significant, which supports H1. According to Model 3 of Table 4, the coefficient of login*online reputation ($B = 0.217$, $T = 6.80$, $P < 0.01$) is positive and statistically significant, which supports H3a. According to Model 4 of Table 4, the coefficient of login*offline reputation ($B = 0.345$, $T = 10.58$, $P < 0.01$) is positive and statistically significant, which supports H4a. The moderation of online reputation and offline reputation in the search stage are presented in Figs. 2 and 3. According to Model 5 of Table 4, the coefficient of login*online reputation ($B = 0.110$, $T = 3.13$, $P < 0.01$) is smaller than login*offline reputation ($B = 0.324$, $T = 9.66$, $P < 0.01$), which contradicts H5a. And the *lincom* function is used to test the moderation of online reputation versus offline reputation in the search stage (Eq. (5))

$$sig\ B_{Login*Online\ reputation} - B_{Login*Offline\ reputation} = 0.000 \qquad (5)$$

Table 5 presents the results of the decision equation, shows the results with only control variables in Model 1, and then adds the independent variables and moderators in Model 2–5. The R^2, Adjust -R^2 and F are reasonable and significant, and VIF statistics are also reasonable. According to Model 2 of Table 5, we found evidence to support H2, because the coefficient of login ($B = 1.538$, $T = 61.46$, $P < 0.01$) is positive and statistically significant. According to Model 3 of Table 5, we found evidence to support H3b, because the coefficient of login*online reputation ($B = 0.682$, $T = 31.59$, $P < 0.01$) is positive and statistically significant. According to Model 4 of Table 5, we found evidence to support H4b, because the coefficient of login*offline reputation ($B = 0.243$, $T = 9.91$, $P < 0.01$) is positive and statistically significant. According to Model 5 of Table 5, the coefficient of login*online reputation ($B = 0.679$,

Table 4. Parameter estimates of search equation (N = 5758)

Variable	Model 1	Model 2	Model 3	Model 4	Model 5
Constant	7.104** (56.62)	6.537** (62.59)	7.256** (72.22)	6.695** (65.50)	7.286** (73.18)
Gender	−0.383** (−8.00)	−0.217** (−5.46)	−0.269** (−7.32)	−0.295** (−7.56)	−0.292** (−7.98)
Hospital level	−0.048 (−1.11)	−0.058 (−1.62)	−0.265** (−7.84)	−0.108** (−3.08)	−0.270** (−8.09)
Login		1.742** (51.42)	1.271** (36.90)	1.763** (53.54)	1.320** (37.99)
Online reputation			0.402** (17.45)		0.430** (16.34)
Login*Online reputation			0.217** (6.80)		0.110** (3.13)
Offline reputation				0.125** (6.61)	−0.040* (−1.97)
Login*Offline reputation				0.345** (10.55)	0.324** (9.66)
R^2	0.011	0.323	0.426	0.361	0.438
Adjust -R^2	0.011**	0.322**	0.426**	0.361**	0.437**
F	33.33	913.59	854.64	650.21	639.50

T statistics in parentheses; ** Correlation is significant at the 0.01 level (2-tailed); * Correlation is significant at the 0.05 level (2-tailed).

Table 5. Parameter estimates of decision equation (N = 5758)

Variable	Model 1	Model 2	Model 3	Model 4	Model 5
Constant	0.221^*(2.24)	-0.279^{**}(−3.61)	0.064(0.94)	-0.227^{**}(−2.97)	0.065(0.95)
Gender	-0.156^{**}(−4.14)	−0.010(−0.33)	−0.011(−0.43)	−0.038(−1.29)	−0.009(−0.35)
Hospital level	0.127^{**}(3.74)	0.118^{**}(4.48)	0.004(0.18)	0.102^{**}(3.91)	0.004(0.19)
Login		1.538^{**}(61.46)	1.100^{**}(47.11)	1.549^{**}(62.69)	1.097^{**}(46.12)
Online reputation			0.052^{**}(3.36)		0.057^{**}(3.19)
Login*Online reputation			0.682^{**}(31.59)		0.679^{**}(28.33)
Offline reputation				0.011(0.78)	−0.008(−0.57)
Login*Offline reputation				0.243^{**}(9.91)	0.001(0.04)
R^2	0.005	0.399	0.572	0.416	0.572
Adjust -R^2	0.005^{**}	0.399^{**}	0.572^{**}	0.415^{**}	0.572^{**}
F	14.59	1275.03	1537.52	817.64	1098.01

T statistics in parentheses; ** Correlation is significant at the 0.01 level (2-tailed); * Correlation is significant at the 0.05 level (2-tailed).

$T = 28.33$, $P < 0.01$) is positive and statistically significant, which supports H5b. And the *lincom* function is used to test the moderation of online reputation versus offline reputation in the decision stage (Eq. (6)).

$$sig\ B_{Login*Online\ reputation} - B_{Login*Offline\ reputation} = 0.000 \tag{6}$$

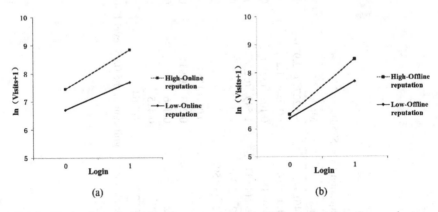

(a)   (b)

Fig. 2. Moderation effects of online reputation and offline reputation in the search stage

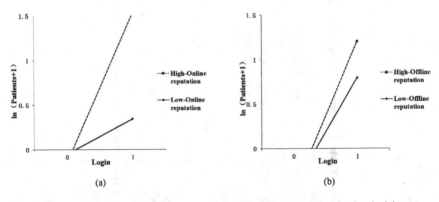

(a)   (b)

Fig. 3. Moderation effects of online reputation and offline reputation in the decision stage

5   Discussion and Conclusion

Drawing on signaling theory, this study proposes a research model to explore the effects of physician's login behavior on patients' search and decision, and the moderations of physician's online reputation and offline reputation. The results indicate that physician's login behavior has positive effects on patients' search and decision. Furthermore, the physician's online reputation and offline reputation moderate these positive relationships. Especially, the moderation of online reputation is higher than offline reputation in the decision stage and lower in the search stage (Fig. 2).

This study extends our understanding of physicians' login behavior in OHCs. By exploring the effects of physician's login behavior on patient's search and decision, this study adds to online healthcare literature. The results show that physicians' reputation not only has a direct impact on patients' search and decision, but also has moderation effects on the relationship between physician' login behavior and patients' search and decision. Findings of this study also suggest differences between the roles of online reputation and offline reputation in patients' search and decision stages. Overall, this study provides a comprehensive and in-depth analyses of physician's reputation (Fig. 3).

However, this study has certain limitations. First, the interpretation of the findings is limited by using data from only one OHC, Haodf.com, and one type of physicians who are expert in coronary heart disease. Therefore, collecting data that are from various platforms simultaneously to further verify the research model is necessary. Second, this study used cross-sectional data to test hypotheses, which lacks of dynamic information to investigate these hypotheses. Therefore, in-depth longitudinal research is needed in this field.

References

1. Wang, X., Zuo, Z., Zhao, K.: The Evolution of User Roles in Online Health Communities – A Social Support Perspective (2015)
2. Song, X.: Research on Social Relationships and Competition Behavior of Patient in Online Health Communities, Harbin Institute of Technology (2015)
3. Marx, G.T.: So surveillance: e growth of mandatory volunteerism in collecting personal information—"Hey buddy can you spare a DNA?". In: Surveillance and Security, pp. 49–68. Routledge (2006)
4. Fichman, R.G., Kohli, R., Krishnan, R.: Editorial overview—the role of information systems in healthcare: current research and future trends. Inf. Syst. Res. **22**(3), 419–428 (2011)
5. Akçura, M.T., Ozdemir, Z.D.: A strategic analysis of multi-channel expert services. J. Manage. Inf. Syst. **34**(1), 206–231 (2017)
6. Yang, H., Guo, X., Wu, T.: Exploring the Influence of the online physician service delivery process on patient satisfaction. Decis. Support Syst. **78**, 113–121 (2015)
7. Yang, H., et al.: Exploring the effects of patient-generated and system-generated information on patients' online search, evaluation and decision. Electron. Commer. Res. Appl. **14**(3), 192–203 (2015)
8. Li, Y., Wu, T., Wu, H.: The impact of reviews of physicians on patient choice (2016)
9. Lu, N., Wu, H.: Exploring the impact of word-of-mouth about physicians' service quality on patient choice based on online health communities. BMC Med. Inform. Decis. Mak. **16**(1), 151 (2016)
10. Cao, X., et al.: Online selection of a physician by patients: empirical study from elaboration likelihood perspective. Comput. Hum. Behav. **73**, 403–412 (2017)
11. Lagu, T., et al.: Patients' evaluations of health care providers in the era of social networking: an analysis of physician-rating websites. J. Gen. Intern. Med. **25**(9), 942–946 (2010)
12. Zhou, J., et al.: Using Reputation to Predict Online Psychological Counselor Appointment: Evidence from a Chinese Website. ACM (2018)
13. Liu, X., et al.: The impact of individual and organizational reputation on physicians' appointments online. Int. J. Electron. Commer. **20**(4), 551–577 (2016)

14. Liu, F., Li, Y., Ju, X.: Exploring patients' consultation behaviors in the online health community: the role of disease risk. Telemedicine e-Health 25(3), 213–220 (2019)
15. Wu, H., Lu, N.: Service provision, pricing, and patient satisfaction in online health communities. Int. J. Med. Informatics 110, 77–89 (2018)
16. Liu, F., Guo, X., Ju, X., Han, X.: Exploring the effects of different incentives on doctors' contribution behaviors in online health communities. In: Chen, H., Fang, Q., Zeng, D., Wu, J. (eds.) ICSH 2018. LNCS, vol. 10983, pp. 90–95. Springer, Cham (2018). https://doi.org/10.1007/978-3-030-03649-2_9
17. Guo, S., et al.: How doctors gain social and economic returns in online health-care communities: a professional capital perspective. J. Manage. Inf. Syst. 34(2), 487–519 (2017)
18. Wu, H., Lu, N.: How your colleagues' reputation impact your patients' odds of posting experiences: evidence from an online health community. Electron. Commer. Res. Appl. 16, 7–17 (2016)
19. Wang, J., Xiao, N., Rao, H.R.: An exploration of risk information search via a search engine: queries and clicks in healthcare and information security. Decis. Support Syst. 52(2), 395–405 (2012)
20. Liu, G., Zhou, L., Wu, J.: What affects patients' online decisions: an empirical study of online appointment service based on text mining. In: Chen, H., Fang, Q., Zeng, D., Wu, J. (eds.) ICSH 2018. LNCS, vol. 10983, pp. 204–210. Springer, Cham (2018). https://doi.org/10.1007/978-3-030-03649-2_20
21. Wang, X., Zhao, K., Street, N.: Analyzing and predicting user participations in online health communities: a social support perspective. J. Med. Internet Res. 19(4), e130 (2017)
22. Wang, L., et al.: Modeling physicians' dynamic behaviors in an online healthcare community: an empirical study using a vector autoregression approach (2017)
23. Yan, Z., et al.: Knowledge sharing in online health communities: a social exchange theory perspective. Inf. Manage. 53(5), 643–653 (2016)
24. Yu, H., Xiang, K., Yu, J.: Understanding a moderating effect of physicians' endorsement to online workload: an empirical study in online health-care communities. IEEE (2017)
25. Gao, G.G., et al.: A digital soapbox? the information value of online physician ratings (2011)
26. Guo, S., et al.: Doctor–patient relationship strength's impact in an online healthcare community. Inf. Technol. Develop. 24(2), 279–300 (2018)
27. Gregg, D.G., Scott, J.E.: The role of reputation systems in reducing on-line auction fraud. Int. J. Electron. Commer. 10(3), 95–120 (2006)
28. Liu, X.-X.: The impact of online doctor reputation and doctor effort on consultation amount, Harbin Institute of Technology (2014)
29. Liang, Q., Luo, F., Wu, Y.: The impact of doctor's efforts and reputation on the number of new patients in online health community. Chin. J. Health Policy 10(10), 63–71 (2017)
30. Stiglitz, J.E.: Information and the change in the paradigm in economics. Am. Econ. Rev. 92(3), 460–501 (2002)
31. Spence, M.: Signaling in retrospect and the informational structure of markets. Am. Econ. Rev. 92(3), 434–459 (2002)
32. Evans, R.G.: Supplier-induced demand: some empirical evidence and implications. In: Perlman, M. (ed.) The Economics of Health and Medical Care. IEAS, pp. 162–173. Palgrave Macmillan UK, London (1974). https://doi.org/10.1007/978-1-349-63660-0_10
33. Ba, S., Pavlou, P.A.: Evidence of the effect of trust building technology in electronic markets: price premiums and buyer behavior. MIS Q. 26(3), 243–268 (2002)

34. Shapiro, C.: Premiums for high quality products as returns to reputations. Q. J. Econ. **98**(4), 659–679 (1983)
35. Gao, G., et al.: The information value of online physician ratings. Working Paper (2011)
36. Li, Y., et al.: Exploring the effects of online rating and the activeness of physicians on the number of patients in an online health community. Telemedicine e-Health (2019)

Dynamic Evolution of Social Network in OHCs Based on Stochastic Actor-Based Model: A Case Study of WeChat Group

Chengkun Wang, Jingxuan Cai, Jiahui Gao, and Jiang Wu[✉]

School of Information Management, Center for E-Commerce Research and Development, Wuhan University, Wuhan 430072, Hubei, China
jiangw@whu.edu.cn

Abstract. With the seamless integration of Internet technology and medical industry, the online health community (OHC), transcending the restrictions of time and geo-graphical distances, provides users with rich and customized information services as well as emotional support. By studying user behavior and the social network evolution in the online health community, it can effectively improve the user activity of the online health community and the efficiency of users' access to information. In this paper, the online health WeChat group is taken as the research object to established a social network based on the @ relationship among users. It explores the influence of individual behaviors on the evolution of network structure through the Stochastic Actor Model. Results show that the user behaviors in the online health WeChat group are of periodicity and turnover. The frequency of speech works differently for the overall and individual network structure changes. It promotes the enrichment of overall network structure while impede the @ relationships among individuals. This paper, exploring the network structure evolution in online health community, carries guiding suggestions concerning the management and maintenance of the online health community.

Keywords: Social network analysis · WeChat group · Online health community · Net evolution

1 Introduction

The OHC is the online platform that can transcend the restrictions of time and geographical distances and bring patients and doctors together, from which participants can seek information, share experience, and gain emotional supports [1]. With the gradual development of people's health awareness, a large number of online health communities, such as eHealth Forum, haodf.com, chunyuyisheng.com, and 39.net, have flourished vigorously. They effectively integrate various medical resources, improves the overall medical level, at the same time provides patients with communication platforms to meet their urgent needs for information and emotional support.

As an instant message software, WeChat has thoroughly integrated into people's daily life [2]. The combination of the WeChat group and the OHC provides participants with a more convenient environment to communicate with each other. Compare with

H. Chen et al. (Eds.): ICSH 2019, LNCS 11924, pp. 170–176, 2019.
https://doi.org/10.1007/978-3-030-34482-5_15

regular BBS OHCs, the online health WeChat group is of more flexibility and instantaneity due to the characteristics of WeChat, which is much closer to daily communication habits. Unlike the broadcast speeches in WeChat groups, the users in the online health WeChat group, in order to convey information accurately, prefer to @ other participants and set up a strong relationship. Accordingly, for the sake of analyzing the role transformation and information dissemination in the online health WeChat group, it is crucial to explore the evolution of the social network based on the @ relationship.

This paper collects the real message records from an online health WeChat Group. A social network is established through the mutual relationship between the participants. Social network analysis method and the Stochastic Actor-based Model are used to explore the evolution of the @ relationship network structure in the online health WeChat group. From the perspective of participants, this paper analyzes the impact of network structure and network location on user behavior. It carries guiding significance for the daily operation and maintenance of the online health community.

2   Related Work

In the existing research on online health community, researchers used topic analysis and machine learning methods to analyze the participants' communication content. Topics discussed in the community mainly include disease prevention, diagnose, treatment, pharmacological function, disease care, etc. [3]. According to the Social Support Theory, the online health community can provide effective social support for participants, including information support, emotional support, and companionship. Different types of social support also affect participants' behavior in the community [4]. In addition, information support from OHCs can also derive emotional support for participants. And negative emotions can be significantly released.

As WeChat has thoroughly integrated into people's daily lives, researchers attach importance to the impact of WeChat groups on the online health community. The motivation for users to participate in the online health community is for seeking health information or emotional support [5]. Their behavior would be influenced by social motivation, information acquisition motivation, and trust. The perceived value of the online health community also has a positive impact on users' continued use intention [6]. At the same time, the social value and information acquisition would also promote users' 'like' behavior [7]. The online health WeChat group satisfies users' need for an online health community and serves the patients as well as their families and friends.

To sum up, previous studies mainly focus on the doctor-driven OHCs. Few scholars combine the online health community with the WeChat group. Meanwhile, most researchers study the user-generated content and users' role classification in the OHCs. There is still a gap in the evolution and transformation of user behavior in the community. Thus, this paper conducts a social network analysis to the Medulloblastoma WeChat group to explore the evolution of the relationship between participants in the online health community.

3 Methodology

3.1 Data Collection

The paper takes the Convey-Love WeChat group as the research object. The Convey-Love is the largest OHC of central nervous system tumor patients in China, founded by cancer patients and their families. This paper collects 49180 messages from the Medulloblastoma WeChat group in the Convey-Love Community from March 20, 2018 to March 14, 2019. After data cleaning, there are 45968 text messages from 563 users. Among all the messages, there are 11777 @ relationships. To reveal the evolution of user social connection, the whole sample is classified into four periods, with 3 months for each. The statistic descriptions for all periods are presented in Table 1.

Table 1. Basic information of WeChat groups in different periods

Period	Number of participants	Number of messages	Number of @
2018.04–2018.07	140	6897	1452
2018.07–2018.10	244	11520	2487
2018.10–2019.01	352	16137	3237
2019.01–2019.04	317	10391	2254

Since the Medulloblastoma WeChat group is an OHC made up of strangers with an administrator as its core, the @ relationships with the administrator take a relatively considerable proportion. To explore the network evolution of users rather than that of the administrator, this paper removes nodes and edges related to the administrator from the entire network.

3.2 Research Methods

This paper analyzes the social network of @ relationship from two aspects. (1) It explores the evolution of online health WeChat group from the overall network structure, taking participants as nodes and the @ relationship between participants as edges, establishing a two-way social network, and analyzing the evolution of social network through the parameters of node input, output, and centrality; (2) Based on the Stochastic Actor Model, it uses the commonly-used social network dynamic analyzing method RSIENA - a R package for SIENA estimation- to explore the dynamic change of the network. The network will influence the dynamics of the behavior, and the behavior will influence the dynamics of the network. In other words, the co-evolution of networks and behavior is studies within the online health WeChat group.

4   Data Analyses and Results

4.1   The Evolution of the Network

In order to present the evolution of the social network of the online health WeChat group, this paper adopts Gephi to visualize the network. Results are shown in Fig. 1. Each node stands for a certain user. The size of the node indicates its speech frequency. The thickness of the edges represents the number of @ the user received.

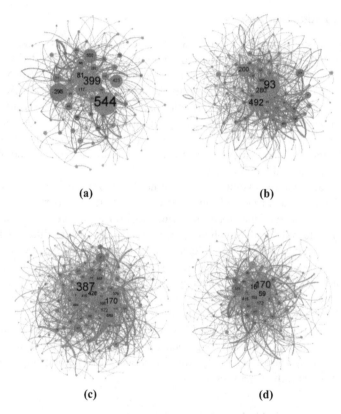

(a)   (b)

(c)   (d)

Fig. 1. Online health WeChat group social relationship evolution

As it is shown in Fig. 1, the social network shows a trend of sustained expansion over time. When the online health WeChat group firstly established, only a few nodes participate in the network. And the network structure is relatively simple. The speech frequency and centrality of several core nodes are much higher than that of other nodes. With the gradual development of the community and the improvement of community management, the social network continues to expand. However, in the fourth period, due to the traditional holiday- Spring Festival – in China, the number of speeches and @ messages in the WeChat group displays an obvious declining trend, as shown in

Fig. 1(c). As a consequence of that, the social network shrank. And the edges were sparser compared with the former period.

From the aspect of individuals, few nodes exist in all four periods, while some nodes exist in the two of them, indicating that the Medulloblastoma WeChat group is of periodicity and turnover. The reason may be that Medulloblastoma has a relatively short treatment cycle and a lower cure rate. Patients will participate in the online health WeChat group during the treatment and withdraw from it after the end of the treatment or the death of the patient.

4.2 SIENA Estimation Results

The formation of social networks is a dynamic and complex process. In addition to the influence of individual basic attributes and randomness, it is also affected by network structure effects, such as reciprocity, balance, and ternary closure [8]. SIENA mainly analyzes the dynamic changes of the network based on the Stochastic Actor-based Model. The model believes that the formation and evolution of the network is determined by actions of the nodes in the network. Each node decides to establish or break off the relationships with other nodes by controlling its own output. In the process of network evolution, each node tries its best to optimize its social structure and ultimately bring about changes to the entire network [9].

In order to describe the evolution of social networks, RSIENA is used to estimate the user speech frequency, triadic closure, participant activity, and participant similarity and test the significance of the stochastic actor model. Results are shown in Table 2. Rate function Rate reflects the evolution speed of the network at different intervals. Rate parameter period 1, rate parameter period 2, and rate parameter period 3 respectively represent the average change degree of the edge of each node in three evolution intervals. The speech frequency has a significant positive impact on the formation of the network. In other words, there are more active participants are in the community. The reason may by lied in the truth that there are massive participants in the communities and users have to use @ to convey information to each other accurately. The frequency similarity has a significant positive impact on the formation of the links in the network. The stronger the similarity between two participants, the easier it is to establish a connection between them.

Table 2. SIENA model estimation results

Variable	Estimate	Standard error	t-ration
Rate parameter period 1	2.1597	0.0613	–
Rate parameter period 2	3.2117	0.0754	–
Rate parameter period 3	3.0679	0.0741	–
Rate effect frequency on rate	0.0006	0.0001	0.0261
Eval transitive triplets	−5.6995	0.5203	−0.0486
Eval frequency ego	−0.0029	0.0003	0.0930
Eval frequency similarity	0.1263	0.1371	−0.0361

Note: $|t| < 0.1$ indicates that the parameter converges during the estimation process.

In addition, for individuals, the impact of frequency ego and transitive triplets on the formation of relationship in the network are significantly negative. The high frequency infers that the participant is in the center of the conversations. There is no need to @ him/her specifically to attract his/her notice. The transitive triplets indicates that the evolution of social network will not promote the formation of triadic closures. In other words, even if two people @ the same person, the chance that they @ each other would not boost, which is consistent with the actual situation.

5   Conclusions

Based on the Social Support Theory and the Stochastic Actor Model, this paper studies the @ relationship network in a Medulloblastoma WeChat group and its evolution in one year after it is been launched. Findings show that, in an online health WeChat group, the @ network would expand over time. And the network structure is of periodicity and turnover. Results from the SIENA explores the factors affecting the evolution of the social network. The more active the WeChat group is, the more @ relationships between participants would developed. However, it would not promote the formation of triadic closure. For individuals, the more the number of speeches, the fewer times it been @. And similar participants are easier to form the @ link. However, this paper still suffers from limitations. Firstly, it merely takes one online health WeChat group as the research object. More samples could be analyzed to avoid contingency. Besides, due to the information disclose policy of WeChat, detailed information about the user is missing. Accordingly, this paper does not take into consideration the unique characteristics of users. The future study could be done on the impact of personal information on the evolution of social networks.

Acknowledgments. This research is supported by the National Natural Science Foundation of China (No. 71573197).

References

1. Martijn, V.D.E., Faber, M.J., Aarts, J.W.M., Kremer, J.A.M., Marten, M., Bloem, B.R.: Using online health communities to deliver patient-centered care to people with chronic conditions. J. Med. Internet Res. **15**(6), e115 (2013)
2. Qiu, J., Li, Y., Jie, T., Zheng, L., Hopcroft, J.E.: The lifecycle and cascade of WeChat social messaging groups. In: International Conference on World Wide Web (2016)
3. Macias, W., Lewis, L.S., Smith, T.L.: Health-related message boards/chat rooms on the Web: discussion content and implications for pharmaceutical sponsorships. J Health Commun. **10** (3), 209–223 (2005)
4. Wang, X., Zhao, K., Street, N.: Social support and user engagement in online health communities. In: Zheng, X., Zeng, D., Chen, H., Zhang, Y., Xing, C., Neill, D.B. (eds.) ICSH 2014. LNCS, vol. 8549, pp. 97–110. Springer, Cham (2014). https://doi.org/10.1007/978-3-319-08416-9_10
5. Che, H.L., Cao, Y.: Examining WeChat users' motivations, trust, attitudes, and positive word-of-mouth: evidence from China. Comput. Hum. Behav. **41**, 104–111 (2014)

6. Gan, C.: Understanding WeChat users' liking behavior: an empirical study in China. Comput. Hum. Behav. **68**, 30–39 (2017)
7. Bambina, A.: Online Social Support: The Interplay of Social Networks and Computer-Mediated Communication. Cambria Press, Youngstown (2007)
8. Snijders, T.A.B., Steglich, C.E.G., Schweinberger, M.: Manual for SIENA version 3. Times Literary Supplement TLS, vol. 14, no. 2, pp. 257–258 (2005)
9. Snijders, T.A.B., Bunt, G.G.V.D., Steglich, C.E.G.: Introduction to stochastic actor-based for network dynamics. Soc. Netw. **32**(1), 44–60 (2010)

Understanding WeChat Users' Herd Behavior in Forwarding Health Information: An Empirical Study in China

Juan Wang[1] and Kunfeng Liu[2(✉)]

[1] School of Information Management, Wuhan University, Wuhan, China
565480204@qq.com
[2] School of Information Management, Zhengzhou University of Aeronautics,
Zhengzhou, China
liukunfeng_zzia@163.com

Abstract. This paper attempts to examine the impacts of social influence factors and herd effect on the herd behavior on forwarding health information of WeChat users. The results of data analysis show that social influence factors have a significant impact on the herd behavior on forwarding health information of WeChat users through two mechanisms, namely, normative social influence and informational social influence. And herd effect factor has a positive impact on the herd behavior in forwarding health information. Especially, the impacts of informational social influence factors are greater, which had been ignored by previous literature. Implications for research and practice are also discussed.

Keywords: Herd behavior · Health information forwarding · Social influence · Normative social influence · Informational social influence

1 Introduction

With the rapid development of the social media applications, people move social networks from offline to online and expand into new social networks. However, social media not only provides social support, but also provides information support for users [1–3], social media has become an important information source for people [4]. The retweeting or sharing behavior of social media user is the main way of information dissemination. From the microscopic point of view, information dissemination in social networks is the process of information passing from one node to another, forming a certain information cascade [5]. In social media, the user's information forwarding behavior is very common [6–8]. The herd behavior in the information forwarding of social media users is the behavior that the user observes the information forwarded by many other users then forwards the same information as well. However, herd behavior in the health information forwarding in social media has brought considerable uncertainty influence to the society [9, 10].

In order to better guide and optimize the herd behavior in the health information forwarding, help users reduce or even eliminate the user' blindness and spontaneity on herding information behavior, enhance users' autonomy and selectivity on herding

© Springer Nature Switzerland AG 2019
H. Chen et al. (Eds.): ICSH 2019, LNCS 11924, pp. 177–188, 2019.
https://doi.org/10.1007/978-3-030-34482-5_16

information behavior. It is necessary to study the factors that influence the herd behavior in health information.

Since WeChat has become the fastest growing social media platform [11]. WeChat is set as the research context. Compared to other social media, the distinctive characteristic of WeChat lies to the familiarity among users: most of the WeChat "friends" recognize each other in the reality. Thus, the following research question is put forward: In the context of WeChat, what factors affect users' herd behavior in health information forwarding?

To approach above research question, this paper will present a research model based on the social influence theory and herd effect. In this study, we examine how the social influence factors affect WeChat users' herd behavior in forwarding health information. The proposed research model was empirically tested via 236 WeChat users collected through an online survey. In doing so, this study offers several contributions.

2 Theoretical Background

2.1 Herd Information Forwarding Behavior

Herd behavior, refers to the tendency of individuals to do what most people do, even if they think they should do something different [12, 13]. The traditional interpretation of herd behavior is manifested in; firstly, imitating the behavior of others, imitating the behavior of others means firstly observing the behavior or decision of others and following the actions or decisions of others; secondly, neglecting the information that they have, as When a person is conducting a herd behavior, first of all, he does not care much about and believes in the private information he owns, and secondly, he is more willing to trust others' information and appreciate others' behavior. Herd behavior is widespread in all areas of society, mainly in the pursuit of shopping behavior [14, 15], herd investment behavior [16, 17], herd entertainment behavior [18, 19] and herd information system adoption and use behavior [12, 20]. The herd behavior in the information forwarding of social media users is the behavior that the user observes the information forwarded by many other users then forwards the same information as well.

2.2 Social Influence Theory

Social influence is defined in psychology as a phenomenon that causes changes in individual perceptions, attitudes, emotions, and behaviors under the influence of the social environment. When a person's behavior (or opinion or emotion) is influenced by others in the social network, there is a social influence [21].

Deutsch and Gerard divide social influence into normative and informational social influence from the perspective of social psychology [12]. Normative social influence refers to the performance that an individual in order to obtain the approval of other people in the reference group or to meet the expectations of others. Informational social influence refers to the fact that an individual obtains information from reference groups as their basis for judging the authenticity of things.

Similar views have been studied in existing literature. In prior research, Venkatesh et al. found that subjective norms, social factors and images are three important dimensions of social influence when constructing UTAUT model [18]. Dholakia et al. argued that group norms and social identity are two key group-level determinants by examining the social influence model of users' participation in virtual community based on network and small groups [19]. Cheung and Lee found that subjective norms and social identity significantly influence the we-intention to use social networking sites [20]. Chen et al. revealed that four social factors which influence Web 2.0 users' intention of continued use are subjective norms, images, key groups, and electronic word of mouth [22]. Tsai and Bagozzi argued that group norms and social identity are effective factors which influence users' contribution behavior on virtual community based on social influence model [23]. When Zhao et al. examined sources and impacts of social influence from online anonymous user, it was found that perceived review quality positively affected informational influences, while informational influences positively affected the perceived decisions quality and the perceived usefulness of websites [24]. Chung and Han revealed that information source credibility combined with network externalities significantly affect the informational and normative social influence of tourism information social media combined social influence theory and ELM theory [25]. Chou found that information quality and source credibility are important influence factors from the social influence perspective through investigating the influencing factors of knowledge adoption behavior of virtual community users [26].

Based on the above analysis, it can be summarized that there are two mechanisms of social influence underlying the social media behavior, one is the normative social influence, which mainly reflects the influence of subjective norms, group norms and social identity on individual behaviors; the other one is informational social influence, which mainly reflects the influence of information quality and source credibility.

3 Research Model and Hypotheses Development

3.1 Research Model

The research model shown in Fig. 1, the current research takes subjective norms as the embodiment of normative social influence, while information quality and source credibility are the embodiment of informational social influence, and takes imitating others as the herd effect factor.

3.2 Hypotheses

3.2.1 Normative Social Influence

Subjective norms refer to the social pressures that individuals feel about whether to adopt a particular behavior. The subjective norms in this study refer to the influence of WeChat users to meet the expectations of others who wish to follow others to forward health information. Lots of previous research indicate that, subjective norm is an important external factor which affects the behavior of social media users. Lu and Hsiao found that blog users continue to update blog content with the encouragement of

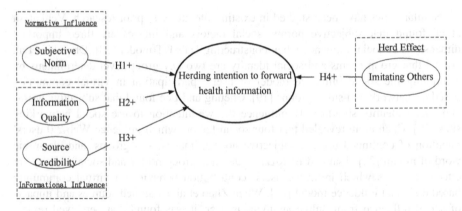

Fig. 1. Research model

those who are important to them [27]. Pelling and White showed that social media users tend to keep their words and deeds consistent with important others [28]. In a social media environment, users are more likely to be socially stressed by others due to they are more likely to be influenced by others through social interactions [20, 29].

In the current research, the users' herd behavior in health information forwarding in the context of WeChat emphasize that individuals observe the health information from the WeChat Moments or WeChat group forwarded by others, then guided by others who have influence on their behavioral decisions and forward the same information. Hence, the following hypothesis is posited:

H1: Subjective norm is positively associated with herding intention to forward health information.

3.2.2 Informational Social Influence

In addition to the above-mentioned normative social influence factors, people are affected by the informational social influence factors inevitably when they use the social media. Due to the lack of corresponding quality assurance mechanisms for online social media information, there are tremendous of information generated by users with uncertainty quality and source credibility, also causing information overload for users.

Forwarding information on social media is also an expression of the individual's self-concept and the sharing and interaction with other users. Compared to other social media, the distinctive characteristic of WeChat lies to the familiarity among users: most of the WeChat "friends" recognize each other in the reality. Since WeChat is a social media with strong tie, the recipients of user generated information are generally acquaintances with certain social relationships, maintaining social image and reputation is an essential consideration [11]. So an individual observes that other WeChat users are forwarding health information. In General, the health information will be reasonably evaluated by users, while checking the quality of the information and the credibility of the information sources.

In the context of WeChat users' herd behavior in forwarding health information, information quality is one construct defined as the quality of outputs shared by other user, which refers to completeness, accuracy and currency. Source credibility is defined as the extent to which the persons generating information in social media are perceived to be trustworthy, knowledgeable, and convincing [30, 31]. Zhang and Watts (2008) argued that "argument quality and source credibility are often consistent across the online community." In current research, information quality and source credibility may be intertwined [32].

From persuasion view, recipients' adoption behaviors are governed by argument quality of information, which refers to the persuasive power of the arguments embedded in the provided information [43]. Cheung et al. found that the strength of the argument and the credibility of the source are important information determinants of the user's perception of the credibility of the electronic word-of-mouth, and thus positively influence the user's adoption of online comments [33]. Zhang argued that information quality and source credibility positively affect consumers' participation in brand loyalty [34]. Zha's study may demonstrate that the information quality and source credibility of social media positively affect the user's perception of the information fit-to-task [30]. Hu and Sundar argue that individuals have different opinions about online health information when information sources come from professionals rather than laymen [35]. It may indicate it is important for Internet users to assess online health information that whether the source of information is authoritative and credible. Lee and Sundar showed that the trustworthiness of health tweets significantly affects the forwarding behavior of Twitter users [36]. Therefore, an individual tends to be more likely to accept and adopt higher credibility information source rather than lower credibility information source [37, 38].

In the context of WeChat, it is reasonable to suggest that if users perceive information quality, source credibility to be higher, they would be likely to follow other users to repost the same information. Therefore, the authors make the following hypothese:

H2: Information quality is positively associated with herding intention to forward health information.

H3: Source credibility is positively associated with herding intention to forward health information.

3.2.3 Impact of Herd Behavior on Health Information Forwarding

The herd behavior is derived from the study of animal clustering behavior. It is extended to user behavior research, which mainly means that in the incomplete information environment, people will be influenced by most people in the selection process. The result of independent thinking, and the decision-making behavior that imitates the actions of others [3]. The herding effect emphasizes that followers often have a wider range of sources of information, and their motivation to obtain information is often to reduce costs and avoid wrong choices. The way in which information is obtained often depends on the observation of the others' behavior [12]. The behavior of forwarding health information in the public is affected by the herd effect. It mainly refers to the incompleteness of the health knowledge in the process of forwarding health information by the WeChat users, causing the user to follow the imitation of others. Herd behavior can effectively reduce the after-sales regret of user participation, and follow-up is the best choice strategy. Therefore, the research hypothesis is proposed:

H4: Imitating others is positively associated with herding intention to forward health information.

4 Measurement Development and Data Collection

4.1 Measures

All of the constructs and the corresponding measure items were adapted from the previous literature to fit the context of this study. Specifically, the items measuring subjective norm were adapted from Yoo et al. and Venkatesh et al. [18, 39]; the items measuring information quality and source credibility were adapted from Bhattacherjee, Sanford and Zha et al. [30, 31]; the items measuring the imitating others and herding intention to forward health information were adapted from Sun [40].

4.2 Data Collection

All items were measured with a seven-point Likert scale, ranging from strongly disagree (1) to strongly agree (7). When the initial questionnaire was developed, 18 users with rich experience of WeChat were invited for a pilot survey. Based on their feedback, the authors adjusted the wording of several items to improve readability and clarity.

This study aims to explore the factors affecting users' herding intention to forward health information. The empirical data in this study were collected an online survey. Consequently, a total of 236 respondents were used for the following data analysis. Table 1 shows the demographic information of the samples.

5 Data Analysis and Results

5.1 Measurement Model Validation

Measurement validity can be assessed in terms of content validity, convergent validity and discriminant validity, which can be tested by the combination of potential variables (Composite Reliability, CR) and internal consistency coefficients (Cronbach's Alpha). In general, the CR value and Cronbach's Alpha value of the latent variable reach 0.7 [41], which means that the model has higher reliability. Table 2 presents the average variance extracted (AVE), composite reliability (CR) and Cronbach's alpha of each construct. It can be seen that all the values of CR and AVE exceed the threshold value. It indicates that the measurement model has a sound reliability and convergent validity.

Table 1. Demographic information of respondents.

Category	Item	Frequency	Percent (%)
Gender	Male	85	36.02
	Female	151	63.98
Age	18–25	100	42.37
	26–35	92	38.98
	36–45	23	9.74
	>45	21	8.91
Position	Undergraduate	107	45.34
	Master student	79	33.47
	Doctoral student	50	21.19
Field	Natural Sciences	33	13.98
	Social Sciences	102	43.22
	Arts and Humanities	39	16.53
	Others	62	26.27
Occupation	Student	129	54.66
	Staff in Institution	45	19.07
	Staff in Enterprise	37	15.68
	Self-employment	8	3.39
	Others	17	7.2
Experience with WeChat (years)	1–2	9	3.81
	2–3	16	6.78
	3–4	48	20.34
	>4	163	69.07

If all square roots of AVE for each construct are greater than all of the inter-construct correlations, sufficient discriminant validity can be established. As shown in Table 3, the square root of each construct's AVE is larger than its correlations with other constructs, exhibiting sufficient discriminant validity of the measurement model [42].

Table 2. Overview of the measurement model

Constructs	Items	AVE	CR	Cronbach's Alpha
Subjective norms (SN)	4	0.757	0.926	0.893
Information quality (INFQ)	3	0.886	0.959	0.936
Source credibility (SCRE)	3	0.908	0.967	0.949
Imitation (IMI)	3	0.820	0.932	0.890
Herding intention to forward information (HINT)	3	0.904	0.966	0.947

Table 3. Correlations between constructs and square roots of AVEs

	SN	INFQ	SCRE	IMI	HINT
SN	**0.870**				
INFQ	0.493	**0.941**			
SCRE	0.503	0.645	**0.953**		
IMI	0.569	0.481	0.430	**0.906**	
HINT	0.608	0.500	0.535	0.524	**0.951**

5.2   Structural Model with Results and Hypotheses Testing

The structural model with results is presented in Fig. 2 where p is based on the two-tailed t value. Following Zha et al. [30], tests of significance were performed using the bootstrap resampling procedure with 1000 samples so as to obtain the t values of the estimates. The R^2 of herding intention to forward health information is 0.518, suggesting good predictive validity of the model.

It can be seen from Fig. 2 that three out of four hypotheses were supported. Except for subjective norm (b = 0.210, t = 1.023), all other factors significantly affect users' herding intention to forward health information, thus H1, H3 and H4 are supported, while H2 is not supported.

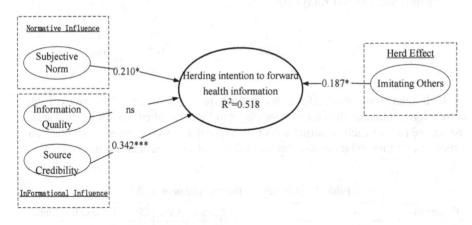

***p<0.001; **p<0.01; *p<0.05 ns: non-significant

Fig. 2. Research model with results

6 Discussion and Conclusion

6.1 Discussion of Findings

From Fig. 2, both the normative social influence factor (subjective norm), informational social influence factors (source credibility) and herd effect (imitating others) have significant positive effects on herding intention to forward health information. In addition, Fig. 2 suggests that the effect of source credibility is the largest one, whereas information quality has insignificant impact on WeChat users' herd behavior on forwarding health information. This result is consistent with Hu and Sundar (2010).

Zha's research shows that it would involve users of social media different level cognitive effort on central route (information quality) and peripheral route (source credibility), respectively [30]. When user involve more focused immersion and more cognitive effort, they depend on central route (information quality) greater than peripheral route (source credibility). However, in the current research, the explanatory impact of the source credibility is greater than other factors, while the impact of information quality is negative, indicating that the WeChat user's herd behavior on forwarding health information is greatly affected by the peripheral route, WeChat user's efforts involved are not so deep. Hence, source credibility has more effect on users' herding intention to forward health information, compared with information quality.

6.2 Implications for Research

Several implications for theory can be derived from the study.

First, This study proposes to analyze the factors that affect herd behavior on forwarding health information from the perspective of social influence combined with the herding effect in the context of WeChat which is a high-sociability social media. Therefore, this study empirically examines a research model that takes herd behavior on forwarding health information as a result of social influence factors and herd effect, enriching related literature about herd behavior on information in social media, contribute to figure out the mechanism of WeChat users' herd behavior on forwarding health information.

Second, based on two dimensions of social influence factors, namely normative social influence and informational social influence proposed by Deutsch and Gerard [12], this study examines the impacts on herding intention to forward health information of these factors in the context of WeChat. Most of the previous literature only noticed normative social influence factors impact on users' behavior in social media [20, 29], while the dimension of informational social influence is largely ignored by previous literature.

Third, ELM has been applied and extended in many existing studies, but it is rarely used for the research of information sharing and forwarding behavior of social media users. Social media with unique characteristics has become a new and important source of information. Based on the normative social influence and information social influence, this research perceives Central and peripheral routes borrowed from ELM theory to explain how information characteristics affect individual attitudes and behavioral changes, with information quality and source credibility as informational social influence factors, to better understand what affect users' herding behavior on forwarding health information.

6.3 Implications for Practice

As mentioned above, the herd behavior on forwarding health information in social media is quite common. It is a double-edged sword which may cause positive or negative effects in different situations. The findings of the study also provide some insights to practitioners.

First, this study shows that both normative social influence factors and informational social influence factors can affect social media users' herding intention to forward health information. Among them, the impact of informational social influence factors on social media users' herding intention to forward information is greater, and the effect of source credibility is the largest one. Thus, the network governance department can develop convincing windows on different social media, make full use of the wisdom of medical health experts, create trustworthy information spokespersons, publish and disseminate correct health information in time, make effort to become a credible health information source on social media.

In addition, this research conclusion also suggests that social media health information content providers such as WeChat Subscription, etc., should strive to improve their professional level and ability, try to improve their credibility, make users rely on their output of information content, so that the providers could expand the impact of their health information WeChat Subscription.

7 Limitations and Future Research

This study explores the impact of normative social influence factors (subjective norm), informational social influence factors (information quality and source credibility) and the herd effect (imitating others) on WeChat users' herd behavior on forwarding health information.

There are several limitations to be noted when applying the findings in future research. First, this paper takes WeChat which is a high-sociability application as the research context. Whether or not the conclusions can be applied for other social media with different sociability in other countries should be further tested in future research. Second, this study focuses on social influence factors and herd behavior factor, several other factors, such as reciprocity norm, perceived usefulness, perceived ease of use, and other factors have not been considered in this study. Thus, future research can further include other important factors to examine the robustness of our study.

References

1. Kane, G.C., Alavi, M., Labianca, G., et al.: What's different about social media networks? A framework and research agenda. MIS Q. **38**(1), 275–304 (2014)
2. Hanna, R., Rohm, A., Crittenden, V.L.: We're all connected: the power of the social media ecosystem. Bus. Horiz. **54**(3), 265–273 (2011)

3. Kaplan, A.M., Haenlein, M.: Users of the world, unite! the challenges and opportunities of social media. Bus. Horiz. **53**(1), 59–68 (2010)
4. Kim, K.S., Sin, S.C.J., Yoo-lee, E.Y.: Undergraduates' use of social media as information sources. Coll. Res. Libr. **75**(4), 442–457 (2014)
5. Hu, C., Xu, W., Hu, Y., et al.: Review of information diffusion in online social networks. J. Electron. Inf. Technol. **39**(4), 794–804 (2017). (in Chinese)
6. Pramanik, S., Wang, Q., Danisch, M., et al.: Modeling cascade formation in Twitter amidst mentions and retweets. Soc. Netw. Anal. Min. **7**(1), 41 (2017)
7. Bakshy, E., Hofman, J.M., Mason, W.A., et al.: Everyone's an Influencer: Quantifying Influence on Twitter. https://dl.acm.org/citation.cfm?id=1935845
8. Taxidou, I., Fischer, P.M., Nies, T.D., et al.: Information diffusion and provenance of interactions in twitter: is it only about retweets? Inf. Syst. Res. **2**(2), 87–115 (2016)
9. Kim, K.S., Sin, S.C.J.: Selecting quality sources: bridging the gap between the perception and use of information sources. J. Inf. Sci. **37**(2), 178–188 (2011)
10. Arazy, O., Kopak, R.: On the measurability of information quality. J. Am. Soc. Inf. Sci. Technol. **62**(1), 89–99 (2011)
11. Ihm, J., Kim, E.: The hidden side of news diffusion: understanding online news sharing as an interpersonal behavior. New Media Soc. **20**(11), 4346–4365 (2018)
12. Deutsch, M., Gerard, H.B.: A study of normative and informational social influences upon individual judgement. J. Abnorm. Soc. Psychol. **51**(3), 629–636 (1955)
13. Kelman, H.C.: Compliance, identification, and internalization: three processes of attitude change. J. Conflict Resolut. **2**(1), 51–60 (1958)
14. Bagozzi, R.P., Lee, K.H.: Multiple routes for social influence: the role of compliance, internalization, and social identity. Soc. Psychol. Q. **65**(3), 226 (2002)
15. Zhao, K., Stylianou, A.C., Zheng, Y.: Sources and impacts of social influence from online anonymous user reviews. Inf. Manage. **55**(1), 16–30 (2017). S1008924400
16. Hsu, C.L., Lu, H.P.: Why do people play on-line games? an extended TAM with social influences and flow experience. Inf. Manage. **41**(7), 853–868 (2004)
17. Kelman, H.C.: Processes of opinion change. Publ. Opin. Q. **25**(1), 57–78 (1961)
18. Venkatesh, V., Morris, M.G., Davis, G.B., et al.: User acceptance of information technology: toward a unified view. MIS Q. **27**(3), 425–478 (2003)
19. Dholakia, U.M., Bagozzi, R.P., Pearo, L.K.: A social influence model of consumer participation in network- and small-group-based virtual communities. Int. J. Res. Mark. **21**(3), 241–263 (2004)
20. Cheung, C.M.K., Lee, M.K.O.: A theoretical model of intentional social action in online social networks. Decis. Support Syst. **49**(1), 24–30 (2010)
21. Zhang, J., Tang, J., Li, J., et al.: Who influenced you-predicting retweet via social influence locality. ACM Trans. Knowl. Disc. Data **9**(3), 1–26 (2015)
22. Chen, S.C., Yen, D.C., Hwang, M.I.: Factors influencing the continuance intention to the usage of web 2.0: an empirical study. Comput. Hum. Behav. **28**(3), 933–941 (2012)
23. Tsai, H.T., Bagozzi, R.P.: Contribution behavior in virtual communities: cognitive, emotional, and social influences. MIS Q. **38**(1), 143–163 (2014)
24. Zhao, K., Stylianou, A.C., Zheng, Y.: Sources and impacts of social influence from online anonymous user reviews. Inf. Manage. **55**(1), 16–30 (2018)
25. Chung, N., Han, H.: The relationship among tourists' persuasion, attachment and behavioral changes in social media. Technol. Forecast. Soc. Change **123**(10), 370–380 (2016)
26. Chou, C.H., Wang, Y.S., Tang, T.I.: Exploring the determinants of knowledge adoption in virtual communities: a social influence perspective. Int. J. Inf. Manage. **35**(3), 364–376 (2015)

27. Lu, H.P., Hsiao, K.L.: Understanding intention to continuously share information on weblogs. Internet Res. **17**(4), 345–361 (2007)
28. Pelling, E.L., White, K.M.: The theory of planned behavior applied to young people's use of social networking web sites. CyberPsychol. Behav. **12**(6), 755–759 (2009)
29. Cheung, C.M.K., Chiu, P.Y., Lee, M.K.O.: Online social networks: Why do students use facebook? Comput. Hum. Behav. **27**(4), 1337–1343 (2011)
30. Zha, X., Yang, H., Yan, Y., et al.: Exploring the effect of social media information quality, source credibility and reputation on informational fit-to-task: moderating role of focused immersion. Comput. Hum. Behav. **79**(2), 227–237 (2018)
31. Bhattacherjee, A., Sanford, C.: Influence processes for information technology acceptance: an elaboration likelihood model. MIS Q. **30**(4), 805–825 (2006)
32. Watts, S.A., Wei, Z.: Capitalizing on content: information adoption in two online communities. J. Assoc. Inf. Syst. **9**(2), 73–94 (2008)
33. Cheung, M.Y., Luo, C., Sia, C.L., et al.: Credibility of electronic word-of-mouth: informational and normative determinants of on-line consumer recommendations. Int. J. Electron. Commer. **13**(4), 9–38 (2009)
34. Zhang, K.Z.K., Barnes, S.J., Zhao, S.J., et al.: Can consumers be persuaded on brand microblogs? an empirical study. Inf. Manage. **55**(1), 1–15 (2017)
35. Hu, Y., Sundar, S.S.: Effects of online health sources on credibility and behavioral intentions. Commun. Res. **37**(1), 105–132 (2010)
36. Lee, J.Y., Sundar, S.S.: To tweet or to retweet? that is the question for health professionals on twitter. Health Commun. **28**(5), 509–524 (2013)
37. Cheung, C.M.K., Lee, M.K.O., Rabjohn, N.: The impact of electronic word-of-mouth. Internet Res. **18**(3), 229–247 (2008)
38. Grewal, D., Gotlieb, J., Marmorstein, H.: The moderating effects of message framing and source credibility on the price-perceived risk relationship. J. Consum. Res. **21**(1), 145–153 (1994)
39. Yoo, J., Choi, S., Choi, M., et al.: Why people use Twitter: social conformity and social value perspectives. Online Inf. Rev. **38**(2), 265–283 (2014)
40. Sun, H.: A longitudinal study of herd behavior in the adoption and continued use of technology. MIS Q. **37**(4), 1013–1041 (2013)
41. Segars, A.H.: Assessing the unidimensionality of measurement: a paradigm and illustration within the context of information systems research. Omega **25**(1), 107–121 (1997)
42. Fornell, C., Larcker, D.F.: Evaluating structural equation models with unobservable variables and measurement error. J. Mark. Res. **18**(1), 39–50 (1981)

How Does Health Knowledge Sharing Affect Patient Perceived Value in Online Health Communities? A Social Capital Perspective

Cui Guo, Zhen Zhang, and Junjie Zhou[(✉)]

Business School, Shantou University, Shantou, China
jjzhou@stu.edu.cn

Abstract. The purpose of this paper is to explore the relationship between health knowledge sharing and patient perceived value in online health communities (OHCs). It is also aimed at explaining the disparity of patient perceived value among different patients by testing the moderating effect of patient social capital on the above relationship in OHCs. A total of 352 valid samples are collected in mainland China while adopting structural equation model (SEM) approach. The empirical results indicate that both aspects of health knowledge sharing, namely health knowledge seeking and health knowledge contribution, have significantly positive influences on patient perceived value in OHCs. Moreover, the effect of health knowledge seeking on patient perceived value is stronger than the effect of health knowledge contribution. Besides this, the moderating effects of patient social capital on the relationship between health knowledge sharing and patient perceived value are significant. Specifically, patient social capital strengthens the relationship between health knowledge contribution and patient perceived value, while it weakens the relationship between health knowledge seeking and patient perceived value in OHCs.

Keywords: Health knowledge sharing · Patient perceived value · Patient social capital · Online health communities

1 Introduction

With rapid development of internet technology, patients are increasingly participating in online health communities (OHCs). In America, nearly 80% of adult users have searched for health information on internet [1]. In China, health websites have more than 100 million visits per month from January 2011 to January 2012 [2]. OHCs are online communities where users share health knowledge, consult experts and communicate with members on health or treatment issues through Internet [3]. There are many well-known OHCs including GoodDoctor in China and PatientsLikeMe in the US, which have achieved great success [4].

OHCs can help connect many users with each other having similar health conditions efficiently. At this platform, patients can have access to health information and support beyond the restrictions of time and space, and obtain more personalized health information. Meanwhile, OHCs can help patients to reduce the cost of health information search and improve the efficiency of the search while protecting patients'

© Springer Nature Switzerland AG 2019
H. Chen et al. (Eds.): ICSH 2019, LNCS 11924, pp. 189–197, 2019.
https://doi.org/10.1007/978-3-030-34482-5_17

privacy [5]. The above advantages make OHCs more and more popular with every passing day. However, due to the open and voluntary nature of using OHCs, patients can easily quit or choose to use other OHCs at any time, which enable few OHCs to achieve success and ensure sustainability [6]. The sustainable development of OHCs is always paid a lot of attention by scholars and OHCs managers.

Perceived value plays a great role in user continuance to intention to online communities (OCs) [7]. In other words, patient perceived value is crucial to the sustainable development and success of OHCs [8]. Undoubtedly, studying perceived value may contribute to attracting users to continue to use OHCs and promoting the sustainable development of OHCs. Thus, the antecedents of perceived value are worth studying. When participating in OHCs, patients can obtain value. For one thing, patients can obtain health knowledge to improve their health conditions when seeking knowledge in OHCs. For another, patients may receive the appreciation from others, build close relationships and improve their status when contributing health knowledge in OHCs. Thus, there is an unclear relationship between health knowledge sharing and patient perceived value in OHCs. We focus on the question, "How does health knowledge sharing affect patient perceived value within OHCs?"

To answer the question above, we propose a theoretical model including health knowledge sharing, patient perceived value and patient social capital. First, we study both aspects of health knowledge sharing, namely knowledge seeking and knowledge contributing. Previous studies pay a little attention to both knowledge seeking and knowledge contributing within OHCs. Analyzing both aspects of health knowledge sharing simultaneously may contribute to understanding the similarity and difference in their effects on patient perceived value in OHCs. Second, patients usually perceive different value although they go through the same health knowledge sharing. Prior studies provide a little knowledge about this phenomenon. To explain this phenomenon, this paper validates the moderating role of patient social capital in the relationship between health knowledge sharing and patient perceived value in OHCs.

This paper is organized as follows. In Sect. 2, the literature associated with patient perceived value, health knowledge sharing, and patient social capital will be reviewed. In Sect. 3, we will present our research model and develop the hypotheses. In Sect. 4, we will describe the development of questionnaire, the process of data collection and empirical results. In Sect. 5, we will point out the conclusions, contributions of this study, and end our work with limitation and future research.

2   Literature Review

2.1   Knowledge Sharing

Knowledge sharing can enrich the resource of OHCs and bring the traffic for OHCs. It can promote the sustainable development of OHCs. Previous studies have not fully considered knowledge sharing behaviors in OHCs. Thus, this study reviews previous research on knowledge sharing in OCs.

Prior studies have seldom analyzed both knowledge seeking and knowledge contribution in one model. Knowledge sharing refers to individuals posting and viewing posts in OCs and should involves knowledge seeking and knowledge contribution [9, 10]. Knowledge seeking refers to the search or acquisition of knowledge [9, 11]. Knowledge contribution is considered as knowledge presenting or sending to others [12]. Knowledge seeking and knowledge contribution are inseparable behaviors. Analyzing knowledge seeking and knowledge contribution simultaneously contributes to our understanding of the similarity and difference of the two aspects of knowledge sharing in OCs.

Existing literature has concentrated on the drivers of knowledge sharing in OCs. Scholars explores knowledge sharing from the perspectives of social capital [13], social cognitive theory [14] and so on. For example, Wasko and Faraj integrate social capital and motivation factors to study knowledge contribution. They discover that reputation positively influences the helpfulness and volume of knowledge contribution, while reciprocity has a negative effect on volume of knowledge contribution [13]. However, previous studies pay a few attentions on the consequences of knowledge sharing.

Based on previous research, this study aims to simultaneously explore how the two behaviors influence patient perceived value in OHCs. Prior studies have shown that patients often encounter a lot of obstacles and perceive various costs when participating in OHCs [15, 16]. The obstacles involve technical barriers related to website design, and non-technical barriers associated with their own abilities [16]. Moreover, The perceived cost of health knowledge contribution in OHCs is mainly divided into cognitive cost and execution cost [15]. Cognitive cost refers to the negative emotions associated with recalling painful experiences, while execution cost refers to the time and effort spent on contributing knowledge in OHCs.

2.2 Patient Social Capital

Social capital is the foundation of trust, cooperation and group activities which plays an important role in the function and continuity of the community. Social capital is defined from different perspectives. For example, from the perspective of network resources, Bourdieu considers it to be the aggregate of actual and potential resources associated with a durable network based on an institutionalized relationship of mutual under-standing and recognition [17].

Based on previous studies, Nahapiet and Ghoshal define social capital as the sum of actual and potential resources derived from and embedded in the network of rela-tionships possessed by an individual or social unit. It involved three dimensions of structure, relationship and cognition [18]. Structural capital is the overall pattern of connections between actors [18]. Social capital is often measured by the form of social interaction with respect to the strength of connection and frequency of communication among community members [19]. Relational capital is defined as the asset created and utilized by social relations, including trust, respect and a norm of reciprocity [18]. These forms of assets are rooted in interpersonal relationships and generated by interactions between actors. Cognitive capital refers to the resources that enable shared interpretation and representations among group members [20]. It focuses on a common understanding which can promote interaction among members. This study also assumes that patient social capital involves structural, relational and cognitive capital in OHCs.

3 Hypotheses Development

3.1 Health Knowledge Sharing and Patient Perceived Value

The health knowledge sharing is divided into health knowledge seeking and health knowledge contribution [9, 10]. As open platforms for the exchange and dissemination of health information, OHCs enable patients to obtain health information support and emotional support [21]. While searching for health knowledge, patients can obtain relevant health information to meet their needs for promoting health and reducing disease risk [22]. Patients also conduct information seeking to kill time and relax mood. Besides, patients often conduct health knowledge seeking to provide support to family or friends [23]. It can enhance the relationship among patients and improve the status of patients. In conclusion, patients can perceive value through health knowledge seeking. The more frequently patients conduct health knowledge seeking, the higher value they obtain. Hence, we hypothesize as:

H1a: Health knowledge seeking positively influences patient perceived value in OHCs.

Health knowledge contribution refers to the behavior involving sending or presenting health knowledge to others who post for help. When the health knowledge contributors answer other patients' health questions, the contributors need to integrate and reconsider health knowledge to provide a correct answer. This process can enhance their understanding of previous knowledge. Besides, the knowledge recipient may express their gratitude to the contributors. It enables knowledge contributors to improve their status [24], and to obtain psychological satisfaction and self-worth [15]. It also contributes to helping contributors to develop close relationships with others [15]. In conclusion, patients can perceive value through health knowledge contribution. The more frequently patients conduct health knowledge contribution, the higher value they get. Hence, we hypothesize as:

H1b: Health knowledge contribution positively influences patient perceived value in OHCs.

3.2 The Moderating Effect of Patient Social Capital

Patient social capital in OHCs is generated through social interactions among patients, especially by responding to others' post for help. Providing help can enables patients build close relationships with other patients. As active participants, patients with high level of social capital in OHCs are those who are more inclined to help others and contribute health knowledge. They might have more health knowledge than other patients, thus they do not have much need to search for health knowledge. Even though they ask health questions in OHCs, other patient with less health knowledge cannot answer the questions effectively. Above all, when the social capital of patients is high (low), patients might perceive less (more) value for a given level of health knowledge seeking. Hence, we hypothesize as:

H2a: Patient social capital weakens relationship between health knowledge seeking and patient perceived value in OHCs.

Health knowledge contributors with high social capital have high level of social capital ties referring to paths of health information and resource flow [25]. They have also high level of shared language which represents the overlap of health knowledge among patients [26]. Moreover, they also enjoy high level of trust, reciprocity and respect contributing to their "insiders" perception of each other in OHCs [19]. Compared to patients with low social capital, these health knowledge contributors with high social capital perceive more benefits including more positive appraise and gratitude, and closer relationship in the same contribution process. Furthermore, they perceive lower costs, such as lower transaction cost and lower execution costs such as time and effort [15] in the same contribution process. Therefore, when the level of social capital is high (low), patients might perceive more (less) value for a given level of health knowledge contribution.

H2b: Patient social capital strengthens relationship between health knowledge contribution and patient perceived value in OHCs.

4 Methodology

4.1 Constructs and Scales

We developed a questionnaire to collect data. The questionnaire included 6 constructs. This study adopted items for health knowledge seeking from Yan and Davison [11]; items for health knowledge contribution from Davenport and Prusak [12]; items for patient social capital from Sun et al. [27]; items for patient perceived value from Wang [28]. All measurement items were answered by a 5-point Likert-type scale, with 1 representing completely disagree and 5 completely agree. We further included 4 demographic items on respondents' gender, age, education and tenure level.

4.2 Data Collection

We conducted an online survey via wjx.cn. The questionnaire link was presented among OHCs forums. The survey lasted from January 28 to March 10, 2019. We collected 352 valid samples with the help of OHCs, especially Mijian OHCs.

4.3 Measurement Model Assessment

We conducted explorative factor analysis and confirmative factor analysis based on SPSS 20.0 and Mplus 7.4. The results were as follows. The Cronbach's α of all constructs were greater than 0.6, and all CR value were greater than 0.7, indicating a good reliability. All factor loading values were greater than 0.6 and all AVE values were greater than 0.5, indicating an adequate convergent validity. The values of AVE square root are higher than the correlation values among different constructs, showing good discriminant validity. Furthermore, Harman's single-factor method was used to test the common method bias. The first factor is lower than the suggested value of 50%. Overall, the data did not have a severe problem of common method bias.

4.4 Hypothesis Testing

This study used Mplus7.4 to test the main effect and the moderating effect by Latent Moderated Structural Equations (LMS) approach in the hypothesis model. The results for hypothesis testing are shown in Table 1.

Table 1. Results for the hypothesis testing

Hypothesis	Path description	Std. β value	Result
H1a	HKS → PPV	0.341***	Supported
H1b	HKC → PPV	0.219***	Supported
H2a	HKS*SoC → PPV	−0.119**	Supported
H2b	HKC*SoC → PPV	0.098**	Supported

Note: HKS, HKC, SoC and PPV respectively, are short for health knowledge seeking, health knowledge contribution, patient social capital and patient perceived value.; * $p < 0.05$, ** $p < 0.01$, *** $p < 0.001$.

First, the significant impacts of health knowledge sharing on patient perceived value were observed. Specifically, health knowledge seeking ($\beta = 0.341$, $p < 0.001$) and health knowledge contribution ($\beta = 0.219$, $p < 0.001$) had significant positive impacts on patient perceived value. Therefore, H1a and H1b were supported. Besides, it is found that health knowledge seeking has stronger predictive power than health knowledge contribution ($F = 3.16$, $p < 0.1$). This means that patients perceive more value when seeking health knowledge in OHCs. It is because their main need to participate in OHCs is to obtain health knowledge to improve health conditions [29]. Hence, the perceived value of patients who conduct health knowledge seeking is more than that of patients conducting health knowledge contribution.

Second, the moderating effects of social capital on relationship between health knowledge sharing and patient perceived value were significant. Specifically, social capital has a positive moderating effect on the relationship between health knowledge contribution and patient social capital ($\beta = 0.098$, $p < 0.01$), while social capital has a negative moderating effect on the relationship between health knowledge seeking and patient social capital ($\beta = -0.119$, $p < 0.01$). Therefore, H2a and H2b were supported.

5 Conclusions and Contributions

5.1 Conclusions

This paper finds that health knowledge seeking and health knowledge contribution significantly influence patient perceived value in OHCs. Moreover, health knowledge seeking has a stronger effect on patient perceived value. Besides, the moderating effects of patient social capital on the relationship between health knowledge sharing and patient perceived value are significant. Specifically, patient social capital strengthens the relationship between health knowledge contribution and patient perceived value, while it weakens the relationship between health knowledge seeking and patient perceived value in OHCs.

5.2 Contributions for Research

This study has two significant theoretical contributions. First, it explores the positive effects of health knowledge sharing on patient perceived value in OHCs. This study finds that both health knowledge seeking and contribution positively affect patient perceived value, and knowledge seeking has a stronger influence on patient perceived value in OHCs. This study extends the research on perceived value in OHCs, explores how knowledge sharing influence perceived value in OHCs and contributes to understanding of similarity and difference of two aspects of health knowledge sharing in OHCs.

Second, we explain the disparity of perceived value among patients by studying the moderating effects of patient social capital. The empirical results indicate that patient social capital strengthens the positive relationship between health knowledge contribution and patient perceived value, while it weakens the positive relationship between health knowledge seeking and patient perceived value. This novel finding extends understanding of social capital and enriched the research on social capital in OHCs.

5.3 Implications for Practice

This study explores the effects of health knowledge sharing on patient perceived value in OHCs and showed its practical implications for OHCs administrators. First, OHCs administrators should devote to facilitate health knowledge sharing activities. They can provide the orientation of new users and help patients to participate in interaction in OHCs. Second, OHCs administrators should take measures to help patients build close relationship and increase their patient social capital. For example, OHCs can give knowledge contributors honorary titles and improve their reputation. It contributes to helping them to increase their social capital.

5.4 Limitations and Future Research

This study analyzes the knowledge sharing behaviors of Chinese patients in OHCs and we do not know whether the model and findings can be applied to patients of other culture. Future studies can explore our model in different culture context. Moreover, this study focuses on OHCs and do not test the model in other OCs. Thus, we can analyze the model in other OC in the future.

Acknowledgements. This study was supported by the following grants: National Natural Science Foundation of China (71501062), Natural Science Foundation of Guangdong Province (China) (2017A030307026), Guangdong Provincial Key Research Project for Universities (2016WQNCX036), National Foundation raising project of Shantou University (NFC16002), Scientific Research Startup Funding Project of Shantou University (STF15003), and STU Scientific Research Initiation Grant (STF18011).

References

1. Fox, S., Duggan, M.: Health Online 2013. Pew Research Center Internet & American Life Project, pp. 1–55 (2013)
2. iResearch, iUserTracker: The Bright Prospect of Social Life Service Websites in China (2012). http://service.iresearch.cn/72/20120503/171329.shtml
3. Demiris, G.: The diffusion of virtual communities in health care: concepts and challenges. Patient Educ. Couns. 62(2), 178–188 (2006)
4. Zhou, J.: Factors influencing people's personal information disclosure behaviors in online health communities: a pilot study. Asia Pac. J. Public Health 30(3), 286–295 (2018)
5. Ybarra, M., Michael, S.: Reasons, assessments and actions taken: sex and age differences in uses of Internet health information. Health Educ. Res. 23(3), 512–521 (2008)
6. Ma, M., Agarwal, R.: Through a glass darkly: information technology design, identity verification, and knowledge contribution in online communities. Inf. Syst. Res. 18(1), 42–67 (2007)
7. Zheng, Y., Zhao, K., Stylianou, A.: The impacts of information quality and system quality on users' continuance intention in information-exchange virtual communities: An empirical investigation. Decis. Support Syst. 56, 513–524 (2013)
8. Wang, Y., Lo, H.P., Yang, Y.: An integrated framework for service quality, customer value, satisfaction: evidence from China's telecommunication industry. Inf. Syst. Front. 6(4), 325–340 (2004)
9. Chen, C.J., Hung, S.W.: To give or to receive? factors influencing members' knowledge sharing and community promotion in professional virtual communities. Inf. Manage. 47(4), 226–236 (2010)
10. Zhou, J., Zuo, M., Yu, Y., et al.: How fundamental and supplemental interactions affect users' knowledge sharing in virtual communities? a social cognitive perspective. Internet Res. 24(5), 566–586 (2014)
11. Yan, Y., Davison, R.M.: Exploring behavioral transfer from knowledge seeking to knowledge contributing: the mediating role of intrinsic motivation. J. Assoc. Inf. Sci. Technol. 64(6), 1144–1157 (2013)
12. Davenport, T.H., Prusak, L.: Working Knowledge: How Organizations Manage What They Know. Harvard Business Press, Boston (1998)
13. Wasko, M.M., Faraj, S.: Why should I share? examining social capital and knowledge contribution in electronic networks of practice. MIS Q. 29(1), 35–57 (2005)
14. Park, J., Gabbard, J.L.: Factors that affect scientists' knowledge sharing behavior in health and life sciences research communities: differences between explicit and implicit knowledge. Comput. Hum. Behav. 78, 326–335 (2018)
15. Yan, Z., Wang, T., Yi, C., et al.: Knowledge sharing in online health communities: a social exchange theory perspective. Inf. Manage. 53(5), 643–653 (2016)
16. Mu, X., Lu, K., Ryu, H.: Explicitly integrating MeSH thesaurus help into health information retrieval systems: an empirical user study. Inf. Process. Manage. 50(1), 24–40 (2014)
17. Bourdieu, P.: The forms of capital. In: Richardson, J.G. (ed.) Handbook of Theory and Research for the Sociology of Education, pp. 241–258. Greenwood, New York (1986)
18. Nahapiet, J., Ghoshal, S.: Social capital, intellectual capital, and the organizational advantage. Acad. Manage. Rev. 23(2), 242–266 (1998)
19. Sun, Y., Fang, Y., Kai, H.L., et al.: User satisfaction with information technology services: a social capital perspective. Inf. Syst. Res. 23(4), 1195–1211 (2012)
20. Cicourel, A.: Cognitive Sociology: Language and Meaning in Social Interaction. Penguin Education, Harmondsworth, London (1974)

21. Yan, L., Tan, Y.: Feeling blue? go online: an empirical study of social support among patients. Inf. Syst. Res. **25**(4), 690–709 (2014)
22. Poortaghi, S., Raiesifar, A., Bozorgzad, P., et al.: Evolutionary concept analysis of health seeking behavior in nursing: a systematic review. BMC Health Serv. Res. **15**(1), 523 (2015)
23. Veinot, T.C.E., Kim, Y.M., Meadowbrooke, C.C.: Health information behavior in families: Supportive or irritating? Proc. Am. Soc. Inf. Sci. Technol. **48**(1), 1–10 (2012)
24. Zhang, X., Liu, S., Deng, Z., et al.: Knowledge sharing motivations in online health communities: a comparative study of health professionals and normal users. Comput. Hum. Behav. **75**, 797–810 (2017)
25. Tsai, W., Ghoshal, S.: Social capital and value creation: the role of intrafirm networks. Acad. Manage. J. **41**(4), 464–476 (1998)
26. Chiu, C.M., Hsu, M.H., Wang, E.T.G.: Understanding knowledge sharing in virtual communities: an integration of social capital and social cognitive theories. Decis. Support Syst. **42**(3), 1872–1888 (2007)
27. Sun, Y., Fang, Y., Lim, K.H.: Understanding knowledge contributors' satisfaction in transactional virtual communities: a cost–benefit trade-off perspective. Inf. Manage. **51**(4), 441–450 (2014)
28. Wang, Y.S.: Assessing e-commerce systems success: a respecification and validation of the DeLone and McLean model of IS success. Inf. Syst. J. **18**(5), 529–557 (2008)
29. Inkpen, A.C., Tsang, E.W.: Social capital, networks, and knowledge transfer. Acad. Manage. Rev. **30**(1), 146–165 (2005)

Health Information Seeking Behaviours of the Elderly in a Technology-Amplified Social Environment

Minglei Ying, Rui Lei, Longqi Chen, and Lihong Zhou[⊠]

School of Information Management, Wuhan University, Wuhan,
People's Republic of China
L.zhou@whu.edu.cn

Abstract. This paper reports on a literature review, which aims to understand, analyse and provide a perspective on mechanisms influence the health information seeking behaviours (HISB) of the elderly in a technology-amplified social environment. This study adopted a literature analysis approach, for the analysis of articles retrieved from Web of Science and PubMed academic databases. Based on the "Technology Amplification Theory" proposed by Toyama, the literature analysis pointed to four mechanisms: the intention of the technology products, the access to health information, the capability of the elderly to apply information technology, and the motivation of the elderly's HISB. Although this study focuses on the elderly, the research findings also provide useful implications and insights for researches on other age groups faced with the digital divide.

Keywords: Health information seeking behaviours · Technology amplification theory · Elderly · Literature review

1 Introduction

Benefiting from the unceasing progress of the social economy condition and the medical service and technology, the average human lifespan has been prolonged gradually, and the world's population is aging [1]. In order to take a positive role in maintaining physical and mental health, it is necessary for people, especially the elderly, to access, understand, and utilise health information. Health information, or consumer health information, refers to any information that enables individuals to understand their health and make health-related decisions for themselves or their families [2]. Similarly, Sangl and Wolf [3] regard it as consumer needs-oriented information that is useable for decision-making and facilitating active involvement of consumers in their own health care and the health care system. Rees [4] defines it as medical topic information relevant and appropriate for the general public, including not only information on signs and symptoms, diagnosis, treatment and prognosis of diseases, but also the access, quality and utilisation of health care services. In the past, access to health information was mainly through professional medical personnel, lectures, or traditional media (newspapers, radio, television). With the development of

© Springer Nature Switzerland AG 2019
H. Chen et al. (Eds.): ICSH 2019, LNCS 11924, pp. 198–206, 2019.
https://doi.org/10.1007/978-3-030-34482-5_18

information technology, new media based on the Internet are increasingly becoming essential source of health information [5]. In China, health information can be accessed from WeChat, health applications, online health communities, health information portals, etc.

It is almost universally believed that technologies are essential to the promotion and sustaining health and well-being of the elderly [6–8]. According to the 43rd statistical report on Internet development in China [9], China's Internet penetration rate has reached 59.6% by December 2018, and the proportion of netizens aged 50 and above has increased from 10.5% at the end of 2017 to 12.5%. It is pleased to find that the popularity of the Internet has gradually penetrated into the elderly. However, as shown in Fig. 1, the proportion is still very small when compared with other age groups. The data suggest that while other age groups are enjoying the benefits of the Internet, the elderly are still isolated from it.

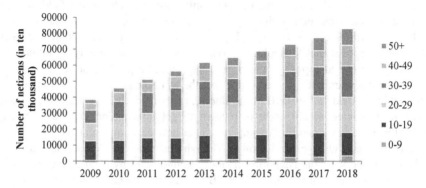

Fig. 1. Number of netizens in China by age from 2009 to 2018 [9]

Health information seeking behaviours (HISB) was first proposed by Lenz [10]. She believes that HISB is a series of interrelated behaviours that can vary along two main dimensions: extent (scope and depth of search) and method (information source used). Lambert and Loiselle [11] define HISB more broadly relate to the ways in which individuals go about obtaining information, including information about their health, health promotion activities, risks to one's health, and illness.

However, despite really wide research attentions on HISB, there is a lack of focus on the elderly. In fact, the current situation of the elderly's HISB is not optimistic [12–14]. It can be found that many of them are still in a predicament [15]. Compared with other age groups, the adoption of technology by the elderly remains limited [16, 17]. And the digital divide has not narrowed over time [13, 18].

Seeing the great social and economic changes after technological innovation, many researchers state in their studies that technologies can contribute to digital equality and play a positive role in improving the lives of the elderly [19–21]. However, there are finds show that the digital divide between the elderly and the young is gradually widening and the influence of technologies is rather limited [22, 23]. Furthermore, previous studies have generally analyzed the factors affecting the elderly's HISB from the perspective of social demographic factors, social cognitive factors and other individual factors of the elderly, but the research on the impact of the technical and social environment is slightly insufficient. Thus, it is necessary to reconsider the impact that technologies truly have. Toyama's technology amplification theory provides a more critical perspective in which technologies only act as amplifier of human intent and capacity. Based on Toyama's theory, we are able to explore the HISB of the elderly in a technological society from a new perspective.

This research aims to understand, analyse and provide a perspective on mechanisms influence the elderly's HISB in a technology-amplified social environment.

2   Theoretical Basis: Technology Amplification Theory

By generalizing and extending the above ideas in politics, education, and mass media, Toyama comes up with one of the currently influential models for the field of information and communication technologies for development, which is the so-called "Technology Amplification Theory". Toyama focuses on the social context of technology and proposes that technology is only an amplifier of underlying human and institutional intent and capacity, which can themselves be positive or negative [24].

As for our research, it is the first time that the technology amplification theory has been used in the field of the HISB of the elderly. Global elderly have seen an explosion of new technologies which might help them to get information in areas including health. However, as warned by Toyama, no matter how dazzling technology is, it could not lead to social change on its own. Though technologies enrich the ways and accelerate the speed to find health information, technologies by itself cannot guarantee or promote the success of the elderly's HISB. A well-intentioned, competent elderly is more likely to benefit from technology, successfully find the targeted health information and thus improve his health conditions than someone who are not. In other words, only when the elderly have positive intent, technology can help to against the digital divide and initiate a virtuous spiral of change [25, 26].

While technology cannot substitute for the human intent or capacity where it is lacking, it tends to amplify existing inequalities [27]. For example, rich and powerful elderly in development countries or regions have better access than those who are not. Also, even if there are no differences in socioeconomic conditions, an elderly who is capable and skilled enough to connect, compare and organize the information can benefit more from the same technology [26]. In a word, the better intent and capacity an elderly have, the more useful health information he will find. Therefore, technology is the amplifier but not the solver of inherent inequalities if without any human intervention.

3   Methodology

A literature review aims to achieve conceptual development and innovation through systematically retrieving, selecting, analysing, and synthesising existing literature [28]. For this reason, the literature review approach was employed as the main methodology in this research. Two databases—Web of Science and PubMed—were used to find relevant literature on the topic of the elderly's HISB. The database search was performed in April 2019, using the search strategy presented below:

(health* or medical) and ("information retrieval" or "information seeking" or "information search") and (old* or elder* or aged or aging or senior*).

4 Findings and Discussion

The data analysis showed that the elderly's HISB is largely different from that of the younger generations. In fact, using technology amplification theory, it can be perceived that in the current healthcare service provision and digital world, it is very difficult for the elderly to search, identify and locate health information. This section presents the findings of the analysis in four subsections, namely: intention of technology products, access to health information, capability of the elderly to apply information technology, and the motivation of the elderly's HISB.

4.1 Intention of the Technology Products

With the intention of more profits, technology product manufacturers tend to design their products and edit the information content catering to the needs of customers with higher income, stronger desire to explore and consume [27]. Therefore, as the system designers are most likely driven by the purpose of maximising financial profit, technology most probably fails to take factors which greatly matter to the elderly such as vision loss, hearing impairment, loss of tactile senses or loss of balance into consideration [29].

Moreover, while the elderly is more suitable for technology products with appropriate front size, clear content structure and less terminology [30], they have to adapt to the unfriendly design of the health information platforms, which in most cases are designed for younger generations. Hence, as discussed in Fischer et al. [31] and Kim and Xie [15], if the elderly need to find health information they need, they have to deal with inadequate readability of the content, poor usability of the online health services, and high complexity of the navigation structure design.

Consequently, it is evident and really not surprising that the current technologies used for health information provision and service amplify difficulties the elderly have in searching for health information. Moreover, due to the technology amplification, it is much easier for younger generations to access health information, since the technologies are mostly designed for them, not the elderly. Technologies enlarge and reinforce the gap of technology utilisation and information accessibility between the two groups.

4.2 Access to Health Information

It is valuable not only for health information providers but also for the elderly to identify which access the elderly utilise to seek health information. As reported in past studies [32–34], the elderly's access to health information was mainly through professional medical personnel, relatives, friends or traditional media (newspapers, radio, television). Yet, the growing personalized and diversified needs of the elderly cannot be adequately catered for by these access [35]. Due to the ubiquitous application of the Internet, some studies have revealed that a lot of new access, such as WhatsApp, WeChat, and public health websites have been offered to the elderly and are gradually becoming the most commonly used electronic access to health information [36, 37].

It should be noted that the elderly rely primarily on face-to-face communication with medical professionals, relatives and friends to obtain health information, rather than the nonliving sources such as the Internet [38]. Thus, medical professionals and individual social networks (relatives, friends, etc.) are listed as their preferred sources of health information. Only when these access are not supportive of the elderly's HISB, or when the elderly want to learn more about health information, the elderly will consider other ways to obtain health information, such as using the Internet.

4.3   Capability of the Elderly

Because of the lack of self-cognitive capability and skills, the elderly have relatively poor capability to search health information, making it impossible for the elderly to effectively use the health information provided by various platforms. HISB can be divided into "information browsing behaviour" and "information retrieval behaviour" [39].

In terms of information browsing behaviour, the physical capabilities of the elderly are declining compared with younger generations, such as cognitive decline, deterioration of memory effects [40], vision aging [41] and so on. Due to the lack of domain knowledge [42], technical operation experience [43] and language capability [44], the elderly are slow to master some new technologies. The low willingness to ask for help [31] makes the situation of the elderly's information browsing behaviour worse.

In terms of information retrieval behaviour, the elderly are not only limited by the retrieval rules but also by their own capabilities. The elderly lack conceptual knowledge related to information retrieval [45] and experience in constructing effective search terms, and cannot clearly distinguish between different browsers and search tools. As a result, the elderly often face the contradiction of lexical mismatch, semantic mismatch, and non-compliance with psychological expectations [40], which may eventually lead to search failure. Similarly, the lack of capability to evaluate online health information [46] also leads to unsatisfactory search results.

4.4   Motivation of the Elderly's HISB

The elderly's behaviours of not only seeking health information from medical professionals but also from the Internet are resulted by multiple motivations. Being in a different state of health means that one will have different motivations. For the ordinary elderly, they often seek information on disease prevention, nutritional diet, exercise regimen, etc., to stay healthy [47]. For the elderly with specific diseases, their motivation varied with the treatment process. Before the appointment with a doctor, motivated by the desire of getting better medical resources and more effective treatment, they may seek information about the credentials and reputation of the healthcare service provider [48]. Medlock et al. [36] show that the elderly most frequently search for health information after an appointment rather than to prepare for an appointment, which may imply that the lack of knowledge or dissatisfaction with the information provided by the doctor will prompt them to seek more comprehensive information [49]. In addition, the desire to understand examination results, to examine the doctor's diagnosis, to make treatment decisions [48, 50], or even the low trust in their treatment [51] also induces the elderly's HISB.

It should be highlighted that the eagerness to heal will motivate the elderly patients, especially those reporting difficulties in accessing medical care when needed, to seek online health information more urgently than the healthy ones [52]. Furthermore, a recent research empirically demonstrates that higher health information need corresponds to higher technology usage of older adults [50].

5   Conclusions

Based on technology amplification theory, the literature analysis revealed four mechanisms influence the elderly's HISB in a technology-amplified social environment: the intention of the technology products, the access to health information, the capability of the elderly to apply information technology, and the motivation of the elderly's HISB. It can be found that there is a contradiction between the intention of technology products and the capability of the elderly. In order to enable older people to obtain more and higher quality health information, we should not only promote technology product manufacturers to adhere to the "elderly-based" design intention, but also help the elderly improve their capability to apply information technology. We believe that only if the both work jointly, the digital divide in the elderly in such technology-amplified social environment can be narrowed. Although this study focuses on the elderly, the research findings also provide useful implications and insights for researches on other age groups faced with the digital divide. Since it is a preliminary study, it should be highlted that the research findings can only be viewed as tentative and need to be further explored in future works.

References

1. United Nations: World population ageing 2017 Report. https://www.un.org/en/development/desa/population/publications/pdf/ageing/WPA2017_Report.pdf. Accessed 16 Apr 2019
2. Patrick, K., Koss, S., Deering, M.J., Harris, L.: Consumer health information: a federal perspective on a important aspect of the national information infrastructure. In: Proceedings of the Second International Workshop on Community Networking 'Integrated Multimedia Services to the Home', Princeton, pp. 261–267. IEEE (1995)
3. Sangl, J.A., Wolf, L.F.: Role of consumer information in today's health care system. Health Care Financ. Rev. 18(1), 1 (1996)
4. Rees, A.M.: Consumer Health Information Source Book, 5th edn. Oryx, Phoenix (1998)
5. Fiksdal, A.S., Kumbamu, A., Jadhav, A.S., et al.: Evaluating the process of online health information searching: a qualitative approach to exploring consumer perspectives. J. Med. Internet Res. 16(10), e224 (2014)

6. Norgall, T.: Fit and independent in the aging population using technology. From concept to reality? Bundesgesundheitsblatt Gesundheitsforschung Gesundheitsschutz 52(3), 297–305 (2009)
7. Satariano, W.A., Scharlach, A.E., Lindeman, D.: Aging, place, and technology: toward improving access and wellness in older populations. J. Aging Health 26(8), 1373–1389 (2014)
8. Garçon, L., Khasnabis, C., Walker, L., et al.: Medical and assistive health technology: meeting the needs of aging populations. Gerontologist 56(Suppl. 2), S293–S302 (2016)
9. China Internet Network Information Center: The 43rd statistical report on Internet development in China. http://www.cac.gov.cn/2019-02/28/c_1124175677.htm. Accessed 15 May 2019
10. Lenz, E.R.: Information seeking: a component of client decisions and health behavior. Adv. Nurs. Sci. 6(3), 59–72 (1984)
11. Lambert, S.D., Loiselle, C.G.: Health information seeking behavior. Qual. Health Res. 17(8), 1006–1019 (2007)
12. Heart, T., Kalderon, E.: Older adults: are they ready to adopt health-related ICT? Int. J. Med. Inf. 82(11), e209–e231 (2013)
13. Vroman, K.G., Arthanat, S., Lysack, C.: "Who over 65 is online?" older adults' dispositions toward information communication technology. Comput. Hum. Behav. 43, 156–166 (2015)
14. Leung, D., Chow, T., Wong, E.: Cancer-related information seeking and scanning behaviors among older Chinese adults: examining the roles of fatalistic beliefs and fear. Geriatrics 2(4), 38 (2017)
15. Kim, H., Xie, B.: Health literacy in the eHealth era: a systematic review of the literature. Patient Educ. Couns. 100(6), 1073–1082 (2017)
16. Choi, N.G., Dinitto, D.M.: The digital divide among low-income homebound older adults: internet use patterns, eHealth literacy, and attitudes toward computer/Internet use. J. Med. Internet Res. 15(5), e93 (2013)
17. Zhang, Y., Lin, Z., Li, X., Xiaoming, T., Zhou, Y., Zhang, X.: Factors affecting ICT use in health communication among the older population in Jiangsu, China. Libri 69(1), 41–53 (2019)
18. Nguyen, A., Mosadeghi, S., Almario, C.V.: Persistent digital divide in access to and use of the Internet as a resource for health information: results from a California population-based study. Int. J. Med. Inf. 103, 49–54 (2017)
19. Torp, S., Hanson, E., Hauge, S., Ulstein, I., Magnusson, L.: A pilot study of how information and communication technology may contribute to health promotion among elderly spousal carers in Norway. Health Soc. Care Commun. 16(1), 75–85 (2010)
20. Gabner, K., Connad, M.: ICT enabled independent living for elderly: a status-quo analysis on product and the research landscape in the field of Ambient Assisted Living (AAL) in EU-27. Institute for Innovation and Technology (2010)
21. Chaumon, M.E.B., Michel, C., Bernard, F.T., Croisile, B.: Can ICT improve the quality of life of elderly adults living in residential home care units? From actual impacts to hidden artefacts. Behav. Inf. Technol. 33(6), 574–590 (2014)
22. Lorence, D.P., Park, H.: New technology and old habits: the role of age as a technology chasm. Technol. Health Care 14(2), 91–96 (2006)
23. Hallows, K.M.: Health information literacy and the elderly: has the internet had an impact? Serials Librarian 61(1), 39–55 (2013)
24. Toyama, K.: Teaching how to fish: lessons from information and communication technologies for international development. J. Mark. Manag. 30, 5–6 (2014)

25. Marais, M.A.: Analysis of the factors affecting the sustainability of ICT4D initiatives. In: Proceedings of IDIA2011, the 5th International Development Informatics Conference on ICT for Development: People, Policy and Practice, Lima, Peru, pp. 100–120 (2011)
26. Toyama, K.: The internet and inequality. Commun. ACM **59**(4), 28–30 (2016)
27. Toyama, K.: Technology as amplifier in international development. In: Proceedings of the 2011 iConference, pp. 75–82. ACM, New York (2011)
28. Grant, M.J., Booth, A.: A typology of reviews: an analysis of 14 review types and associated methologies. Health Inf. Libr. J. **26**(2), 91–108 (2009)
29. Demiris, G.: Home based E-health applications. Stud. Health Technol. Inf. **106**, 15–24 (2004)
30. Schwender, C., Köhler, C.: Introducing seniors to new media technology: new ways of thinking for a new target group. Tech. Commun. **53**(4), 464–470 (2006)
31. Fischer, S.H., David, D., Crotty, B.H., Dierks, M., Safran, C.: Acceptance and use of health information technology by community-dwelling elders. Int. J. Med. Inf. **83**(9), 624–635 (2014)
32. Mann, W.C.: Common telecommunications technology for promoting safety, independence, and social interaction for older people with disabilities. Generations **21**(3), 28–29 (1997)
33. Hirakawa, Y., Kuzuya, M., Enoki, H., Uemura, K.: Information needs and sources of family caregivers of home elderly patients. Arch. Gerontol. Geriatr. **52**(2), 202–205 (2011)
34. Altizer, K.P., Grzywacz, J.G., Quandt, S.A., Bell, R., Arcury, T.A.: A qualitative analysis of how elders seek and disseminate health information. Gerontol. Geriatr. Educ. **35**(4), 337–353 (2014)
35. Raynor, D.K., Savage, I., Knapp, P., Henley, J.: We are the experts: people with asthma talk about their medicine information needs. Patient Educ. Couns. **53**(2), 167–174 (2004)
36. Medlock, S., Eslami, S., Askari, M., et al.: Health information-seeking behavior of seniors who use the internet: a survey. J. Med. Internet Res. **17**(1), e10 (2015)
37. Sultan, K., Joshua, V.R., Misra, U.: Health information seeking behavior of college students in the Sultanate of Oman. Khyber Med. Univ. J. **9**(1), 8–14 (2017)
38. Chaudhuri, S., Le, T., White, C., Thompson, H., Demiris, G.: Examining health information-seeking behaviors of older adults. CIN: Comput. Inf. Nurs. **31**(11), 547–553 (2013)
39. Zhu, S., Deng, X.: Study on influencing factors of internet health information search behavior of the elderly. Libr. Inf. Serv. **59**(5), 60–67, 93 (2015)
40. Stronger, A.J., Rogers, W.A., Fisk, A.D.: Web-based information search and retrieval: effects of strategy use and age on search success. Hum. Factors **48**(3), 434 (2006)
41. Chen, R., Wang, T.: Analysis of Internet use behavior of the elderly. News World **2**, 89–90 (2010)
42. Peter, A.B., Barbara, A.S., Dimitri, A.R., Tobias, M.: International perspectives on how information and ICT can support healthcare. Health Inf. J. **18**(2), 79–82 (2009)
43. Waterworth, S., Honey, M.: On-line health seeking activity of older adults: an integrative review of the literature. Geriatr. Nurs. **39**(3), 310–317 (2018)
44. Flynn, K.E., Smith, M.A., Freese, J.: When do older adults turn to the Internet for health information? Findings from the Wisconsin longitudinal study. J. Gen. Intern. Med. **21**(12), 1295–1301 (2006)
45. Sit, R.A.: Online library catalog search performance by older adult users. Libr. Inf. Sci. Res. **20**(2), 115–131 (1998)
46. Huang, M., Hansen, D., Xie, B.: Older adults' online health information seeking behavior. In: Proceedings of the 2012 iConference, pp. 338–345. ACM, New York (2012)
47. Manafo, E., Wong, S.: Exploring older adults' health information seeking behaviors. J. Nutr. Educ. Behav. **44**(1), 85–89 (2012)

48. Xie, B.: Older adults' health information wants in the internet age: implications for patient–provider relationships. J. Health Commun. **14**(6), 510–524 (2009)
49. McMullan, M.: Patients using the Internet to obtain health information: how this affects the patient–health professional relationship. Patient Educ. Couns. **63**(1–2), 24–28 (2006)
50. Theis, S., Schaefer, D., Broehl, C., et al.: Predicting technology usage by health information need of older adults: Implications for eHealth technology. WORK **62**(3), 443–457 (2019)
51. Bell, R.A., Hu, X., Orrange, S.E., Kravitz, R.L.: Lingering questions and doubts: online information-seeking of support forum members following their medical visits. Patient Educ. Couns. **85**(3), 525–528 (2011)
52. Waring, M.E., McManus, D.D., Amante, D.J., Darling, C.E., Kiefe, C.I.: Online health information seeking by adults hospitalized for acute coronary syndromes: who looks for information, and who discusses it with healthcare providers? Patient Educ. Couns. **101**(11), 1973–1981 (2018)

Data science/Analytics/Clinical and Business Intelligence

Application of Hidden Markov Model on the Prediction of Hepatitis B Incidences

Qiong Liu and Jianhua Yang[(✉)]

School of Economics and Management, University of Science and Technology Beijing, 30 Xueyuan Road, Haidian District, Beijing 100083, China
yangjh@ustb.edu.cn

Abstract. In this study, we apply a hidden Markov model (HMM) to the hepatitis B incidences series published by Chinese Center for Disease Control and Prevention. A two-univariate normal distribution is specified and estimated, where the number of states of the Markov chain is implied by maximum likelihood estimation. These two states, corresponding to different distribution laws, are interpreted as low incidence state and high incidence state accordingly. The probability of state transition is positive, albeit small. The historical states series can be inferred from the estimated HMM. We find that hepatitis B incidence is in low incidence state currently. Based on the estimation result, we predict that hepatitis B incidence will be in low incidence state in the future ten years.

Keywords: Hepatitis B · Disease incidence prediction · Hidden Markov model

1 Introduction

The hepatitis B virus (HBV) is a significant threat to global public health with HBV-related diseases ranking ninth among causes of mortality worldwide [1]. According to [2], HBV is considered the fifth most significant infectious agent that leads to death, with approximately one million HBV-related deaths occurring per year. The application of mathematical statistical methods on modeling, monitoring, and predicting population health data effectively accelerates the formulation, implementation, and improvement of population health management. Appropriate validated statistical models may play an even greater role in obtaining useful information and further assisting in decision making, especially under the current situation of expanding healthcare coverage and population health.

In China, monitoring of HBV and other infectious diseases has been a continual objective since 2004, with participation of both regional and national agencies [3]. Some published studies have proposed frameworks and methods in the context of infectious disease informatics for large-scale detection of HBV [4]. Some methods have been proposed for the automated detection of infectious disease outbreaks [5], such as the Farrington algorithm and the hierarchical time-series algorithm. In addition, other methods for the detection and surveillance of HBV outbreaks exist [6].

In this paper, the hidden Markov model (HMM) is applied in the study of the hepatitis B epidemic. By modeling and estimating the incidences of hepatitis B, we can

© Springer Nature Switzerland AG 2019
H. Chen et al. (Eds.): ICSH 2019, LNCS 11924, pp. 209–221, 2019.
https://doi.org/10.1007/978-3-030-34482-5_19

identify possible outbreaks of hepatitis B in China and their distributions under a particular situation.

2 Literature Review

Studies [7–9] have demonstrated that HMM is suitable for modeling the progression of the infectious and non-infectious disease numbers. These works focus on the modeling and prediction of hepatitis B incidences within a specific region and constant time period using HMM. HMM has also been used in the identification of virus mutations and evolutions [10]. According to [10], the state of the hepatitis C virus evolution can be identified based on the total sequence of the hepatitis C virus and its mutations. In terms of studies on China's hepatitis B epidemic, most Chinese researchers, such as [11–15], have used relatively simple linear time-series analysis methods on modeling and forecasting the incidences of hepatitis B. However, no in-depth study using these time-series analysis methods employs a model with certain limitations. For example, the non-negative and integer condition of the incidence of hepatitis B is not consistent with the time-series analysis of the normal distribution assumption. Only under certain circumstances can it be used for approximations. Nevertheless, existing studies do not discuss these limitations; rather, they are directly applied to time-series models, such as the autoregressive integrated moving average (ARIMA) model.

Furthermore, some studies employed more complex non-linear models to model the number of hepatitis B outbreaks [16–20]. Although this type of model may provide better fitting results, its non-linear characteristics make it unable to analyze the meaning of the model parameters in terms of infectious disease. It is therefore not favorable for guiding further decisions.

Based on our study, we determined that a relatively good balance exists between linear and nonlinear models for the HMM model. This enables better fit and prediction methods as well as a meaningful epidemiological interpretation in the model parameters. Specifically, according to the estimation result of the HMM, the incidence of the hepatitis B epidemic can be respectively divided into low and high states, and the numbers of hepatitis B incidences in subjects of different states have different distributions. By using HMM, it is possible to predict the hepatitis B epidemic state, as well as the distribution and number of incidences. This information can assist decision makers in preventing and controlling outbreaks.

3 Model

In a hidden Markov model (HMM), the distribution function of observed values at each time is controlled by an unobservable finite-state discrete Markov chain. The HMM consists of two parts. The first part is an observable state-dependent process denoted by $\{X_t : t \in \mathbb{N}\}$, where t represents time, and X_t represents the observed value at time t. The second part is an unobservable homogeneous Markov chain with a finite state, i.e., a parameter process, which is denoted by $\{C_t : t \in \mathbb{N}\}$. We use $\mathbf{X}^{(t)}$ to represent the observed series from time 1 to t, and $\mathbf{C}^{(t)}$ to represent the unobservable state sequence of the same period. Therefore, an HMM can be defined as in [21],

$$\Pr\left(C_t \middle| \mathbf{C}^{(t-1)}\right) = \Pr(C_t | C_{t-1}), t = 2, 3, \dots \tag{1}$$

$$\Pr\left(X_t \middle| \mathbf{X}^{(t-1)}, \mathbf{C}^{(t)}\right) = \Pr(X_t | C_t), t \in \mathbb{N} \tag{2}$$

where $\Pr\left(C_t \middle| \mathbf{C}^{(t-1)}\right)$ represents the distribution function of the random variable C_t conditioned on the history up to $t - 1$. The meaning of the above equation is that, at time $t > 1$, the distribution of C_t depends on the last state only, rather than on the entire history. $\Pr\left(X_t \middle| \mathbf{X}^{(t-1)}, \mathbf{C}^{(t)}\right)$ refers to the probability distribution of observable X_t given the previous observations and state sequence, as well as the current state. Equation (2) means that the current distribution of X_t depends only on the current state of the Markov chain. The basic structure of the HMM is illustrated in Fig. 1.

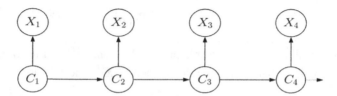

Fig. 1. Basic structure of the HMM

In HMM, the observable variable X_t conditional distribution can be either a discrete or continuous distribution. For the discrete distribution, we use $p_i(x) = \Pr(X_t = x | C_t = i)$ to describe the probability mass function of X_t when the unobservable Markov chain is in the ith state at time t ($i = 1, 2, \dots$, m). For the continuous distribution, $p_i(x)$ is defined as the probability density function of X_t when the unobservable Markov chain is in the ith state at time t ($i = 1, 2, \dots$, m).

The HMM structure can balance the linear and nonlinear models. The unobservable Markov chain of HMM can model correlations between different observations through the Markov property, which is similar to the modeling of correlations in the ARIMA models. Moreover, the unconditional distribution of observations at each time interval consists of m components of probability distributions, thereby making it a mixture, which can achieve a better fit to linear models for the multi-modal time series.

The HMM model parameters are comprised of three parts. The first part is the initial probability of the unobservable (homogeneous Markov chain) parameter process, as expressed by δ. The second part is the transition probability matrix of the process parameter, which is a square matrix with the dimension equal to the square of the number of states of the Markov chain represented by $\mathbf{\Gamma}$, whose elements $\gamma_{ij} = \Pr(C_t = j | C_{t-1} = i)$. The third part is comprised of the parameters in the probability of each state, which is dependent on the state of the process of the distribution function and is represented by θ.

Three problems must be solved for the application of HMM in the prediction of hepatitis B incidences. The first problem is to set the type of distribution and the number of states in the HMM Markov chain and to estimate the model parameters of the three parts. The second problem is the state recognition, namely to identify the state of the hepatitis B epidemic in a specific period and the probability distribution of the incidence number. The third problem is the prediction of the state and distribution of the hepatitis B epidemic under the current state and the number of hepatitis B incidences.

In terms of the estimation problem of an HMM, the number of states of the Markov chain can be estimated by maximizing the log-likelihood function of the HMM. Owing to the complexity of the HMM likelihood function, an expectation-maximization (EM) algorithm is often used in the literature to estimate the HMM parameters [22]. In the case of discrete state-dependent distributions, and given observation sequence $x_1, x_2, \cdots, x_T$, the likelihood function, which is denoted by L_T, can be expressed in the form of Eq. (3).

$$L_T = \Pr\left(\mathbf{X}^{(T)} = \mathbf{x}^{(T)}\right) = \sum_{c_1, c_2, \cdots, c_T = 1}^{m} \Pr\left(\mathbf{X}^{(T)} = \mathbf{x}^{(T)}, \mathbf{C}^{(T)} = \mathbf{c}^{(T)}\right) \qquad (3)$$

where $\mathbf{x}^{(T)}$ is a realization of observable process $\mathbf{X}^{(T)}$ and $\mathbf{c}^{(T)}$ is a realization of the unobservable Markov chain. The joint distribution of $\mathbf{X}^{(T)}$ and $\mathbf{C}^{(T)}$ is

$$\Pr\left(\mathbf{X}^{(T)}, \mathbf{C}^{(T)}\right) = \Pr(C_1) \prod_{k=2}^{T} \Pr(C_k | C_{k-1}) \prod_{k=2}^{T} \Pr(X_k | C_k) \qquad (4)$$

Therefore, the likelihood function can be expressed as Eq. (5).

$$L_T = \sum_{c_1, c_2, \dots, c_T = 1}^{m} \left(\delta_{c_1} \gamma_{c_1, c_2} \gamma_{c_2, c_3} \cdots \gamma_{c_{T-1}, c_T}\right) \left(p_{c_1}(x_1) p_{c_2}(x_2) \cdots p_{c_T}(x_T)\right) \qquad (5)$$

The likelihood function can be written in matrix form, as in Eq. (6),

$$L_T = \delta \mathbf{P}(x_1) \mathbf{\Gamma} \mathbf{P}(x_2) \mathbf{\Gamma} \mathbf{P}(x_3) \cdots \mathbf{\Gamma} \mathbf{P}(x_T) \mathbf{1}' \qquad (6)$$

where δ is a row vector representing the initial probabilities of the Markov chain in different states. $\mathbf{P}(x_t) = diag(p_1(x_t), \cdots, p_m(x_t))$ is a diagonal matrix, where the diagonal entry $p_i(x_t)$ is the probability density or probability mass of observation x_t given that the unobservable Markov chain is in the ith state at time t. $\mathbf{\Gamma}$ is the one-step transition probability matrix of the Markov chain. $\mathbf{1}$ represents a row vector of 1 s with m entries.

Forward and backward probabilities can be defined based on the likelihood function. The forward probabilities, denoted by a vector $\alpha_t, t = 1, 2, \ldots, T$, which is a vector, are defined by

$$\alpha_t = \delta P(x_1)\Gamma P(x_2)\Gamma P(x_3)\cdots\Gamma P(x_t) = \delta P(x_1)\prod_{s=2}^{t}\Gamma P(x_s) \tag{7}$$

The forward probabilities, denoted by $\beta_t, t = 1, 2, \cdots, T$, take the following form:

$$\beta_t' = \Gamma P(x_{t+1})\Gamma P(x_{t+2})\cdots\Gamma P(x_T)\mathbf{1}' = \left(\prod_{s=t+1}^{T}\Gamma P(x_s)\right)\mathbf{1}' \tag{8}$$

Each entry in forward probability $\alpha_t(j), j = 1, 2, \cdots, m$ can be written as $\alpha_t(j) = \Pr(\mathbf{X}^{(t)} = \mathbf{x}^{(t)}, C_t = j)$. Each entry in backward probability $\beta_t(i), i = 1, 2, \cdots, m$ can be written as $\beta_t(i) = \Pr(X_{t+1} = x_{t+1}, X_{t+2} = x_{t+2}, \cdots, X_T = x_T | C_t = i)$.

To estimate HMM using the EM algorithm, we define two zero–one random variables as follows: $u_j(t) = 1$ if and only if $c_t = j, t = 1, 2, \cdots, T$, and $v_{jk}(t) = 1$ if and only if $c_{t-1} = j$ and $c_t = k, t = 2, 3, \cdots, T$. With this notation, the complete-data log-likelihood of an HMM, i.e., the log-likelihood of the observations plus the unobservable state sequence, is given by (9).

$$\log\left(\Pr\left(\mathbf{x}^{(T)}, \mathbf{c}^{(T)}\right)\right) = \log\delta_{c_1} + \sum_{t=2}^{T}\log\left(\gamma_{c_{t-1},c_t}\right) + \sum_{t=1}^{T}\log(p_{c_t}(x_t)) \tag{9}$$

The EM algorithm for HMM proceeds as follows:

E Step: Replace all quantities $v_{jk}(t)$ and $u_j(t)$ by their conditional expectations given the observations $\mathbf{x}^{(T)}$ (and given the current parameter estimates):

$$\hat{u}_j(t) = \Pr\left(C_t = j | \mathbf{x}^{(T)}\right) = \alpha_t(j)\beta_t(j)/L_T \tag{10}$$

$$\hat{v}_{jk}(t) = \Pr\left(C_{t-1} = j, C_t = k | \mathbf{x}^{(T)}\right) = \alpha_{t-1}(j)\gamma_{jk}p_k(x_t)\beta_t(k)/L_T \tag{11}$$

M Step: Replace $v_{jk}(t)$ and $u_j(t)$ by $\hat{v}_{jk}(t)$ and $\hat{u}_j(t)$ and maximize the complete data log-likelihood function with respect to the three sets of parameters: the initial distribution δ, transition probability matrix Γ, and parameter of the state-dependent distribution.

Repeat the EM algorithm until the log-likelihood function converges. Regarding the state identification problem, the Viterbi algorithm can be used to calculate the probability that the Markov chain will appear in a specific state at each time interval. By choosing the state with the largest probability, the identification problem can be solved [23]. In mathematical form, we begin by defining

$$\xi_{1i} = \Pr(C_1 = i, X_1 = x_1) = \delta_i p_i(x_1) \tag{12}$$

and, for $t = 2, \cdots, T$,

$$\xi_{ti} = \max_{c_1, c_2, \ldots, c_{t-1}} \Pr\left(\mathbf{C}^{(T-1)} = \mathbf{c}^{(T-1)}, C_t = i, \mathbf{X}^{(T)} = \mathbf{x}^{(T)}\right) \tag{13}$$

It can then be verified that the probabilities ξ_{tj} satisfy the following recursion, for $t = 2, \cdots, T$ and $i = 1, 2, \cdots, m$

$$\xi_{tj} = \left(\max_{i} (\xi_{t-1,i}\gamma_{ij}) \right) p_j(x_t) \tag{14}$$

The required maximizing sequence of states $i_1, i_2 \cdots, i_T$ can then be recursively determined from $i_T = \underset{i=1,\ldots,m}{\text{argmax}}\, \xi_{Ti}$, and, for $t = T - 1, T - 2, \cdots, 1$, from $i_t = \underset{i=1,\ldots,m}{\text{argmax}}(\xi_{ti}\gamma_{i,i_{t+1}})$.

In terms of the prediction problem, we begin by denoting $\mathbf{X}^{(-t)}$ as Eq. (15).

$$\mathbf{X}^{(-t)} = (\mathbf{X}_1, \cdots, \mathbf{X}_{t-1}, \mathbf{X}_{t+1}, \cdots, \mathbf{X}_T) \tag{15}$$

Using the likelihood of an HMM and the definition of the forward and backward probabilities, it immediately follows that for, $t = 2, 3, \cdots, T$,

$$\Pr\left(X_t = x | \mathbf{X}^{(-t)} = \mathbf{x}^{(-t)} \right) \tag{16}$$

Here, $\mathbf{B}_t$ is defined as $\mathbf{\Gamma P}(x_t)$. For discrete-valued observations, the forecast distribution $\Pr(X_{T+h} = x | \mathbf{X}^{(T)} = \mathbf{x}^{(T)}), h > 0$ of an HMM can be computed as a ratio of likelihoods:

$$\Pr\left(X_{T+h} = x | \mathbf{X}^{(T)} = \mathbf{x}^{(T)} \right) \tag{17}$$

defining $\boldsymbol{\phi}_T = \boldsymbol{\alpha}_T / \boldsymbol{\alpha}_T \mathbf{1}'$, we have

$$\Pr\left(X_{T+h} = x | \mathbf{X}^{(T)} = \mathbf{x}^{(T)} \right) = \boldsymbol{\phi}_T \mathbf{\Gamma}^h \mathbf{P}(x) \mathbf{1}' \tag{18}$$

This conditional probability function can be used to forecast future observations.

For the state prediction of HBV incidences, given the definition of forward and backward probabilities, it follows that

$$\alpha_t(i)\beta_t(i) = \Pr\left(\mathbf{X}^{(T)} = \mathbf{x}^{(T)}, C_t = i \right) \tag{19}$$

Therefore, the conditional distribution of state, given the observation series, can be obtained as

$$\Pr\left(C_t = i | \mathbf{X}^{(T)} = \mathbf{x}^{(T)} \right) = \frac{\Pr\left(\mathbf{X}^{(T)} = \mathbf{x}^{(T)}, C_t = i \right)}{\Pr\left(\mathbf{X}^{(T)} = \mathbf{x}^{(T)} \right)} = \frac{\alpha_t(i)\beta_t(i)}{L_T} \tag{20}$$

Consequently, for $t > T$, a similar form of conditional distribution can be used for state prediction. It can be verified that, for $h \in \mathbb{N}$ and $i = 1, 2, \ldots, m$,

$$\Pr\left(C_{T+h} = i \middle| \mathbf{X}^{(T)} = \mathbf{x}^{(T)}\right) = \frac{\boldsymbol{\alpha}_T \boldsymbol{\Gamma}^h(,i)}{L_T} = \boldsymbol{\phi}_T \boldsymbol{\Gamma}^h(,i) \tag{21}$$

where $\boldsymbol{\Gamma}^h(,i)$ is the ith column of $\boldsymbol{\Gamma}^h$, and $\boldsymbol{\phi}_T = \boldsymbol{\alpha}_T / \boldsymbol{\alpha}_T \mathbf{1}'$. This equation shows that the probability that future HBV incidences will be in a specific state is primarily determined in accordance with the HMM transition probability matrix.

4 Empirical Analysis

4.1 Data and Distribution Assumption

In January 2004, the Chinese Center for Disease Control and Prevention began publishing on a monthly basis its notifiable infectious disease report. The general situation of statutory infectious diseases of the previous month is documented, including the incidences of death and the number of various types of viral hepatitis. In the A, B, C, D, and E categories of hepatitis, as well as in its unclassified categories, the incidences of hepatitis B consistently comprised the highest number. Unlike other types of hepatitis, hepatitis B does not demonstrate a clear dependence on seasonal or trend changes. Therefore, the reaction of the statistical modeling on hepatitis B incidences is more complex than the number of other types of hepatitis models.

In this study, we employed the number of monthly incidences of hepatitis B from January 2004 to March 2016 as a sample (147 observations in total). The basic statistical indicators of the sample are shown in Table 1.

Table 1. Statistics of hepatitis B incidences

Max	Min	Mean	Std	Skew	kurts	JB	p-value
125427	36301	99910.65	13122.87	−0.7050	5.7918	59.9211	0.0000

Based on the preliminary findings in Table 1, the Jarque–Bera statistical incidences of the hepatitis B number of samples reach 59.9, and the corresponding p-value is close to 0. This indicates that the probability distribution of the number of hepatitis B incidences does not exhibit the characteristic of normal distribution. Under the normal situation, the hepatitis B incidences are the number of non-zero integers; i.e., the number is a counter variable. Therefore, the Poisson distribution is more reasonable. However, an apparent feature of the Poisson distribution is that the mean and variance values are equal.

In contrast, in the number of samples of hepatitis B incidences, the mean value is 99910.65 and the variance value is 172209759. It is obvious that the degree of dispersion is significantly greater than the Poisson distribution. In this case, it is very likely that the incidence of hepatitis B at each time point is a mixture of many Poisson distributions. This situation is more favorable to setting the state-dependent HMM to a Poisson process.

However, the average number of hepatitis B incidences reaches 99,910 with a minimum of 36,301. If the number of incidences is assumed to be a mixed Poisson distribution, a barrier will exist for the actual estimation model; i.e., some of the occurrence probabilities at some observation points will be very close to zero and stored as 0s instead of floating-point numbers in the computer. This problem is known as numerical underflow. In this case, it will not work when running the EM algorithm to estimate the parameters.

To solve this problem, we herein assume that hepatitis B incidences comprise a mixture of normal distributions. The rationale for this assumption is that, when the sample observations are relatively large (e.g., larger than 1,000), the Poisson distribution is very close to the normal distribution [24]. Moreover, the EM algorithm can bypass the problem of numerical underflow by using normal distribution function.

In addition, for the normal distribution mixture, which corresponds to different parameters in different states of the Markov chain distribution functions, it is not necessary to follow a normal distribution. Consequently, the assumption is not contrary to the basic statistical characteristics of the incidences of hepatitis B.

4.2   Parameter Estimation and State Identification

By calculating the log-likelihood and Akaike information criterion (AIC) values of the samples of hepatitis B incidences at different states and numbers, it can be found that two states of HMM are the most appropriate. In this case, the three HMM model parameters are the initial probability vector (δ_1, δ_2) of the unobservable Markov chain and the state transition matrix, $\begin{bmatrix} \gamma_{11} & \gamma_{12} \\ \gamma_{21} & \gamma_{22} \end{bmatrix}$.

Additionally, the normal distribution parameters (μ_1, σ_1) correspond to state 1, and the normal distribution parameters (μ_2, σ_2) correspond to state 2. The corresponding HMM model is a normal distribution covering the HMM model with two states.

In this model, we can obtain the estimated values and basic statistics based on the parameters of the above-mentioned EM algorithm, as shown in Table 2.

Table 2. Estimation result of a two-state uni-variate normal HMM based on hepatitis B incidences

	Coefficient	Std. error	t-statistics	p-value
δ_1	0.0000	1.0020	0.000	1.000
δ_2	1.0000	1.0020	0.998	0.318
γ_{11}	0.9784	0.0211	46.340	0.000***
γ_{12}	0.0216	0.0211	1.022	0.307
γ_{21}	0.0279	0.0203	1.375	0.169
γ_{22}	0.9721	0.0203	47.981	0.000***
μ_1	92000	1118.2	82.318	0.000***
σ_1	64380	100.8	63.847	0.000***
μ_2	106100	1621.3	65.445	0.000***
σ_2	16730	86.32	193.832	0.000***

***Significant at the 99% confidence level

As shown in Table 2, most of the parameters of a two-state uni-variate normal HMM for hepatitis B incidences are statistically significant. Among them, the initial probability vector of the Markov chain is not apparent; however, this parameter does not have a significant effect on the application of HMM for forecasting. For the four elements of the Markov chain transition matrix, γ_{11} and γ_{22} are significant; moreover, the corresponding estimates are 0.9784 and 0.9721, respectively. This indicates the high likelihood that the hepatitis B epidemic will spread when the epidemic is in a particular state.

Nevertheless, a state change may still occur. For example, the possibility of a transition from state 1 to state 2 is 0.0216, and the possibility of a transition from state 2 to state 1 is 0.0279, while the two parameters are very similar to each other. In general, the probability of a state transition is not zero, indicating the possibility that an outbreak of a hepatitis B state is possible but relatively low. In most cases, the hepatitis B epidemic will remain unchanged.

For different epidemic states, some differences exist for the distribution of hepatitis B incidences. From Table 2, we can determine that the parameters of the normal distribution of the two states are statistically significant. For the first epidemic, the probability of the incidence of hepatitis B is subject to the normal distribution with the mean value of 92,000 and the standard deviation of 64,380. In contrast, for the second epidemic, the probability of hepatitis B incidences is subject to the normal distribution with the mean value of 106,100 and the standard deviation of 16,730.

In the context of infectious disease informatics, the outbreaks and incidence of a specific infectious disease within a region and period depend on the initial state. The difference in previous states could lead to different probability distributions of incidences. Given the estimation result showing different distribution parameters at different states, we interpret the estimation result as follows: the first one is in a low state, with a lower mean value. However, the standard deviation is large. Consequently, the prediction accuracy of the number of incidences of hepatitis B will be relatively low. In contrast, the second one is in a high state with a higher mean value. The standard deviation is relatively low, and the prediction accuracy is relatively high.

After obtaining the model parameters, the Viterbi algorithm can be used to identify a specific moment of the hepatitis B epidemic state. Identification of the hepatitis B epidemic state is based on the probability of an epidemic in a specific state calculated from the HMM model, namely $\Pr(C_t = i)$. In this study, there are only two states for the hepatitis B epidemic. The state recognition is derived from the comparison of $\Pr(C_t = 1)$ and $\Pr(C_t = 2)$. That is, if the former is relatively large, the incidence of the hepatitis B epidemic is in a low state; otherwise, it is in a high state. Based on the estimated HMM model, we can calculate the sequence of the two above-mentioned probabilities, as shown in Fig. 2.

According to the probabilities shown in Fig. 2, we can identify the state of the epidemic of hepatitis B, as shown in Fig. 3. It is clearly evident that, from January 2004 to March 2006, there is a low incidence of a hepatitis B epidemic in China. In this state, the average number of hepatitis B incidences is relatively low, but it fluctuates. In April 2006, the state of the hepatitis B incident epidemic changes and the outbreak occurs until August 2012. In this state, the average number of incidents is relatively high;

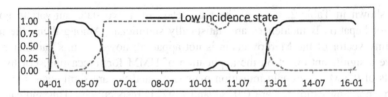

Fig. 2. Probabilities of hepatitis B occurring in different states.

however, it shows a small fluctuation. In September 2012, the hepatitis B epidemic state transitions from a high to a low incidence state.

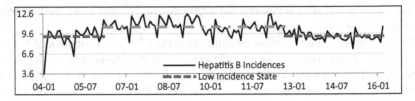

Fig. 3. Chinese hepatitis B incidents and state identifications

4.3   Prediction Application

According to the estimated HMM model, the incidence of a hepatitis B epidemic is in a low state for the last item in the sample. In the next period, on the other hand, the probability of the epidemic in the low incidence state is 0.9784, and the probability in the high state is 0.0216. Therefore, according to the probability distribution, we can calculate the probability of the incidence of hepatitis B in a specific interval (a, b), namely,

$$\Pr(a \le x \le b) = \int_a^b f(u)du \qquad (22)$$

Based on the nature of normal distribution moments, we may additionally obtain the number of hepatitis B incidents of the next period to be 92,305 cases with a standard deviation of 65,173 cases. The probability of hepatitis B incidents occurring in a specific state in the future could be calculated according to the state prediction Eq. (21). Based on the estimation results, these probabilities are calculated and presented as in Fig. 4.

As shown in Fig. 4, the probabilities of hepatitis B incidents occurring in low incidence states are all greater than 0.5 for each month ten years in the future, while the probabilities of hepatitis B incidents in high incidence states are all less than 0.5. These probabilities converge to 0.5 as the predicting horizon expands. This prediction, as shown in Fig. 4, implies that hepatitis B outbreaks in China would remain in a low incidence state for a relatively long time in the future. Note that the standard deviation of the hepatitis B incidence distribution in a low incidence state is larger than that of the

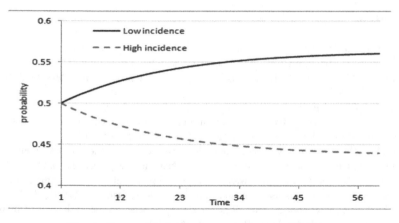

Fig. 4. State predicting horizons and state probabilities

high incidence state, which means that the probability of a high incidence at some month in the future is likewise high.

5 Conclusion

Hepatitis B is one of the most frequently occurring diseases in China. Scientific modeling for the incidence number is an important issue in public health management. An accurate model with a good fitting, robust parameters, and high prediction accuracy is important for early prevention of a hepatitis B epidemic, vaccine preparations, and medical staffing. Based on the HMM combined with hepatitis B Chinese Center for Disease Control and Prevention data, wherein established a normal distribution HMM with two states.

We estimated the parameters based on an EM algorithm and divided the states of a hepatitis B epidemic into low and high incidents. The two states correspond to the different distributions of incidences. For a low incidence state, the mean value is small; however, it significantly fluctuates. For a high incidence state, the mean value is large; however, it weakly fluctuates. With HMM, we can identify and predict the distribution and state of a hepatitis B epidemic outbreak at a specific time period. For infectious diseases other than HBV, HMM can be used to model their incidences as long as the time series observations show some degree of autocorrelation and multimodality.

Acknowledgements. The research was partially supported by National natural science foundation No. 71231001, Fundamental Research Funds for the Central Universities project TW2018009/NTUT-USTB-107-01.

References

1. Lavanchy, D.: Worldwide epidemiology of HBV infection, disease burden, and vaccine prevention. J. Clin. Virol. Off. Publ. Pan Am. Soc. Clin. Virol. **34**(4), 1–3 (2005)
2. Szmaragd, C., Balloux, F.: The population genomics of hepatitis b virus. Mol. Ecol. **16**(22), 4747–4758 (2007)
3. Liu, X., Chongsuvivatwong, V., Jiraphongsa, C., et al.: Evaluation of hepatitis A surveillance data and outbreak detection in Yunnan province, China, from 2004 through 2009. SE Asian J. Trop. Med. Public Health **42**(4), 839–850 (2011)
4. Yan, W., Zhou, Y., Wei, S., et al.: The difficulties of early detection for infectious disease outbreak in China: a qualitative investigation. J. Nanjing Med. Univ. **22**(1), 66–70 (2008)
5. Unkel, S., Farrington, C.P., Garthwaite, P.H., et al.: Statistical methods for the prospective detection of infectious disease outbreaks: a review. J. Roy. Stat. Soc. **175**(1), 49–82 (2012)
6. Watkins, R.E., Eagleson, S., Hall, R.G., et al.: Approaches to the evaluation of outbreak detection methods. BMC Public Health **6**(1), 263 (2006)
7. Strat, Y.L., Carrat, F.: Monitoring epidemiologic surveillance data using hidden Markov models. Stat. Med. **18**(24), 3463–3478 (1999)
8. Watkins, R.E., Eagleson, S., Veenendaal, B., et al.: Disease surveillance using a hidden Markov model. BMC Med. Inform. Decis. Mak. **9**(1), 1–12 (2009)
9. Lu, H.M., Zeng, D., Chen, H.: Markov switching models for outbreak detection. In: Castillo-Chavez, C., Chen, H., Lober, W., Thurmond, M., Zeng, D. (eds.) Infectious Disease Informatics and Biosurveillance. Integrated Series in Information Systems, vol. 27, pp. 111–144. Springer, Boston (2011). https://doi.org/10.1007/978-1-4419-6892-0_6
10. Nahas, M.E., Kassim, S., Shikoun, N.: Profile hidden Markov model for detection and Nahas prediction of hepatitis C virus mutation. Int. J. Comput. Sci. Issues **9**(5), 1694–1814 (2012)
11. Yu, L.F., Wu, A.P., Zhou, S.L., et al.: Application of seasonal ARIMA model in forecasting incidence of hepatitis C in China. J. Zhengzhou Univ. (Med. Sci.) **3**, 344–348 (2014)
12. Wu, A.P., Chen, Y.P., Zhang, T.Z., et al.: Application of ARIMA model on prediction of hepatitis B incidence. China J. Mod. Med. **22**(22), 78–82 (2012)
13. Wang, T., Yan, X.H., Zhu, Z.L.: Application of ARIMA model on prediction of hepatitis B incidence. Chin. J. Health Stat. **31**(4), 646–647 (2014)
14. Zheng, Y.L., Zhang, L.P., Zhang, X.L., et al.: SARIMA model for the prediction of hepatitis B incidence in Xinjiang. Mod. Prev. Med. **42**(22), 4033–4035 (2015)
15. Liu, T., Yao, M.L., Huang, J.G., et al.: Application of combined prediction model in prediction of incidence of hepatitis C. Chin. J. Vaccines Immun. **24**(06), 674–679 (2018)
16. Yang, D.Z.: Application of general regression neural network in hepatitis B incident cases time series forecasting. Comput. Appl. Softw. **30**(4), 217–219 (2013)
17. Chen, Y.F., Zhang, M., Wang, X.L., et al.: Application of ARIMA model and BP neural network model on prediction of hepatitis B incidence in China. Jiangsu J. Prev. Med. **3**, 23–26 (2015)
18. Chen, Y.P., Wu, A.P., Fan, H.M., et al.: Application of grey system on prediction of viral hepatitis B incidence. Chin. J. Health Stat. **24**(24), 77–81 (2014)
19. Zhang, Q., Chen, C.: Application of improved GM(1,1) model in prediction of hepatitis B incidence in Hengshui. Mod. Prev. Med. **44**(11), 1925–1928 (2017)
20. Xu, X.S., Sun, N., Du, Y.C., et al.: Optimization of GM(1,1) model and its application in prediction of hepatitis B incidence. Chin. J. Health Stat. **35**(05), 772–774+778 (2018)
21. Zucchini, W., Macdonald, I.L.: Hidden Markov models for time series: an introduction using R, pp. 29–100. CRC Press, Boca Raton; London; New York (2009)

22. Welch, Lloyd R.: Hidden Markov models and the Baum-Welch algorithm. IEEE Inf. Theory Soc. Newsl. **53**(2), 194–211 (2003)
23. Viterbi, A.J.: Error bounds for convolution codes and an asymptotically optimal decoding algorithm. IEEE Trans. Inf. Theory **13**, 260–269 (1967)
24. Feller, W.: An Introduction to Probability Theory and Its Applications, pp. 420–421. Wiley, New York; London; Sydney (1967)

Identifying Physician Fraud in Healthcare with Open Data

Brandon Fan[1,4(✉)] ⓘ, Xuan Zhang[2,4] ⓘ, and Weiguo Fan[3,4] ⓘ

[1] Blacksburg High School, Blacksburg, VA 24060, USA
brandonfan1256@gmail.com
[2] Virginia Tech, Blacksburg, VA 24060, USA
xuancs@vt.edu
[3] Tippie College of Business, University of Iowa, Iowa City, IA 52242, USA
weiguo-fan@uiowa.edu
[4] Tianjin University, Tianjin, China

Abstract. Health care fraud is a serious problem that impacts every patient and consumer. This fraudulent behavior causes excessive financial losses every year and causes significant patient harm. Healthcare fraud includes health insurance fraud, fraudulent billing of insurers for services not provided, and exaggeration of medical services, etc. To identify healthcare fraud thus becomes an urgent task to avoid the abuse and waste of public funds. Existing methods in this research field usually use classified data from governments, which greatly compromises the generalizability and scope of application. This paper introduces a methodology to use publicly available data sources to identify potentially fraudulent behavior among physicians. The research involved data pairing of multiple datasets, selection of useful features, comparisons of classification models, and analysis of useful predictors. Our performance evaluation results clearly demonstrate the efficacy of the proposed method.

Keywords: Healthcare · Fraud prediction · Machine learning · Imbalanced data · Entity matching

1 Introduction

Healthcare fraud encompasses multiple fraudulent activities including health insurance fraud, fraudulent billing of insurers for services not provided, and exaggeration of medical services [8]. This fraudulent behavior causes excessive financial losses in the magnitude of billions of dollars of losses every year and significant patient harm. The U.S. national health expenditure, in percent GDP, has increased from 5% to 18.3% between 1960 and 2017[1]. With such an intensive demand for healthcare services, healthcare fraud has become a mainstream issue. About 10% of the U.S. healthcare expenditure is produced by fraud, which represents more than 100 billion dollars per year, according to the General Accounting office in the United States [11]. The requirement for effective and efficient approaches for fud identification is necessary

---

[1] https://www.statista.com/statistics/184968/us-health-expenditure-as-percent-of-gdp-since-1960/.

© Springer Nature Switzerland AG 2019
H. Chen et al. (Eds.): ICSH 2019, LNCS 11924, pp. 222–235, 2019.
https://doi.org/10.1007/978-3-030-34482-5_20

considering the serious consequence of healthcare frauds and increasing demand for high quality healthcare. Current methods rely on the manual review of materials by human experts that is extremely labor-intensive and time-consuming, but is still the major approach for healthcare fraud detection in many places [14]. Another problem is that nonpublic and highly domain-specific data is used in current approaches, which greatly hinders generalizability and extensibility in real world applications [4, 10, 14]. Additionally, most preceding methods implement healthcare fraud identification at the claim level [10, 12, 14], but little work has investigated detection of fraudulent physicians utilizing the aggregated comprehensive records (e.g. prescription, payment, patient reviews, etc.). We believe detecting physician fraud could be more effective when we can leverage information cues from different open sources.

To fill the research gaps above, we are motivated to develop a methodology that uses open datasets to predict healthcare fraud at the physician level and reduce the workload of human experts. In particular, a list of Excluded Individuals and Entities (LEIE) and board actions were used as labels for fraud cases. Different publically available predictor datasets, such as Part D Prescriber, Open Payment, and Social Media datasets, were consolidated and used for building a predictive model to identify potentially fraudulent behavior among physicians. The research involved data pairing and entity matching of multiple datasets, selection of useful features for modeling, imbalanced data analysis, classification model comparisons, and analysis of useful predictors. Experimental results showed that features from the Part D Prescriber dataset produced the best F1 score of 75.59% when doing prediction with the Prescriber dataset. The F1 score increases to 96.1% if we use physician instances occurring in both social media and Prescriber datasets. Our model and results also provide great insights to healthcare regulators for better regulations.

The rest of the paper is organized as follows: the Related Work section reviews related work in healthcare fraud detection and highlight the research gap; the Approach section describes our proposed research framework; the Datasets section introduces the open datasets we have investigated; the Experiment Results section demonstrates the experimental details and related discussions, and the Conclusion section summarizes the paper, discusses the limitations and future work.

2 Related Work

Due to the significance of detecting healthcare fraud and the problems of manually reviewing materials by human experts, researchers have conducted extensive studies in automatic and effective techniques for detecting healthcare fraud. This existing research focuses on multiple types of frauds, collects data from various sources, and proposes diverse features and models to capture fraudulent cases.

When it comes to fraudulent behaviors, there are three primary groups of people according to Yang and Hwang [14]. The first party consists of service providers, such as physicians, hospitals, ambulance companies, and laboratories. The second party consists of insurance subscribers, including patients and patients employers. The final party consists of insurance carriers, who receive regular premiums from their sub-scribers and pay health care costs on behalf of their sub-scribers, such as government departments on healthcare and private insurance companies. This research focuses on the first group of people: the service providers.

Several relevant studies on healthcare fraud prediction have been conducted. Yang and Hwang propose a data-mining framework which utilizes the concept of clinical pathways to develop a healthcare fraud detection model [14]. The proposed approach has been evaluated objectively by a real-world data set gathered from the National Health Insurance (NHI) program in Taiwan. Liou et al. utilize data mining techniques to detect fraudulent or abusive reporting by healthcare providers using invoices for outpatient services. This research was also carried out based on the NHI data [7]. Recently, Thornton et al. built upon the Medicaid environment and developed a Medicaid multidimensional schema that provides a set of multidimensional data models to predict fraudulent activities [12].

The datasets used for fraud identification were collected from insurance carriers [6]. The major government data sources for existing healthcare fraud include: the US Health Care Financing Administration (HCFA) [9], the Bureau of National Health Insurance (NHI) in Taiwan area [1, 5, 13], and the Health Insurance Commission (HIC) in Australia [3, 4].

Although a great deal of effort has been put into developing healthcare fraud detection models, and some progress has been achieved, there are a few limitations. The first and most important one is that most of these datasets are not publicly available and/or are highly domain-specific and require extensive background knowledge to conduct feature engineering. Models developed using these proprietary data sets have limited generalizability and are hard to replicate in reality. Almost no research study explores the usefulness of publicly available datasets, how to extract useful features from these open data sets, and lastly how to combine multiple datasets to improve performance.

3 Datasets

3.1 Fraud Label Datasets

Two datasets were used as fraud labels for fraud prediction in this research design: the LEIE dataset and the Board Action datasets.

LEIE Dataset. The Office of Inspector General (OIG) of the U.S. has the authority to exclude individuals and entities from federally funded health care programs pursuant to sections 1128 and 1156 of the Social Security Act and maintains a list of all currently excluded individuals and entities called the List of Excluded Individuals and Entities (LEIE)[2]. Anyone who hires an individual or entity on the LEIE may be subject to civil monetary penalties (CMP). The physician records present in the LEIE dataset was then combined with the subsequent board action dataset to create a conglomerate fraud label dataset.

---

[2] https://oig.hhs.gov/exclusions/exclusions_list.asp.

Board Action Datasets. Medical Boards are established in many states to properly regulate the practice of medicine and surgery. Every year, these boards take administrative actions to address possible cases of professional misconduct, license term violations, improper prescriptions, etc., and make this information available to the public. As its difficult to collect the board action records of all the 50 states, we chose states with large populations. According to Wikipedia, the top 5 US states with the largest population are CA, TX, FL, NY, and PA. However, its difficult to extract board action records of Texas and Pennsylvania from electronic files, and New York has surprisingly low matches with the payment feature dataset. Therefore, the board action records of California, Florida, and North Carolina were selected for this research.

Thus, our label dataset is a combination of both the LEIE dataset and the Board Action Dataset. These are then matched with predictor dataset records (discussed in the subsequent section) in order to gather features on physicians with labeled fraudulent activities as well as physicians that are considered unfradulent. The predictor dataset features provide us the features for a vector Px where we pass through a function f (x) that produces a fraudulent label of Py $\in$ 0, 1. 0 being non-fraudulent, and 1 being fraudulent.

3.2   Predictor Datasets

Part D Prescriber Dataset. The Part D Prescriber Public Use File (PUF)[3] provides information on prescription drugs prescribed by individual physicians and other health care providers and paid for under the Medicare Part D Prescription Drug Program. The Part D Prescriber PUF is based on information from the Chronic Conditions Data Warehouse of the Centers for Medicare & Medicaid Services (CMS), which contains Prescription Drug Event records submit- ted by Medicare Advantage Prescription Drug (MAPD) plans and by stand-alone Prescription Drug Plans (PDP). The dataset identifies providers by their National Provider Identifier (NPI) and the specific prescriptions that were dispensed at their direction, listed by brand name (if applicable) and generic name. For each prescriber and drug, the dataset includes the total number of prescriptions that were dispensed and the total drug cost. The total drug cost includes the ingredient cost of the medication, dispensing fees, sales tax, and any applicable administration fees and is based on the amount paid by the Part D plan, Medicare beneficiary, government subsidies, and any other third-party payers. The advantage of these data is the fact physicians are mandated to report their Part D prescription activities to the CMS since they have to submit a claim in order to be paid. Therefore, the Prescriber dataset is less biased in contrast to the CMS payment dataset, whose payment records are submitted voluntarily.

---

[3] https://www.cms.gov/Research-Statistics-Data-and-Systems/Statistics-Trends-and-Reports/Medicare-Provider-Charge-Data/Part-D-Prescriber.html.

CMS Open Payment Dataset. Open Payments[4], which is managed by the CMS, is a national disclosure program created by the Affordable Care Act (ACA). The program, promotes transparency and accountability by helping consumers understand the financial relationships between pharmaceutical and medical device industries, and physicians and teaching hospitals. These financial relationships may include consulting fees, research grants, travel reimbursements, and payments made from the industry to medical practitioners. It is important to note that financial ties between the health care industry and health care providers do not necessarily indicate an improper relationship. Applicable manufacturers and applicable GPOs enter detailed information about payments, other transfers of value, or investment interests into CMSs Open Payments system. Among the three types of payments (i.e. General Payments, Research Payments, and Physician Ownership or Investment Interest Information), we used the General Payments in this research, which saves the most common payment records. One concern about this dataset is that the data is self-reported. While there is a great care taken to ensure that the reported payments are correct, there are no checks in place to ensure that ALL payments are reported and database is complete. In addition, Table 4 shows that the fraud prediction accuracy using payment features is lower than using prescription features.

Social Media Dataset. The Healthgrades.com website contains rich information about physicians, hospitals and health care providers. It has amassed information on over 3 million U.S. health care providers, with more than 9 million ratings and reviews over 18-year period of time. Healthgrades has built the first comprehensive physician rating and comparison database. We developed automated crawlers to download the ratings and reviews for all doctors in California, Florida, and North Carolina. The key fields include overall rating, number of ratings, detailed ratings (Trustworthiness, Explains condition well, Answer questions, Time well spent, Scheduling, Office environment, and Staff friendliness), text reviews and corresponding ratings, etc.

4 Methodology

4.1 Feature Extraction from Open Datasets

Using the open datasets discussed in the previous section, we identify and extract primary features from each dataset to utilize as features for the fraud detection framework. These features are determined based on domain knowledge as well as consultation with insurance companies and are further conglomerated into one comprehensive model for physician fraud detection. Each feature, its associated definition, and dataset is shown in Table 1.

---

[4] https://www.cms.gov/openpayments/.

Table 1. Selected features from the three predictor datasets. Bolded features were used in a comprehensive model.

Dataset	Feature	Description
Part D prescriber dataset	**TOTAL_CLAIM_COUNT**	Number of medicare part D claims, including refills
	TOTAL_DAY_SUPPLY	Number of day's supply for all claims
	TOTAL_DRUG_COST	Aggregate cost paid for all terms
	Average_Day_Supply_Per_Claim	Average day supply per claim of physician
	TOTAL_CLAIM_COUNT_DEVIATION	Total sum of deviation from average claim count
	TOTAL_DAY_SUPPLY_DEVIATION	Total sum of deviation from day supply
	TOTAL_DRUG_COST_DEVIATION	Total sum of deviation from drug cost
	Average_Day_Supply_Per_Claim_Deviation	Total sum of deviation from average day supply per claim
	Specialty (dummy variable)	Physician's expertise
	Average_Claim_Count	TOTAL_CLAIM_COUNT / Records per Physician
CMS open payment	Unusual drug prescription	Presence of unusual drug prescription
	Payment count	Total payment count over all records
	Payment amount	Total payment amount over all records
	Primary type (dummy variable)	Primary type of payment
	Unusual device prescriptions	Presence of unusual device prescription
Social media dataset	**Average review rating**	Average user review rating from 1 to 5
	Rating count	Total number of user reviews
	Trustworthiness	A rating from 1 to 5 of physician's trustworthiness
	Explains condition well	A rating from 1 to 5 of physician's clarity
	Answer questions	Properly answers questions of patients
	Time well spent	A rating from 1 to 5 of physician's appointments
	Scheduling	A rating from 1 to 5 of physician's scheduling habits
	Office environment	A rating from 1 to 5 of how physician's office environment
	Staff friendliness	A rating from 1 to 5 of how friendly physician is to staff
	State	State of Physician's Practice

4.2 Physician Fraud Detection Framework

Using the identified features, we then proceed to create a physician fraud detection framework. Our proposed framework for physician fraud detection using open data can be summarized in Fig. 1. The detailed steps are explained below.

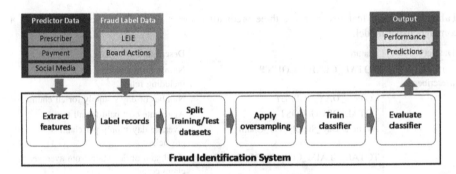

Fig. 1. Fraud detection framework using open datasets

Step 1. First, various features were extracted from multiple predictor datasets. Some features were obtained through special calculation (e.g. deviation features) or data aggregation (e.g. average or sum). Then, logistic regression was conducted to identify the most relevant features for further analysis. In addition, combinations of features from different datasets were performed to do comprehensive fraud prediction.

Step 2. Data pairing and entity matching were performed to match the fraud labels extracted from LEIE (2015–2016) and board actions datasets with data records in the predictor datasets (e.g. Part D Prescriber and open payment datasets). The entire dataset was split into training and test with a ratio of 80:20. The splitting followed a stratified shuffle process, keeping the original class proportions in both training and test datasets.

Step 3. Since the data was extremely imbalanced (e.g. only 0.045% physician records of the LEIE data were fraudulent), SMOTE oversampling [2] was applied to both datasets before training a classifier to prevent the classifier from predicting all physicians in the test set as the major class (Non-Fraud).

Step 4. Next, classifiers were trained using different classification algorithms including Logistic Regression, Naive Bayes, Decision Tree, and SVM.

Step 5. Finally, the classification performance was evaluated on the held-out test dataset, which was balanced dataset after oversampling. The Weighted F1 was used as a comprehensive measure of performance.

5   Experiment Results

5.1   Part D Prescriber Dataset

Since one physician may have multiple drug prescription records in this dataset, we need to aggregate the records and create a single record for each physician, which will be used for classification. In this way, 837,679 physician records were extracted from the Prescriber data for fraudulent behavior prediction.

Because board action data is state-dependent, we were unable to utilize the information to correspond with the prescriber data. In addition, we wished to deliberately test the capability of the prescriber predictor dataset that does not include a state feature, thus reducing a confounding variable. Finally, the LEIE provides the most relevant and reputable source of information that can be easily matched to for prediction. Among this large number of physicians, only 383 (0.045%) matched the LEIE fraud records.

We tried two methods for data aggregation and feature creation:

– Take the factors (e.g. TAL CLAIM COUNT, TOTAL DAY SUPPLY, etc.) related to a drug as features of a physician. If there are M types of drugs and N factors for each drug, a physician will have N * M features. This feature was created to identify which drug prescription is most highly correlated with fraud. A potential problem of this method is, the features of a physician might be very sparse, as one physician only have prescription records on a small number of drugs.
– For the K Prescription records of each physician, mean values were taken on key factors (e.g. TOTAL CLAIM COUNT, TOTAL DAY SUPPLY, etc.). Next, these mean values were added as features of a physician.

For the first data aggregation method, 8 types of features were tried for each drug and the corresponding fraud prediction performance are shown in Table 1. As 873 drugs are related with the prescription records of 383 fraud physicians, which will produce too many features, we used the Chi-Square feature selection algorithm to pick out the top 100 relevant drugs. Together, they will form 8 * 100 = 800 features. The best Weighted F1 was produced by the Nave Bayes classifier.

Among these 8 types of features, half of them were Deviation features, which were calculated as below.

– Calculate the average value of the TOTAL CLAIM COUNT, TOTAL DAY SUPPLY, TOTAL DRUG COST, and Average Day Supply Per Claim of each specialty-drug pair.
– For each of the above features, the difference between each physicians value and the specialty drug average was measured and difference or Deviation was noted.

The performance measure Weighted F1 was calculated as below. Here C is the number of classes, while Wi is the number of true instances of class i.

$$F1 = 2\frac{precision \cdot recall}{precision + recall} \tag{1}$$

$$Weighted\ F1 = \frac{\sum_{i=1}^{C} W_i \cdot F_1}{C} \tag{2}$$

For the second data aggregation method, we calculated the mean value of key factors (e.g. TOTAL CLAIM COUNT, TOTAL DAY SUPPLY, etc.) related to each physician. This research proves the Specialty (as a dummy variable) is an important feature for each physician. Ten features for each physician were extracted, which produced the best fraud prediction performance on the Part D Prescriber data. The performance of fraud prediction with these features are shown in Table 2. Again, the Nave Bayes classifier obtained the best weighted F1 of 75.59%. The Deviation features in Table 2 indicates the difference between a physicians value and the Specialty Average, which is a slightly different from the Deviation features in the previous table. Those deviations mean the difference between a physicians value and the Specialty-Drug Average.

The calculation of the Unusual Drug Prescription feature was accomplished as follows.

Table 2. Classification performance using 800 features of top 100 relevant drugs extracted for physicians

Features (800)	Classifier	Weighted F1
8 Categories of features: TOTAL_CLAIM_COUNT TOTAL DAY SUPPLY TOTAL_DRUG_COST Average_Day_Supply_Per_Claim TOTAL_CLAIM_COUNT_DEVIATION TOTAL DAY SUPPLY DEVIATION TOTAL_DRUG_COST_DEVIATION Average_Day_Supply_Per_Claim_Deviation	Logistic regression	59.04%
	Naïve Bayes	67.69%
	SVM	50.33%

- Find the Unusual Drug Prescription patterns, by identifying the top 5% rare specialty-drug prescription events.
- For each physician, count how many prescription records match those Unusual drug prescription patterns.

Table 3. Classification performance using 10 features extracted for physicians

Features (10)	Classifier	Weighted F1
TOTAL_CLAIM_COUNT TOTAL DAY SUPPLY TOTAL_DRUG_COST Average_Day_Supply_Per_Claim TOTAL_CLAIM_COUNT_DEVIATION TOTAL DAY SUPPLY DEVIATION TOTAL_DRUG_COST_DEVIATION Average_Day_Supply_Per_Claim_Deviation Specialty (dummy variable) Unusual drug prescription	Logistic regression	69.08%
	Naïve Bayes	75.59%
	SVM	44.77%

Most Useful Features: We examined the co-efficient of the 10 features introduced in Table 3 using a logistic regression analysis. To make this analysis fairer, all the numerical features were normalized before running the logistic regression. Since the Specialty was taken as a dummy variable, it produced 191 features during the classification process. Running correlation analysis, high coefficients in the 10 specialties indicate physicians in these specialties are more likely to commit fraud. For example, if a physician practices specialties such as Personal Emergency Response Attendant, Osteopathic Manipulative Medicine, and Neurological Surgery, he or she has a higher fraud probability. Its not surprising to see Legal Medicine here. An unexpected case is Family Medicine. Physicians in this specialty has a positive association with fraud risks. Besides those specialties, other features such as TOTAL CLAIM COUNT, TOTAL CLAIM COUNT DEVIATION, Unusual Drug Prescription, Average Day Supply Per Claim, Unusual Drug Prescription, and Average Day Supply Per Claim Deviation also have high coefficients. For instance, physicians with high TOTAL CLAIM COUNT has a higher fraud probability. In addition, a physician may have a high fraud risk if he or she made a high Average Day Supply Per Claim or an Unusual Drug Prescription. The subsequent classification results are seen in Table 3.

5.2   CMS Open Payment Dataset

The same fraud prediction process used on the Part D Prescriber dataset was applied to the CMS payment datasets. Because CMS is an open, public dataset, we utilized both LEIE and Board Actions to increase the number of matched records in comparison to the previous experiment. Both LEIE and Board Action (records of CA, NC, and FL) were tried as fraud labels in this research.

1. Take LEIE records as fraud labels

In this experiment, 233 matches were made with physicians in the LEIE data using First Name, Last Name and State. If stricter matching conditions were applied, such as First Name, Last Name, State, and City, 28 matched for physicians were attained. Table 4 shows that using more matched cases produces much better prediction performance (Weighted F1 increases from 53.70% to 71.42%) for Naive Bayes classifier.

2. Take Board Action records as fraud labels

In contrast to the LEIE dataset, the Board Action records identified a larger number of matched physicians. As shown in Table 5, 55, 235, and 153 disciplined providers were found in the 2016 board action records of NC, CA, and FL, respectively. The payment datasets of 2013–2015 were used as independent variables. In this experiment, we utilized the "State" feature to see if performance can be improved. First Name, Last Name, State, and City were used as matching condition. Just like the LEIE case, the prediction performance increases along with the number of disciplined providers. California had the best prediction performance.

3. Most useful features

Among the features extracted from the Open Payment datasets, the most relevant features are Unusual Drug Prescription, Payment Amount, and Payment Count, when taking LEIE and Board Action Records as labels, respectively.

5.3 Social Media Dataset

Following the similar procedures introduced earlier, we combined all the cases from LEIE and board actions as healthcare frauds. After conducting data matching based on first name, last name, city and state, only 555 (1.86%) cases out of 29,843 are found fraudulent. Table 6 shows that the classification performance was not satisfactory. The best performance was obtained by using decision tree classifier, which give F1 score of 0.646, indicating the review data can be used to predict healthcare frauds, but this single dataset is not enough for accurate predicting.

Most useful features: Five features (Rating Count, Average Review Rating, Trustworthiness, Explains Condition Well, Answer Questions) were selected based on the p-value in the logistic regression results at significant level of 0.05 for the comprehensive analysis below.

5.4 Comprehensive Datasets

Lastly, all three predictor datasets are merged. Only 265 (1.43%) cases out of 22,770 with complete fields in all three datasets are found fraudulent. Oversampling is applied to both datasets before training classifier to prevent the classifier from predicting all physicians in the test set as the major class (Non-Fraud). The classification performance with high weighted F1 using features from the merged dataset is shown in Table 7. The constraint of this method is that it only works on a very small number of instances with complete fields.

Table 4. Classification performance using 5 features from payment data and LEIE labels

Features	Matching condition	Fraud cases	Classifier	Weighted F1
Specialty (dummy variable)	FN+LN+State	233	Logistic regression	59.01%
Payment count			Naive Bayes	71.42%
Payment amount	FN+LN+State +City	28	Logistic regression	60.13%
Unusual drug prescriptions				
Unusual device prescriptions			Naive Bayes	53.70%

Table 5. Classification performance using 6 features from payment data and board action labels

Features	Fraud dataset	Fraud cases	Classifier	Weighted F1
Primary type (dummy variable)	NC board actions	55	Logistic regression	57.29%
Specialty (dummy variable)			Naive Bayes	54.96%
Payment count	CA board actions	235	Logistic regression	70.31%
Payment amount			Naive Bayes	65.81%
Unusual drug prescriptions Unusual device prescriptions	FL Board Actions	153	Logistic regression	56.55%
			Naive Bayes	56.41%

6 Limitation and Future Work

Identifying healthcare fraud is the primary task of this research, thus we have concentrated on acquiring better fraud prediction accuracy, including the attempts on various features and algorithms. As future work, well investigate potential interesting findings, to find features which are significant indicators of frauds.

Because the data was imbalanced and sparse, it was challenging to make accurate prediction on the complete. More data collection is needed from other states to make the predictive model more robust and general across states for fraud examination. We will leave this for future research as well.

Table 6. Classification performance using 11 features from social media

Features (11)	Classifier	Weighted F1
Average review rating	Decision tree	64.6%
Rating count	Logistic regression	46.6%
Average rating		
Trustworthiness		
Explains condition well		
Answer questions		
Time well spent		
Scheduling		
Office environment		
Staff friendliness State		

Table 7. Classification performance using 8 features from social media, open-payment datasets and prescriber datasets

Features (10)	Classifier	Weighted F1
Average review rating	Decision tree	96.1%
Rating count	Logistic regression	91.5%
Average rating		
Trustworthiness		
Explains condition well		
Payment count		
Total payment amount		
Average claim amount		
Claim count		
State		

7 Conclusion

This paper introduces a methodology to use publically available data sources (e.g. Prescriber, Payment, and Social media) to identify potentially fraudulent behavior among physicians. Fraud and other misconduct records in LEIE and Board action datasets are used as fraud cases. The research involved data pairing and entity matching of multiple datasets, selection of useful features, comparisons of classification models, and analysis of useful predictors. Our performance evaluation results clearly demonstrate the efficacy of the proposed method. The best Weighted F1 score of 96.5% is achieved using the merged datasets, while the best Weighted F1 of 75.59% is obtained using data from single source. Our main findings include the following:

(a) In contrast to the annual CMS open payment datasets, the Part-D Prescriber dataset has more records, more physicians, and more matched excluded physicians. According to these facts, the Part-D Prescriber dataset is more reliable and provides more useful information in term of fraud prediction.

(b) Taking LEIE fraud labels as the dependent variable, the important signals in the Part-D Prescriber dataset that indicate fraud include Physician Specialty, TOTAL CLAIM COUNT, TOTAL CLAIM COUNT DEVIATION, Unusual Drug Prescription, Average Day Supply Per Claim, Unusual Drug Prescription, and Average Day Supply Per Claim.

(c) The important signals in the payment dataset indicating fraud include Physician Specialty such as Hepatology, and other features such as Unusual Drug Prescription and Payment Amount.

(d) The combination of the Part-D prescriber dataset, open-payment dataset, and the social media dataset gives the best performance.

Acknowledgements. This publication was made possible by the support of Dr. Robin Russell, and Dr. Nottingham Quinton from the Pamplin College of Business, Virginia Tech for their help during this research.

References

1. Chan, C., Lan, C.: A data mining technique combining fuzzy sets theory and bayesian classifier—an application of auditing the health insurance fee. In: Proceedings of the International Conference on Artificial Intelligence, vol. 402408 (2001)
2. Chawla, N.V., Bowyer, K.W., Hall, L.O., Kegelmeyer, W.P.: Smote: synthetic minority over-sampling technique. J. Artif. Intell. Res. **16**, 321–357 (2002)
3. He, H., Hawkins, S., Graco, W., Yao, X.: Application of genetic algorithm and k-nearest neighbour method in real world medical fraud detection problem. JACIII **4**(2), 130–137 (2000)
4. He, H., Wang, J., Graco, W., Hawkins, S.: Application of neural networks to detection of medical fraud. Expert Syst. Appl. **13**(4), 329–336 (1997)
5. Hwang, S.Y., Wei, C.P., Yang, W.S.: Discovery of temporal patterns from process instances. Comput. Ind. **53**(3), 345–364 (2004)
6. Li, J., Huang, K.Y., Jin, J., Shi, J.: A survey on statistical methods for health care fraud detection. Health Care Manag. Sci. **11**(3), 275–287 (2008)
7. Liou, F.M., Tang, Y.C., Chen, J.Y.: Detecting hospital fraud and claim abuse through diabetic outpatient services. Health Care Manag. Sci. **11**(4), 353–358 (2008)
8. Rudman, W.J., Eberhardt, J.S., Pierce, W., Hart-Hester, S.: Healthcare fraud and abuse. Perspect. Health Inf. Manag./AHIMA Am. Health Inf. Manag. Assoc. **6**(Fall) (2009)
9. Shapiro, A.F.: The merging of neural networks, fuzzy logic, and genetic algorithms. Insur. Math. Econ. **31**(1), 115–131 (2002)
10. Sokol, L., Garcia, B., Rodriguez, J., West, M., Johnson, K.: Using data mining to find fraud in HCFA health care claims. Top. Health Inf. Manag. **22**(1), 1–13 (2001)
11. Thompson, L.: Health insurance, vulnerable payers lose billions to fraud and abuse. Report to Chairman, Subcommittee on Human Resources and Intergovernmental Operations. United States General Accounting Office, Washington, DC, May 1992
12. Thornton, D., Mueller, R.M., Schoutsen, P., Van Hillegersberg, J.: Predicting healthcare fraud in medicaid: a multidimensional data model and analysis techniques for fraud detection. Procedia Technol. **9**, 1252–1264 (2013)
13. Wei, C., Hwang, S., Yang, W.S.: Mining frequent temporal patterns in process databases. In: Proceedings of International Workshop on Information Technologies and Systems, Australia, vol. 175180 (2000)
14. Yang, W.S., Hwang, S.Y.: A process-mining framework for the detection of healthcare fraud and abuse. Expert Syst. Appl. **31**(1), 56–68 (2006)

Detecting False Information in Medical and Healthcare Domains: A Text Mining Approach

Jiexun Li[✉]

Western Washington University, Bellingham, WA 98225, USA
Jiexun.li@wwu.edu

Abstract. In recent years, a lot of false information in medical and healthcare domains has emerged and spread over the Internet. Such false information has become a big risk to public health and safety. This study investigates this problem by analyzing data collected from two fact-checking websites, 416 medical claims from Snopes.com and 1,692 healthcare-related statements from PolitiFact.com. Topic analysis reveals frequent words and common topics occurring in these claims spread online. Furthermore, using text-mining and machine-learning techniques, this study builds prediction models for detecting false information and shows promising performance. Several textual and source features are identified as good indicators for true or false information in medical and healthcare domains.

Keywords: False information · Medical · Healthcare · Text mining

1 Instruction

People are always looking for new and good information. The internet, especially with the emergence of Web 2.0 and social media, has become the largest repository and platform for people to consuming and spreading information. Particularly, when having medical or health-related questions, many people now like to go to the internet to seek information, as an alternative to seeing a doctor. On websites such as CDC.gov and WebMD, we can get high-quality and reliable information. However, we have to be aware of the fact that the Internet has also become a major origin and channel that spreads false information, including fake news, false beliefs, and hoaxes [1]. For instance, in February 2018, a Facebook post (http://archive.is/ojBBL) blamed the increased deaths of the 2017–2018 flu season on an antiviral drug Tamiflu. Another social media rumor in early 2018 claims that JUULing, or use of a JUUL e-cigarette, has caused cancer in four students. Both claims turned out to be false. Such false beliefs and hoaxes, in the medical and healthcare domains, are often presented in text-based format and can be easily spread through social media like Twitter and Facebook. Some may cause unnecessary panic amongst general public. When people take such false information for granted in making their health-related decisions, their health and even their lives could be put in danger. Due to the vast amount of information online, there is

© Springer Nature Switzerland AG 2019
H. Chen et al. (Eds.): ICSH 2019, LNCS 11924, pp. 236–246, 2019.
https://doi.org/10.1007/978-3-030-34482-5_21

an urgent need to fact-check such information to prevent the spread of false beliefs and hoaxes.

This research is aimed at analyzing health-related claims online using a text mining approach. The goal is to investigate the feasibility of developing predictive models and identifying cues to detect false information in medical and healthcare domains. In particular, this research focuses on addressing the following three questions:

- *Q1: What are the main topics of health-related claims?* By answering this question, we can gain insights into the frequent keywords and topics of health claims widespread over the internet.
- *Q2: Can we use text-mining models for detecting false claims?* While text mining has achieved success in various domains, analyzing medical or health-related hoaxes in that many texts may have convincing content but fabricated facts. These could pose challenges in building predictive models for differentiating false and true information.
- *Q3: What are textual cues that can help to detect false claims?* If we could identify some common cues occurring in the text of false claims, we can educate people to look for these red flags when reading medical and health claims online.

2   Related Work

The amount of false information spread over the internet is on the rise. In recent years, there is a surge of research aimed at identify false information using text-mining techniques. Most related work has focused on two categories of false information: opinion-based (e.g., fake reviews) and fact-based (e.g., fake news) [1]. False information is often created in a way to invoke interest and/or believable to readers, which make detecting them a challenge.

False information is usually spread through social media platforms like Twitter or Facebook and the analysis to detect them should not be limited the text itself but also on how it is presented, by who, and in what format and context [2]. Kumar and Shah review different characteristics of false information [1]. Opinion-based false information often exhibits characteristics such as duplications, short lengths, over-exaggeration, skewed rating distribution, and short inter-arrival times. Fact-based false information often tends to be longer, generates more confusion, and is created by newer accounts that are tightly connected. Luca and Zervas built empirical data models to investigate the economic incentives to commit review fraud [3]. They identified business type, performance, and competition are among the main factors for businesses in committing fake review spam. Shu et al. also demonstrate the predictive power of social context for fake news detection [4]. Hence, when detecting fake information in other domains, we should consider features of the information sources in addition to linguistic features from text.

False information detection algorithms into three categories [1]: (1) feature-based algorithms rely on various types of features aforementioned to differentiate true and false information; (2) graph-based algorithms detect false information by targeting groups of spreaders coordinated in boosting a story; and (3) model-based algorithms emulate information spread patterns based on information propagation models. Among the three categories, feature-based algorithms are mostly common used in that features can be engineered and extracted from information of interest.

In previous studies, fake reviews, due to their big impact on product sales, either positive or negative, have attracted many researchers' attention. Although fake reviews can be deliberately written by either human or machine to sound authentic, there are a number of linguistic cues that can be extracted for detection [5, 6]. Some linguistic classification models can achieve over 90% accuracy in finding fake opinion spam. While the priest climbs a post, the devil climbs ten. New linguistic techniques have emerged to generate fake reviews that stay on topic to fool existing detectors [7]. More studies will continue to improve models for fake information detection using more advanced features and prediction techniques.

In the context of medical and healthcare, false information can be held and distributed by patients, clinicians, as well as general public, deserves special attention because it can cause harm. To my knowledge, compared to studies combatting fake news and fake reviews, research in detecting false information in medical domain is still limited though it is getting more attention recently. Some studies apply features and techniques that achieved success in other domains to detect false medical information [8]. For a different domain, domain-specific feature engineering is critical to have good detection performance. Hence, more in-depth research is needed to develop features and algorithms for detecting false information in such important domains. In November 2018, AMA Journal of Ethics produced a Special Issue on False Belief in Health Care [9], which attempts to address this issues from different perspectives of ethics, including education, law, code, society, policy, etc. This study focuses on the technical aspect and attempts to design prediction models for detecting false medical and healthcare information.

3 Research Design

3.1 Data Collection

In order to investigate false information in medical and healthcare domains, I choose two well-known fact-checking websites: *Snopes.com* and *Politifact.com*. In particular, Snopes has been considered "the internet's definitive fact-checking resource" for a long time. Started in 1994, it investigates urban legends, hoaxes, and folklore in a variety of domains. In Snopes' archive, it divides different claims into over forty categories, including one category named "medical" (URL: https://www.snopes.com/fact-check/category/medical/). For each claim, Snopes fact-checks it and rates if it is true of false. Its current rating system gives a rating out of the following values: true, mostly true, false, mostly false, mixture, unproven, miscaptioned, and outdated. Since the website went through some changes over the years, the formats and templates of webpages are not always consistent, which poses some challenges to web scraping. In total, I collect a total of 416 claims from Snopes.

PolitiFact is a website that focuses on fact-checking US politics. It rates the accuracy of claims by elected officials and others. This website was awarded the

Pulitzer Prize for National Reporting in 2009 for "its fact-checking initiative during the 2008 presidential campaign." PolitiFact uses rate statements on its own trademarked Truth-O-Meter, including the following six levels of truth:

True – The statement is accurate and there is nothing significant missing.

Mostly true – The statement is accurate but needs clarification or additional information.

Half true – The statement is partially accurate but leaves out important details or takes things out of context.

Mostly false – The statement contains an element of truth but ignores critical facts that would give a different impression.

False – The statement is not accurate.

Pants on fire – The statement is not accurate and makes a ridiculous claim.

PolitiFact organizes all statements by subjects and this study focuses on the subject "Health Care" (URL: https://www.politifact.com/subjects/health-care/). From this page, I collect a total of 1692 statements.

In addition, PolitiFact keeps track of the sources of all statements. For individuals with a sufficiently large number of rated statements, the website aggregates all his or her ratings in a "scorecard." Such a scorecard says a lot about one's credibility. I also scrape data about 754 sources of the 1,692 health-care related statements. From each source's page, I scrape data of name, description, and scoreboard if available. Out of the 754 sources, only 194 has sufficient statements to earn a scoreboard on the website.

Table 1. Distribution of statements with different ratings/rulings

Snopes		PolitiFact	
Rating	Count	Ruling	Count
True	48	True	182
Mostly true	8	Mostly true	267
Mixture	43	Half true	343
Mostly false	33	Mostly false	348
False	133	False	371
Others	151	Pants on fire	166
		Others	15
Total	**416**	Total	**1692**

3.2 Topic Analysis

Our first research question is concerned with the topics of medical and health-related claims/statements. Snopes and Politifact collected a variety of statements based on their relevance and popularity. These statements cover the whole spectrum from *true* to *false* in different ratings. In this study, our topic analysis uses all of these claims despite their rating/ruling to gain insights into the overall distribution of topics that attract people's attention. To answer this question, two approaches are used. First, a simple word count on the two datasets can review the most frequent words occurring in these statements. While word count measures the occurrence of each individual words, it cannot reveal the dependency among words and furthermore the topics in a collection of documents. In text mining, topic modeling is a statistical tool for discovering hidden semantic structures from a collection of texts. This study uses a widely used topic model, Latent Dirichlet Analysis (LDA), to identify main topics in the two datasets [10]. Based on the intuition that documents cover a small number of topics and that topics use a certain set of words, LDA can estimate the document-topic and topic-word distributions from a body of text.

3.3 Prediction Models

PolitiFact's Truth-O-Meter contains six levels from "True" to "Pants on fire." Snopes also adopts a similar multi-level rating system. This study defines the field "rating" in both datasets as an ordinal variable rather than a nominal variable in that it indicates different levels of truth. Thurs, I build regression models to predict the rating of a statement based on features from the statements. In both datasets, I convert each rating to a numeric score "*trust*" following Table 1. Claims with a rating not in Table 1 (e.g., *unproven*) are not included in our regression analysis.

Table 2. A mapping table to convert ratings to scores.

Snopes		PolitiFact	
Rating	Score	Ruling	Score
True	1	True	1
Mostly true	0.5	Mostly true	0.5
Mixture	0	Half true	0
Mostly false	−0.5	Mostly false	−0.5
False	−1	False	−1
		Pants on fire	−2

For machine learning in a new domain, feature engineering is critical in that finding relevant features with strong predictive powers largely determines prediction accuracy. For detecting false medical and healthcare information, this study considers two types of features:

- *Textual features*: From each claim/statement, I use a series of standard text-processing operators, including tokenization, stopword removing, transforming to lower case, and generating 2-grams, to extract features. Then, based on mutual information score, top 500 textual features are selected to build prediction models. This feature extraction and selection process is used for both Snopes and Politifact datasets.
- *Source features*: As shown in related work, features other than text can improve false information detection. For the two datasets used in this study, Snopes does not describe the source of each claim in a way that can be easily scraped or extracted.

PolitiFact, on the other hand, provides a profile page for each political figure or group including information such as title, party, and a short description. For those with a large number of rated statements, the website also provides a summary of different ratings as a "scorecard." For these individuals, I define a score named *credibility* by calculating the weighted average of the six ruling scores received (in Table 2) by the percentage of each ruling. For example, if someone's claims include 75% true (1) and 25% false (−1), then his/her credibility score is 75% × 1 + 25% × (−1) = 0.5. Hence, for PolitiFact, I also define and extract the following features for each source: *group* (group or individual), *party* (democrat, republican, or NA), and *credibility*.

4 Results

4.1 Topic Analysis

Figure 1 shows the most frequent words in the two collections of claims i.e., 415 claims from Snopes and 1,692 statements from PolitiFact. Top words in the Snopes data set (e.g., use, cause, cancer, flu, health) seem to be describing negative effects to health, while top words in PolitiFact (e.g., health, care, Obamacare, plan) are mostly related to political aspects of healthcare.

Furthermore, I run LDA using the TF-IDF scores of words on the two datasets and identify the main topics. For the Snopes dataset, the number of topics is set to 10. For the PolitiFact dataset, since the topics seem more monotonically focused on healthcare policies, I only set to find the top five main topics. Table 3 summarizes the main topics and their corresponding top words with high weights. The right column contains interpretation of each topic based on the highly weighted words.

From the medical claims picked and investigated by Snopes, they are often related to people's concerns about causes of illnesses (e.g., cancer, flu). When it comes to potential risks to one's health, especially ones that may lead to cancer and deaths of women and children, people tend to be highly sensitive and alerted, which often leads to widely spread rumors.

For the PolitiFact dataset, however, the most frequent words are quite different. Since PolitiFact.com is a website that focuses on fact-checking statements in US politics, the healthcare-related statements mainly covers the political aspects of health care, evidently from its mostly frequent words, including dataset, including health, care, Obamacare, insurance, plan, etc. The five topics also seem to be correlated to each other. The statements collected from PolitiFact are dated from September 2007 to February 2019. During this past 12 years, the U.S. went through making of Omabacare, the landmark federal health care law passed by Democrats in 2010, to republicans' ongoing attempt to repeal and replace Obamacare with new law. It is no surprise to see that these words frequently mentioned by political figures and groups. Since Obamacare remains a deeply divisive battleground between to the parties, the debate will continue with such related words popping up in both true and false statements.

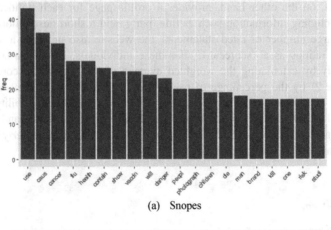

(a)   Snopes

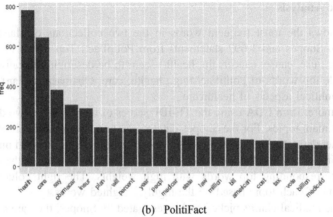

(b)   PolitiFact

Fig. 1. Most frequent words in the two datasets

4.2   Prediction Models

The topic analyses above include all statements regardless their ratings (e.g., true, false, etc.). Hence, although they show the most frequent words and main topics related to medical and health care spread around the Internet, they have not answered the question on how to detect false medical/healthcare information. Furthermore, we build linear regression models to investigate to what extent text and source features can help to detect false information from these two collections of medical and healthcare statements. Table 4 shows the model fitness of linear regression models on the two datasets. For both models, R^2 and mean squared error (MSE) are only at a satisfactory level. Hence, although these features demonstrate some predictive powers on how trustworthy a claim/statement is, they are not strong enough to achieve high accuracy for detecting false information. More advanced features and algorithms should be explored to improve prediction accuracy.

Table 3. Main topics identified in Snopes and PolitiFact datasets

IDs	Words (weights)	Topics
(a) 10 topics in Snopes		
1	cause (0.084) + legend (0.050) + heart (0.036) + children (0.035) + attack (0.034) + product (0.033) + vaccine (0.031) + cancer (0.030) + pain (0.029) + effect (0.026)	Vaccines causing heart attacks
2	kill (0.077) + article (0.074) + drug (0.062) + hand (0.045) + result (0.042) + die (0.040) + leave (0.039) + people (0.034) + person (0.029) + brand (0.027)	Drugs causing deaths
3	water (0.043) + spread (0.043) + burn (0.037) + blood (0.037) + mail (0.035) + hair (0.035) + hospital (0.032) + family (0.027) + vitamin (0.027) + contain (0.027)	Water spread
4	help (0.043) + woman (0.042) + prevent (0.041) + food (0.041) + human (0.034) + cause (0.028) + test (0.027) + baby (0.025) + prove (0.024) + increase (0.023)	Women health
5	disease (0.053) + study (0.047) + medicine (0.041) + risk (0.040) + swine (0.034) + treatment (0.033) + give (0.030) + American (0.027) + children (0.027) + condition (0.024)	Medical study
6	children (0.055) + death (0.053) + year (0.051) + drug (0.051) + cause (0.048) + ingest (0.033) + danger (0.031) + cancer (0.031) + chemical (0.028) + scientist (0.028)	Child death
7	health (0.091) + care (0.077) + patient (0.053) + remove (0.036) + develop (0.032) + cancer (0.032) + abortion (0.028) + brain (0.028) + admit (0.027) + company (0.021)	Health care
8	drink (0.053) + vaccine (0.044) + women (0.036) + health (0.034) + contain (0.032) + danger (0.023) + infant (0.023) + document (0.023) + risk (0.022) + skin (0.022)	Drink affecting women health
9	photograph (0.079) + show (0.077) + level (0.050) + live (0.037) + cure (0.036) + serve (0.034) + legal (0.031) + cause (0.028) + lead (0.027) + danger (0.027)	High lead level causing danger
10	cancer (0.088) + research (0.059) + doctor (0.053) + danger (0.053) + brand (0.046) + patient (0.042) + cure (0.039) + make (0.035) + manufacture (0.032) + avoid (0.029)	Cancer research
(b) Five topics in PolitiFact		
1	Obamacare (0.021) + insurance (0.018) + vote (0.016) + say (0.016) + percent (0.013) + people (0.011) + year (0.010) + Medicare (0.010) + women (0.009) + go (0.009)	Obamacare
2	say (0.018) + spend (0.012) + history (0.012) + country (0.012) + increase (0.011) + Obamacare (0.011) + want (0.011) + Medicare (0.010) + Trump (0.010) + cost (0.009)	Increased cost and spending
3	say (0.016) + Medicare (0.015) + insurance (0.014) + state (0.013) + Obamacare (0.013) + billion (0.013) + plan (0.012) + Obama (0.011) + year (0.011) + cost (0.011)	Medicare insurance

(continued)

Table 3. (*continued*)

IDs	Words (weights)	Topics
4	plan (0.022) + provide (0.014) + current (0.014) + Obamacare (0.014) + insurance (0.011) + abortion (0.011) + people (0.011) + mandatory (0.011) + say (0.011) + individual (0.010)	Mandatory insurance plan
10	percent (0.015) + American (0.015) + year (0.014) + million (0.012) + Obamacare (0.012) + people (0.011) + say (0.011) + insurance (0.010) + major (0.010) + state (0.010)	Insurance coverage

Table 4. Model fitness of regression models

Datasets	Features	R^2	MSE
Snopes	Text	0.5313	0.3305
PolitiFact	Text + source	0.5475	0.2350

4.3   Relevant Features for False Information Detection

Although these regression models are not accurate enough for automatic detection of false information, we can still gain some insights into good indicators for true or false medical or healthcare-related claims/statements. Table 5 lists top 10 words (or phrases) that has a significantly positive or negative relationship with a statement's *trust* score. In particular, among medical claims collected by Snopes, including a *photograph* as evidence should even be considered a red flag because pictures could be fake and deceiving. Statements claimed to be based on "*scientific*" research may be fabricated, too. In statements in PolitiFact, strong words such as *takeover, eliminated, rid, anybody*, and *everybody* are often indicators of over-exaggeration.

Table 5. Top features identified from two datasets

Snopes		PolitiFact	
Positive	Negative	Positive	Negative
#YEAR	Photograph shows	Expectancy	Homes
Researchers	Scientific	Nursing	Charlie
Attack	Abortion	Unelected	Takeover
Year	Plant	Expensive	Eliminated
Blood	Old	Primary	Rid
Flu	Year old	Level	Anybody
Nan	Spread	Counties	Obesity
#NUMBER	Citizens	Mental	Votes
People	Deaths	Lives	Babies
Cancer	Honey	Expanded	Everybody

For PolitiFact dataset, in addition to textual features, I also include features for the source. Regression result shows that:

- Compared to individual politicians, groups (organizations) are more likely to make false statements.
- Political party belonging, i.e., democrat or republican or none, does not seem to be a significant predictor for false statements.
- One's credibility score as calculated based on the scoreboard on PolitiFact does have a significant positive relationship with the trust score of a statement. People who have lied a lot before tend to have low credibility and their statements also tend to be less trustworthy.

5   Concluding Remarks

False medical and healthcare information spread online has become a big risk to public health and safety. This research investigates this problem by analyzing related data collected from two fact-checking websites. Topic analysis reveals frequent words and common topics occurring in these claims spread online. Using feature engineering and machine learning techniques, this study extracts and identifies several key features of text and source for false information detection.

Future work can extend this research from the following directions: (1) *feature engineering*: design and examine a more comprehensive set of features (e.g., textual, source, temporal, graph); (2) *detection algorithms*: apply advanced algorithms such as deep learning and word embedding for detecting false information; and (3) *stance analysis*: analyze and identify the stance of ruler on the claim and supporting evidence to better understand the incentives and techniques in creating false or fake information.

References

1. Kumar, S., Shah, N.: False Information on Web and Social Media: A Survey, April 2018
2. Sloan, L., Quan-Haase, A., Rubin, V.L.: Deception detection and rumor debunking for social media. In: The SAGE Handbook of Social Media Research Methods, pp. 342–363 (2017)
3. Luca, M., Zervas, G.: Fake it till you make it: reputation, competition, and yelp review fraud. Manag. Sci. **62**(12), 3412–3427 (2016)
4. Shu, K., Wang, S., Liu, H.: Beyond news contents: the role of social context for fake news detection. In: Proceedings of the Twelfth ACM International Conference on Web Search and Data Mining, pp. 312–320 (2019)
5. Ott, M., Choi, Y., Cardie, C., Hancock, J.T.: Finding deceptive opinion spam by any stretch of the imagination. In: Proceedings of the 49th Annual Meeting of the Association for Computational Linguistics: Human Language Technologies, vol. 1, pp. 309–319 (2011)
6. Li, J., Ott, M., Cardie, C., Hovy, E.: Towards a general rule for identifying deceptive opinion spam. In: Proceedings of the 52nd Annual Meeting of the Association for Computational Linguistics (vol. 1: Long Papers), pp. 1566–1576 (2014)

7. Juuti, M., Sun, B., Mori, T., Asokan, N.: Stay on-topic: generating context-specific fake restaurant reviews. In: Lopez, J., Zhou, J., Soriano, M. (eds.) ESORICS 2018. LNCS, vol. 11098, pp. 132–151. Springer, Cham (2018). https://doi.org/10.1007/978-3-319-99073-6_7

8. Purnomo, M.H., Sumpeno, S., Setiawan, E.I., Purwitasari, D.: Keynote speaker II: biomedical engineering research in the social network analysis era: stance classification for analysis of hoax medical news in social media. Procedia Comput. Sci. **116**, 3–9 (2017)

9. Tsay, M.A.J.: The internet, ethics, and false beliefs in health care. AMA J. Ethics **20**(11), 1003–1006 (2018)

10. Blei, D.M., Ng, A.Y., Jordan, M.I.: Latent Dirichlet allocation. J. Mach. Learn. Res. **3**(Jan), 993–1022 (2003)

Research on Cerebrovascular Disease Prediction Model Based on the Long Short Term Memory Neural Network

Qiuli Qin[1], Chunxiao Yao[1(✉)], and Yong Jiang[2]

[1] Beijing Jiaotong University, Beijing, China
{qlqin,17125479}@bjtu.edu.cn
[2] China National Clinical Research Center for Neurological Diseases, Beijing, China
jiangyong@ncrcnd.org.cn

Abstract. Aiming at the characteristics of high recurrence rate of cerebrovascular disease and the low prediction accuracy of traditional methods, a prediction model of recurrent risk of cerebrovascular disease based on long-term and short-term memory (LSTM) neural network was proposed. The predictive index of cerebrovascular disease was screened by the forward greedy attribute reduction algorithm based on the domain rough set theory. The long-short memory neural network was used to train and predict the cerebrovascular disease dataset. Through the model simulation, the results show that the proposed method has higher accuracy and better prediction performance than the support vector machine (SVM) method.

Keywords: Cerebrovascular disease · Predictive model · LSTM neural network · Feature selection

1 Introduction

Cerebrovascular disease has the characteristics of acute onset, long course of disease, serious illness and slow recovery. The number of patients is the highest in the world. It is the highest mortality rate in China and an important cause of disability in the elderly and even middle-aged people. At present, the first incidence of cerebrovascular diseases is mostly studied, and there are few studies on the risk of recurrence. After the onset of cerebrovascular disease, the risk of recurrence is 9 times that of the average individual, and the incidence rate is significantly increased. This also emphasizes the importance of secondary prevention of cerebrovascular disease. Constructing a disease recurrence risk prediction model to assess the risk level of cerebrovascular disease, thereby identifying high-risk groups, and taking timely guidance and preventive measures for different patients' physical conditions and appropriate treatment intensity, reducing recurrence, is important for prevention of cerebrovascular diseases means.

Existing disease prediction methods are mostly based on traditional machine learning methods. Malathi [1] constructed a predictive model by combining Fuzzy sety theory, k-nearest neighbor and case-based reasoning. The experimental results reveal

© Springer Nature Switzerland AG 2019
H. Chen et al. (Eds.): ICSH 2019, LNCS 11924, pp. 247–256, 2019.
https://doi.org/10.1007/978-3-030-34482-5_22

that the model can improve the prediction accuracy. Shadman Nashif [2] constructed a heart disease prediction model based on support vector machine. Weng [3] studied four machine learning algorithms (random forest, logistic regression, gradient enhancement machines, neural networks) to predict the risk of cardiovascular disease. Ma [4] constructed a predictive model for the risk of death in patients with severe cerebrovascular disease based on multivariate logistic analysis. Ai [5] constructed support vector machine, decision tree and neural network prediction model respectively, and studied the application effects of different machine learning methods in predicting disease treatment. Chen [6] constructed an artificial neural network prediction model to predict the risk of brain cancer.

Traditional machine learning algorithms have certain defects and limitations. The huge amount of data and the increasing number of data variables make the disease prediction model based on traditional machine learning somewhat lacking in accuracy and calculation speed. In recent years, deep learning has certain applications and development in the fields of disease prediction [7], traffic flow prediction [8], price prediction [9], speech recognition [10], image recognition [11], and natural language processing [12]. At present, domestic and foreign research scholars apply deep learning to disease prediction and achieve certain results. Meyer [13] constructed a deep learning prediction model based on cyclic neural network to predict serious complications during real-time intensive care of cardiothoracic surgery and verified the high accuracy of the predictive model. Lu [14] constructed a cardiovascular and cerebrovascular disease prediction model based on the improved deep belief network. Using the reconstruction error, the model automatically determines the network depth, and the parameter tuning improves the prediction accuracy of the model. Ying [15] constructed a classification prediction model for the severity of chronic obstructive pulmonary disease based on deep belief network. Chen [16] constructed a predictive model of deep belief network for thyroid disease, and the results verified that the prediction model based on deep learning for non-sparse data and sparse data sets has higher accuracy.

Based on the time series characteristics of The China National Stroke Registry (CNSR) data, this paper proposes a prediction method of cerebrovascular disease based on long and short time memory neural network. The attribute reduction algorithm based on domain rough set theory is used to screen prediction indicators and construct LSTM neural network prediction model. Through the cerebrovascular disease data test, the results show that the proposed prediction method has higher accuracy than the SVM prediction method, and it is an effective predictive model for recurrence of cerebrovascular diseases.

2 Basic Theory

2.1 Long and Short Time Memory Neural Network

In traditional neural networks, the output of the model is only related to the current input value. This mechanism makes the model unable to process the sequence data. Recurrent Neural Network (RNN) are often used to process sequence data. The characteristics of sequence data are that there is a strong correlation between the data before and after the sequence. The next value is determined by the current value and the previous value. The internal structure of the RNN can store and store the information before and after the data, and the output of the previous value is saved for each subsequent training. The structure of the RNN is shown in Fig. 1.

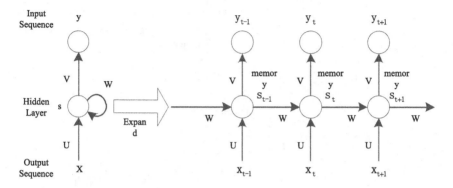

Fig. 1. RNN structure diagram

The LSTM neural network is an improved RNN. It solves the problem that the RNN has low prediction accuracy due to the disappearance or explosion of the gradient and cannot capture the long-term dependency information of the input sequence [17]. Using memory blocks to replace neurons in the hidden layer of traditional neural networks, so that the memory of the neuron is stronger. This method can remember the historical information with very long time interval, and its unique cell control mechanism can solve the gradient explosion and Long-term dependency of time series. The hidden layer structure of the LSTM neural network is shown in Fig. 2.

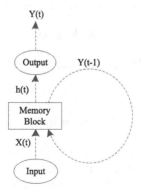

Fig. 2. LSTM neural network hidden layer structure

The memory block of the LSTM neural network consists of three gates: input gate, forgetting gate and output gate. As shown in Fig. 3, the calculation process of a memory block at time t is as follows:

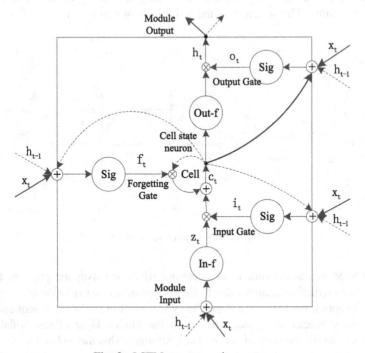

Fig. 3. LSTM memory unit structure

$$c_t = f_t c_{t-1} + i_t \ \tanh(W_{xc}x_t + W_{hc}h_{t-1} + b_c) \tag{1}$$

$$i_t = s(W_{xi}x_t + W_{hi}h_{t-1} + W_{ci}c_{t-1} + b_i) \tag{2}$$

$$f_t = s(W_{xf}x_t + W_{hf}h_{t-1} + W_{cf}c_{t-1} + b_f) \tag{3}$$

$$o_t = s(W_{xo}x_t + W_{ho}h_{t-1} + W_{co}c_t + b_o) \tag{4}$$

$$h_t = o_t \tanh(c_t) \tag{5}$$

c_t, i_t, f_t, o_t, h_t respectively represent the output values of memory cells, input gate, forgetting gate, output gate, and memory modules at time t, s represents the sigmoid function. W_{xi}, W_{xf}, W_{xo} respectively represents the network weight value from the network input layer to the gate corresponding to the module at this time. W_{hi}, W_{hf}, W_{ho} respectively represents the network weight value output from the t-1th LSTM module to the gate corresponding to the moment. W_{ci}, W_{cf}, W_{co} represents the network weight value from the t − 1th cell state neuron to the gate corresponding to the moment, and b represents the deviation vector of the corresponding gate at this time.

2.2 Attribute Reduction Algorithm Based on Domain Rough Set

The rough set of the domain is mainly used to deal with the uncertainty and ambiguity of the data set. It can overcome the shortcomings that the rough set can only deal with the discretized data. It has been proved to be widely used in attribute reduction in various fields [18, 19]. Application domain rough set theory performs attribute reduction on datasets, and provides the same information as the original data by filtering out as few feature indicators as possible, filtering out duplicate, unnecessary, and unrelated indicators, simplifying the number of indicators. To make predictions more efficient, so attribute reduction is the core of the rough set of domains. In this paper, the forward greedy attribute reduction algorithm based on domain rough set is applied to the selection of characteristic indicators for cerebrovascular disease prediction. The algorithm process is shown in Fig. 4:

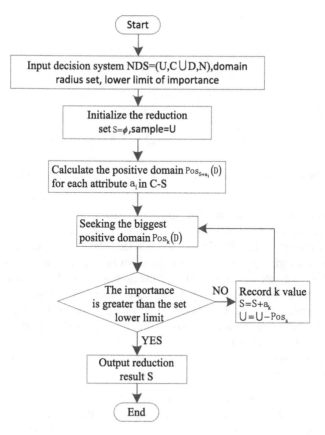

Fig. 4. Forward greedy reduction algorithm

3 Constructing LSTM Memory Neural Network Prediction Model

Based on medical data of cerebrovascular diseases, this paper constructs a predictive model of cerebrovascular disease using LSTM neural network. Figure 5 shows the disease prediction model of the LSTM neural network. In this model, the first layer is the input layer, which is used to receive data, and transform the input data into dimensions, so as to establish contact with the LSTM layer. The middle layer is the LSTM layer, which is used to extract data. The last layer of the feature is the output layer, which outputs the predicted results.

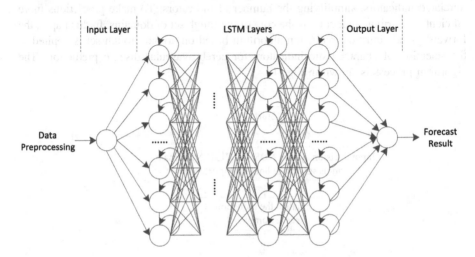

Fig. 5. Disease prediction model based on LSTM neural network

The loss function is a measure function that measures the degree of error between the predicted value and the actual value. It is also the objective function of optimization in the neural network model. The loss function selects the mean square error (MSE). In the LSTM network training process, when the input layer is 1 layer, and the number of cells in the LSTM hidden layer is 200, and the number of LSTM layers is 2, and the number of iterations is 1000, the model prediction effect is the best. In order to avoid the neural network in the training process into the local optimal problem, the Adam optimization algorithm is used to determine the iterative update mode of the weight parameter, so as to optimize the model and make the model prediction effect better.

The implementation process of the disease prediction method based on LSTM neural network is composed of the following five steps:

(1) Construct an LSTM neural network disease prediction model. Set up the LSTM neural network and randomly set the parameters in the model.
(2) Train the LSTM neural network model. Firstly, the data is collected for preprocessing, and the attributes are reduced. The data is divided into training group and

test group. The training group data is used to train the model, the parameters are adjusted, and the loss function of the LSTM neural network is calculated by the forward feedback process. The Adam algorithm is used. Determine the iterative update mode of the weight parameter for the optimization of the LSTM neural network model.

(3) Use the LSTM neural network model for prediction. The test group data is input, and the trained LSTM network model is used for prediction, and the predicted result is output.

(4) Comparative analysis of prediction results. The LSTM neural network model is compared with the predicted results of the SVM model to compare the accuracy of the prediction.

(5) Evaluation prediction model. After the comparative analysis of the predicted results, the validity of the LSTM prediction model is determined.

4   Experimental Analysis

4.1   Data Collection and Preprocessing

The experimental data in this paper is derived from the China National Stroke Registry (CNSR) database. It is based on a standardized follow-up form, which is followed by a follow-up registration of patient information and processing data after stroke patients are admitted to the hospital. A total of 22,538 data were used. Among the attributes in the initial statistics, the index with a deletion rate of 10% was removed, and the attribute columns not related to the prediction of cerebrovascular disease were excluded, leaving 54 related attributes.

Before using experimental data for data analysis, you first need to preprocess the data to obtain data that can be directly analyzed. First, for the data missing of some samples, the attribute average is used to fill in the missing value, that is, the mean of all the statistics of the attribute column in which the missing data is located instead of the missing value. The second is to digitize the data and convert it to a value of 0-5 so that it can directly participate in the numerical calculation. The prediction results of the model are also numerically processed, and the three levels of recurrence rate are normal, non-fatal, and fatal, respectively, represented by 0, 1, and 2.

4.2   Attribute Reduction Results

Attribute reduction is a core part of disease model prediction and a key factor related to the accuracy of prediction results. The construction of predictive index system for cerebrovascular diseases should follow the basic principles of systemic, comprehensive, dynamic, operability and typicality. Forward greedy attribute reduction algorithm based on domain rough set and combined with literature analysis method and comprehensive analysis method for attribute reduction, Finally, there are 18 indicators that can be used to predict cerebrovascular diseases. They are age, smoking, alcohol, hypertension, diabetes, hyperlipidemia, valvular heart disease, atrial fibrillation, transient ischemic attack, ischemic stroke, cerebral hemorrhage, subarachnoid hemorrhage, carotid intima Resection, intracranial angioplasty, peripheral vascular disease, deep venous thrombosis of the lower extremity/pulmonary embolism, family history of stroke, pre-morbid MRS score.

4.3   Analysis of Experimental Results

(1) Evaluation indicators

To assess the effectiveness of the LSTM neural network model in predicting the risk of recurrence of cerebrovascular disease, accuracy and recall were chosen to quantify the performance of the LSTM predictive model. And compare the prediction efficiency of the LSTM network model and the SVM model. The Precision indicates that the correct prediction is positive and the proportion of all predictions is positive. The Recall is also called the true positive rate, indicating that the correct prediction is positive and the proportion is positive. The formula is as follows:

$$Precision = TP/(TP + FP) \tag{6}$$

$$Recall = TP/(TP + FN) \tag{7}$$

TP indicates the number of positive classes that are correctly predicted to be positive, FN indicates the number of positive classes that are incorrectly predicted to be negative, and FP indicates the number of negative classes that are incorrectly predicted to be positive.

(2) Comparative analysis of results

In this paper, the SVM prediction model is selected for comparison. In the traditional machine learning method of disease prediction, the SVM model is the most widely used, and from the prediction effect of the model, the accuracy of the support vector machine is relatively high. Combined with the advantages of SVM with low generalization error rate, the SVM model and the newly constructed LSTM prediction model are selected for comparative analysis of the prediction results to verify the prediction effect of the LSTM prediction model. The prediction results of the two models are shown in Table 1:

Table 1. Comparison of LSTM neural network model and SVM results

Model name	Precision	Recall
LSTM model	0.95	0.97
SVM model	0.93	0.96

As can be seen by observing Table 1, when mainly considering the 18 predictive indicators screened in this paper to predict the risk of cerebrovascular disease, The prediction model of cerebrovascular disease based on LSTM neural network is better than the traditional machine learning method SVM model, and the prediction accuracy is higher. It shows that the model has better adaptability in dealing with the CNSR data of the time series features adopted in this paper. From the prediction results, the accuracy and recall rate of the LSTM network prediction model are slightly larger than the SVM model. The experimental results show that the cerebral vascular disease prediction model based on LSTM neural network has a good effect on both practicability and prediction accuracy. Therefore, the prediction of the risk of cerebrovascular disease is feasible.

5 Conclusion

In this paper, based on CNSR data, a predictive model of recurrent risk of cerebrovascular disease based on long-term and short-term memory (LSTM) neural network is proposed. Firstly, the forward greedy attribute reduction algorithm based on domain rough set theory is used to screen the prediction index. The LSTM prediction model uses the extracted characteristic indicators to predict the risk of recurrence of cerebrovascular disease. The LSTM neural network can solve the defects that traditional neural networks can not use and memorize historical data information, and has good effects on time-series data, which can improve the accuracy of prediction. Experiments show that the LSTM neural network-based cerebrovascular disease prediction model has higher accuracy and higher predictive performance than traditional prediction methods, and provides an effective method for predicting the risk of recurrence of cerebrovascular diseases.

References

1. Malathi, D., Logesh, R., Subramaniyaswamy, V., et al.: Hybrid reasoning-based privacy-aware disease prediction support system. Comput. Electr. Eng. **73**, 114–127 (2019)
2. Shadman Nashif, M., Rakib Raihan, M., Rasedul Islam, M., et al.: Heart disease detection by using machine learning algorithms and a real-time cardiovascular health monitoring system. World J. Eng. Technol. **06**(04), 854–873 (2018)
3. Weng, S.F., Jenna, R., Joe, K., et al.: Can machine-learning improve cardiovascular risk prediction using routine clinical data? PLoS ONE **12**(4), e0174944 (2017)
4. Ma, G., Zhang, D., Peng, C.: Multivariate logistic analysis for predicting the risk of death in patients with acute severe cerebrovascular disease. Chin. J. Pract. Nerv. Dis. **17**(11), 38–41 (2014)
5. Ai, X., Mao, W., Tian, M.: Research on the tendency identification of online disease diagnosis and treatment based on machine learning technology. Chin. J. Med. Libr. Inf. Sci. **27**(07), 1–5 (2018)
6. Chen, G., Jiang, J., Li, F., et al.: Research and application of artificial neural network in lung cancer risk prediction. Comput. Age (11), 56–59+63 (2018)
7. Li, X., Wang, H., Xiong, Y., et al.: Application of convolutional neural network model in pediatric disease prediction. China Digit. Med. **13**(10), 11–13 (2018)
8. Yang, H.J., Hu, X.: Wavelet neural network with improved genetic algorithm for traffic flow time series prediction. Optik – Int. J. Light Electron Opt. **127**(19), 8103–8110 (2016)

9. Chen, J., Hao, Y., Zheng, D., Chen, S.: Modeling and decision of price forecasting in futures market based on DBN deep learning. Comput. Sci. **45**(S1), 75–78+84 (2018)
10. Li, W., Wen, J., Ma, W.: Research on speech recognition system based on deep neural network. Comput. Sci. **43**(z2), 45–49 (2016)
11. Kumar, B.A., Aishik, K., Kumar, B.A., et al.: Script identification in natural scene image and video frames using an attention based convolutional-LSTM network. Pattern Recognit. S0031320318302590 (2018)
12. Lin, Y., Lei, H., Li, X., et al.: Deep learning in natural language processing: methods and applications. J. Univ. Electron. Sci. Technol. China **46**(6), 913–919 (2017)
13. Meyer, A., Zverinski, D., Pfahringer, B., et al.: Machine learning for real-time prediction of complications in critical care: a retrospective study. Lancet Respir. Med. **6**(12), 905–914 (2018)
14. Lu, P., Wang, Y., Li, Q., et al.: Prediction of cardiovascular disease based on improved deep belief network. Appl. Res. Comput. **35**(12), 3668–3672 (2018)
15. Ying, J., Yang, C., Li, Q., et al.: Classification of chronic obstructive pulmonary disease based on deep learning method. J. Biomed. Eng. **34**(06), 842–849 (2017)
16. Chen, D., Zhou, D., Le, J.: Research on predictive methods of benign and malignant thyroid nodules based on deep learning. Microcomput. Appl. **36**(12), 13–15 (2017)
17. Wang, X., Wu, J., Liu, C., et al.: Fault time series prediction based on LSTM cyclic neural network. J. Beijing Univ. Aeronaut. Astronaut. **44**(04), 772–784 (2018)
18. Zhang, Z., Li, D., Li, Y.: Research on audit opinion prediction model based on neighborhood rough set neural network. J. Chongqing Univ. Technol. (Soc. Sci.) **31**(08), 37–43 (2017)
19. Chen, J., Duan, J., Zhang, M.: A comprehensive fault diagnosis model for transformer fault based on neighborhood rough set and correlation vector machine. J. Electric Power System Autom. **28**(11), 117–122 (2016)

Identifying Privacy Leakage from User-Generated Content in an Online Health Community

Yushan Zhu[1], Xing Tong[2], Dan Fan[1], and Xi Wang[1(✉)]

[1] School of Information, Central University of Finance and Economics,
Beijing, China
xiwang@cufe.edu.cn
[2] College of Humanities and Social Sciences, George Mason University,
Fairfax, VA, USA

Abstract. Online Health Communities (OHCs) have become a widely used resource for obtaining and sharing health-related information during the past decade. However, the health information privacy issues of OHCs have not been fully explored. Insufficient attention to personal privacy management may result in intentional or unintentional disclosure of users' sensitive information, and consequently harm the communication environment, as well as individuals' safety. Based on the user-generated content, this preliminary research applies the method of text mining to identify different types of information leakages occur in a breast cancer OHC. The results indicate that approximately 60% of the OHC users are willing to express their emotional feelings, and 10.86% are motivated to disclose their health information. In addition, based on the longitudinal data from 2007 to 2018, we analyzed the OHC user behavior trajectories in private information exposure. The findings of this study have practical implications for OHC users, administers, and website designers.

Keywords: Online Health Community · Privacy leakage · User-generated content · Text mining · User trajectory

1 Introduction

Accelerated by the advancements in the Internet technology, Online Health Communities (OHCs) have become a major source for serving people having health problems and have been frequently reported as an effective platform for people with similar health concerns to communicate [1]. One mechanism that users participate in OHCs is producing large amount of personal information and sharing with other users [2], aiming to get more personalized communications based on individuals' needs [3]. However, as Internet users in increasing number start to actively generate and share information in publicly accessible OHCs, paying insufficient attention to personal privacy management may result in intentional or unintentional disclosure of their private information in the process, such as identity information, insurance information, resident location, health status, and personal feelings. Consequently, it might lead to higher privacy intrusion costs, such as malicious attacks (harassment, human flesh,

© Springer Nature Switzerland AG 2019
H. Chen et al. (Eds.): ICSH 2019, LNCS 11924, pp. 257–268, 2019.
https://doi.org/10.1007/978-3-030-34482-5_23

phishing), illegal interests (trafficking of personal information), and crimes (robbery, extortion, theft) [4]. Privacy leakage has huge potential risks and has become a highly concerned issue in current. In addition, compared with other online communities, the information disclosed on OHCs can be much more sensitive [5]. The benefits that users can get from OHCs is through obtaining social support rather than monetary rewards [6–8]. However, the research on OHC privacy is far from satisfactory.

From the perspective of methodology, as far as we know, most of the research in the past was conducted through questionnaires, in-depth interviews, or obtaining the profile of the community users to analyze their personal information disclosure behaviors. These methods have not fully utilized the actual user-generated content (UGC) on OHCs. In other words, few research directly reveals the relationship between a user's participation and privacy leakage in OHCs based on UGC. Meanwhile, what makes the OHC users to take risks to disclose their sensitive information is open to doubt.

From the perspective of research topic, a critical but understudied theme of OHC privacy is the changes of users' self-disclosure behaviors during a long-term stream. A particular user of an OHC may constantly update medical progression with peers and fill supplemental personal medical information gradually; after becoming a constant user of an OHC, they may be engaged in more daily life topics to keep the bond with other users in this community. Compared with the newly registered users with an aim to get informational, long-term users are more likely to exchange emotional support and companionship in form of off-topic discussions which are rarely about health [1]. In accumulation, chances are that they have disclosed information about themselves more than expected on a platform that is accessible to the public. Under such circumstances, it is unclear whether the OHC users realize the detailed information they disclose about themselves, their important others, or other OHC users may have been sufficient enough for third parties to tailor online services beyond their desire. If so, whether they concern about exceeding the baseline of committing privacy infringement or would be willing to be reminded the potential benefits and risks in practicing such behaviors and accept more user interface features of the website design are practically important questions for OHC users and administers, and designers.

Therefore, we conducted both traditional machine learning approach and a deep learning method to identify users' privacy leakage by automatically text mining UGC from an OHC. At the same time, using the longitudinal data from 2007 to 2018, we are able to summarize UGC privacy leakage trajectories in private information exposure behavior of OHC users over the past eleven years.

There are two primary research questions in this study. First, what kind of private information in OHC is more likely to be leaked through UGC; second, as the users' involvement in the community increase, how will the privacy leakage of users be changed. Through investigating these problems, the OHC administers will better understand the behavior patterns of network users' information leakage and adopt it as a reference for the network construction and management, as well as the improvement of online health communities. At the same time, it may help to generate beneficial guidance for OHC users to help them better protect their own private information, as well as other users' privacy in the community.

2   Theoretical Background

2.1   Users' Privacy in OHCs

Individuals' privacy refers to non-public personal information in the traditional sense. User privacy in the network environment extends the concept to the communication content and digital behavior generated when users participate in network activities. In OHCs, users will disclose their identity information, medical health information, and even personal emotions to varying degrees in order to better participate in information exchange and sharing activities. Therefore, the user privacy leaked in OHCs is not limited to general user information, but also contains a large amount of medical health data. Established on the literature review, this paper labels the OHCs privacy genres into the following five categories:

Identity Information (**II**). Identity information is a descriptive statement about a person's identity, including narrative content such as name, gender, resident location, emails, photos, affiliations, user type (a.k.a. patients and caregivers etc.) etc. Identity information is usually by no means directly relevant to users' knowledge and physical well-being yet imposing high privacy costs.

Detailed Medical Data (**DMD**). Detailed medical data describes clinical information related to cancer history, symptoms, treatments and outcomes (i.e. time of diagnosis, cancer stage, treatment progress and regimen).

Other Medical Related Information (**OMRI**). This type of content is medical-related, such as specific hospital or clinician, insurance information, medication ordering, personal budgets, etc., but not contain the users' detailed medical data.

Emotional Feelings (**EF**). Intimate emotional feelings demonstrate OHC users' inner feelings, such as positive feelings like excitement from survival, gratitude for others' support, or negative feelings like anxiety, anger, discomfort, fear, worrisome, confusion through cancer diagnosis and treatment, etc. This type of information can usually reveal the user's current psychological states.

Daily Life (**DL**). This type of content is about daily routine life that people share in casual communication, such as family life, daily activities, holidays, hobbies and so on. Like identity information, this category of content usually has nothing to do with health status.

2.2   Ways and influencing factors of privacy disclosure

The leakage of medical information may damage the reputation of a patient, expose a patient to discrimination. Leaking patient privacy from the Internet is more common and diverse than the traditional methods. OHC users, with the majority of patients may disclose patients' private information. Chen et al. [9] pointed out that the OHC users' privacy is leaked mainly through 4 channels, including voluntarily self-exposure, websites, third parties, and others. Mulliner et al. [10] found that mobile phone network access also leaks privacy, and HTTP agents operated by mobile phone network operators inject additional headers into HTTP connections, resulting in privacy leakage. All types of unauthorized disclosure or loss of sensitive information bring a lot of trouble to the networking environment, as well the users' safety in real life.

Privacy leakage in the Internet is affected by various factors. To be specific, privacy leakage has different degrees of relevance to privacy information content, user characteristics, technical factors, policy factors, and cultural factors. Ge et al. [11] found that most users are willing to provide hobbies, occupations, residential addresses, birthdays, and affiliation information, but not the detailed mailing address and telephone numbers. In terms of demographic variables, Michalopoulos et al. [12] found that users from different ages did not differ much in accepting friendship requests from unknown users. Du el al. [14] proposed a privacy breach attack defense tree to describe a series of activities initiated by attackers and summarized that a user's own privacy protection awareness is the key to reduce privacy leakage rather than defense technology or economic factors. Zhao et al. [15] built a privacy calculation model to investigate the intent of network users to disclose location-related information and found incentives and interaction promotion would increase the chance of privacy leakage, but privacy control and privacy policies would help to reduce the event.

To sum up, OHC users are likely to disclose sensitive information due to the specific needs and message content features. The threatening of the confidentiality of OHC users' information may not only bring risks to individuals, but also harm the communication environment. To better acknowledge what types of information are more likely to be leaked, and how the amount and type of information leakage will change with users' aggregated involvement over time, the following research was performed.

3 Privacy Leakage Identification

In order to identify privacy leakage from UGC online, we crawled public-access posts from a US breast cancer OHC (Breastcancer.org). There are two reasons for selecting this website as the research target. First, people who have such chronic health conditions need continuous support during their long-term battles with the cancer. As a result, patients and their caregivers might publish a large number of stories about themselves over years. Second, since the OHC has already been launched more than 17 years and holding over 100,000 registered users, huge volume of data would be ready for studying. Our dataset contains 4.3 million public posts, including initial posts and comments, from more than 70,000 registered users during March 2007 and April 2018.

Since it is impossible to manually label 4.3 million posts one by one, we leveraged machine learning techniques to automatically discover privacy related content in each post. Specifically, we built classification models to determine what type(s) of privacy leakage each post contains, including II, DMD, OMRI, EF and DL. Note that a post may contain more than one type of leakage mentioned above. Table 1 shows a set of sample posts for each category.

Table 1. Example posts for different types of privacy leakage.

Privacy leakage category	OHC posts
II	*You sound like a good trooper! You also must be a great nurse! Both my mother and sister are nurses*
DMD	*I have had the lump for 7 weeks and it has gotten a little larger and the needle like pain isn't getting better*
OMRI	*When you mention the internist's ethnicity were you meaning that being Asian she would have a different take? My oncologist is "Asian" and he is very conventional*
EF	*They consider most of these 'benign', however, there could be a small chance it is cancer. I'm even more confused/concerned than I was before*
DL	*Happy birthday Lulu! ?What kind of cake will you have?:) Sending you hugs and kisses on your birthday! Love Bobogirl*
Multiple categories	*I'm a 26 y/o female, married, with one child. About 2 mths ago I went to my primary doctor for an odd swelling under my right armpit. After MUCH worrying and back and forth, an ultrasound was done and everything came back normal. I went to the doctor yesterday for a pea-sized lump felt/found in my right breast, about 2 cm below my nipple. I am scheduled to see a general surgeon tomorrow morning. I am worried about tomorrow's appointment. I think I am more upset and nervous to know that my husband goes back overseas in just days. Any advice would be appreciated! THANK YOU!*

With randomly selecting 4,000 posts as the training set, we implemented the annotation task on the platform of Amazon Mechanical Turk (AMT). We released 1000 AMT HITs (Artificial Intelligence Tasks, one task for a worker) in total, with each HIT consisting of 20 posts and annotated by 5 different online workers. Meanwhile, we set a quality control question during each task to accept the reasonable annotation results only. The reliability of the agreement is 0.80 in average measured by Cronbanch alpha value. Table 2 shows a distribution of classified privacy leakage result of the annotated training set.

In terms of feature engineering, we included two feature sets extracted from the text of training set. One is the bag of words (BOW) features named as Feature-set 1, which is one of the most common used technique in the text mining problems. The other one is the Word2Vec (W2V) features named as Feature-set 2, a word embedding technique that generates vector representations for posts. After varying the size of the vector, we selected 256 as the best performing value. In other words, one post is represented by a vector of length 256 for training the classifier. With these two feature sets, we were able to compare the predictive power of the explicit words and implicit relationship between words in identifying privacy leakage from UGC.

Table 2. Distribution of privacy leakage in the training set.

Privacy leakage	Number	Percentage
II	418	10.45
DMD	1,017	25.43
OMRI	231	5.78
EF	1,403	35.08
DL	549	13.73
Total	4,000	100.00

In terms of the model selection of classification, we compared the traditional machine learning algorithms to a deep-learning model. Specifically, for each type of privacy leakage, we first trained 14 classifiers by using 7 traditional machine learning algorithms (Logistic Regression, Support Vector Machine, Naïve Bayes, K-Nearest Neighbors, Decision Tree, Random Forest, AdaBoost with the Decision Tree as the weak learner) and 2 types of feature sets, and obtained the best performance one by adjusting the parameters. In the left side of Table 3, we list the classifiers with the best performance among 14 classifiers for each privacy leakage. After that, we trained another 2 classifiers for the category by using the Long-Short Term Memory (LSTM). LSTM is an excellent variant of Recurrent Neural Network with a certain memory effect, which can effectively take the advantage of historical information in the context. LSTM is widely used in addressing natural language processing problems for its ability of dealing with time correlated data, as well as the semantic analysis. In the right side of Table 3, we list the classifier with the best performance by LSTM model. We used weighted F1-scores and weighted AUC to evaluate the performance of the classification model. The F1-score is the harmonic mean of the accuracy (the correct predicted number AUC (area under the ROC curve) measures the probability that the positive sample ranks higher than the negative sample and provides a robust measure of classification performance. When dealing with unbalanced types of privacy leakage, such as DL and II which have fewer positive instances in the training set (13.73% and 10.45% positives respectively), we used under sampling to reduce the impact.

It is clear from Table 3 that the introduction of deep learning methods can help to improve the performance of the model significantly. In addition, Feature-set 2 outperforms Feature-set 1 among the majority of the models. It is possible that W2V considers the interaction between words, as a result, it can better express the semantics of text than BOW, which focus only on the frequencies of words. Moreover, we found that when we combined Feature-set 2 with the deep learning classification algorithm LSTM, the performance of all models improved. This is very possible that the memory function of LSTM can learn and preserve information, which makes full use of the semantic features of W2V.

Table 3. Result of Evaluations of classification model for OHC.

Privacy leakage	Traditional machine learning classification			Deep learning classification		
	Algorithm	Features	F1-score AUC	Algorithm	Features	F1-score AUC
II	*Logistic regression*	*Feature-set 2*	*0.832* *0.671*	*LSTM*	*Feature-set 2*	*0.931* *0.859*
DMD	*Random forest*	*Feature-set 1*	*0.674* *0.596*	*LSTM*	*Feature-set 2*	*0.852* *0.828*
OMRI	*Adaboost*	*Feature-set 2*	*0.617* *0.594*	*LSTM*	*Feature-set 2*	*0.724* *0.765*
EF	*Logistic regression*	*Feature-set 1*	*0.632* *0.656*	*LSTM*	*Feature-set 2*	*0.732* *0.824*
DL	*Logistic regression*	*Feature-set 2*	*0.811* *0.694*	*LSTM*	*Feature-set 2*	*0.892* *0.878*

To sum up, we selected LSTM combining Feature-set 2 as the best classification model to assign labels of privacy leakage to the rest of posts in the data set. Table 4 shows the distribution of different types of leakage in the community. Intuitively, EF takes the largest amount (59.64%), indicating that users on the community are very inclined to express emotion feelings. This is followed by DMD (10.86%), suggesting that many users tend to describe their own cancer conditions in the OHC. Although DL only accounts for 1.78%, as the least proportion among all types, the high number 77,707 indicates that many users indeed talk about their private life a lot in this public community. Note that the reason why the sum of the percentages of 5 categories privacy leakage is less than 100 is that not all posts revealing private information.

Table 4. Distribution of each category of privacy leakage posts in OHC.

Privacy leakage	Number	Percentage
II	*320,047*	*7.34*
DMD	*473,902*	*10.86*
OMRI	*129,009*	*2.96*
EF	*2,601,944*	*59.64*
DL	*77,707*	*1.78*

After detecting the type of privacy leakage included in each post, we aggregated user-level posts and categorized users based on their overall privacy disclosure. Specifically, for each user, we first used a privacy profiling vector to indicate her privacy leaking behavior. The vector has five elements, each of which is the percentage of all of the five categories of privacy leakage (II, DMD, OMRI, EF, DL) of the user in the OHC. For example, a user with 50% of her posts being II, 30% being DMD, and 70% being DL would have vector of <0.5, 0.3, 0, 0, 0.7>. Since 68,155 users have exposed privacy online, there are 68,155 privacy entries in total, one per user and aggregated over time. Then, we applied the K-means clustering algorithm to divide the users into K groups, by which users with similar privacy leaking behavior vectors assigned to the same cluster. To find the best user grouping, we evaluated various K values (from 2 to 12) using the Calinski-Harabaz Index (CHI) and selected K = 6 by the highest CHI value.

The centroids of 6 clusters are shown in Table 5. In order to better understand privacy leaking behavior, we defined 6 roles based on the features of centroids: Leaker (s) of identity and emotional information (IEL), who posted an average of 82.73% on identity information posts and an average of 97.02% on emotional feeling posts; Leaker (s) of emotional feelings (EL), who were more likely to express emotional feelings (94.90%); Leaker(s) of medical and emotional information (MIEL), who actively posted posts with detailed medical data (83.55%) and emotional feelings (95.20%); Leaker(s) of medical information (MIL), who were more likely to reveal detail medical data (84.85%) and other medical related information (10.56%); Leaker(s) of all types of information (AL), who consisted the largest group of users with relatively balanced profiles in each privacy leakage category; Leaker(s) of identity information (IIL), who were more likely to reveal identity information (85.32%) than others.

Table 5. Centroids of user clusters based on aggregated privacy leaking entries.

Privacy leakage	All users	IEL	EL	MIEL	MIL	AL	IIL
II	0.4128	*0.8273*	0.0285	0.0246	0.1621	0.0890	*0.8532*
DMD	0.4640	0.2133	0.0345	*0.8355*	*0.8485*	0.1176	0.0190
OMRI	0.1865	0.0107	0.0107	0.0198	*0.1056*	0.0316	0.0293
EF	0.8782	*0.9702*	*0.9490*	*0.9520*	0.0492	0.5654	0.0521
DL	0.1228	0.0066	0.0050	0.0074	0.0224	0.0133	0.0285
%users	100%	35.28%	6.34%	5.62%	3.27%	47.32%	2.17%

4   Privacy Leakage Trajectory

The user roles listed in Table 6 represent only static snapshots based on users' accumulated privacy leakage over time. To capture the dynamics of users' role, we need to determine roles over time. For this reason, we checked roles on monthly basis and calculated monthly privacy leaking entries for each user. With k-nearest neighbor (kNN) classification scheme, we compared users' monthly profiles with the 68,155 aggregated privacy leaking entries for all users.

Based on the user's behavior in each month in the OHC, we were able to get a temporal trajectory of a user's privacy leaking behavior changing over time. Figure 1 shows the role transition network in the OHC, describing how users shift from one status to another. The weighted and directed network has 9 nodes. Six of them correspond to the six roles we listed in Table 5 (IEL, EL, MIEL, MIL, AL, IIL are numbered 0 to 5 respectively). Besides one node for the state of the no activity (numbered 6), we also included Registration status (numbered 7) and Churn status (numbered 8). All users started from registration, but over time, they may move to any other node in this diagram. If the user has no posts in our dataset for the past 3 months, we assumed that the user has left the OHC. According to Fig. 1, we can observe that a user who act as an EL in this OHC is very likely to leave the community in the next month, while AL is more likely to stay in, meanwhile, the IEL tends to transit to AL with time goes by.

Table 6. The distribution of user' roles by their numbers of monthly activities.

Role	Number of monthly privacy profiles
IEL	*105,755*
EL	*13,738*
MIEL	*10,873*
MIL	*7,563*
AL	*138,649*
IIL	*4,309*
LU	*346,292*
Total	*627,179*

In order to further observe the users' privacy leaking behaviors' changing over time, we selected 10 users with longest active time from each role cluster in Table 5. With the representative ones, we were able to draw the trend of their privacy leakage in different categories over time in Figs. 2, 3, 4, 5, 6 and 7. The horizontal axis shows months of the users' involvement in the OHC and the vertical axis shows the percentage of posts containing the privacy leakage posted by the users during that month. The participating trajectories in 5 privacy leakage categories of users belonging to one cluster were displayed on the same image containing 50 thumbnails.

Intuitively, in Figs. 2, 3, 4, 5, 6 and 7, the trajectories of 10 columns as well as 10 users of images have a certain similarity. In other words, users belonging to the same role cluster have similarities in privacy leaking behavior. For example, the DL, II and OMRI leakage of AL users tend to increase over time according Fig. 6.

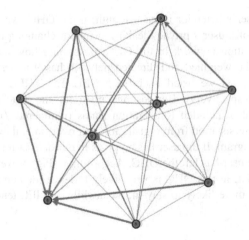

Fig. 1. Transitions of roles in the OHC

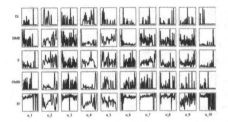

Fig. 2. (left) Privacy leaking trajectory of the 10 most active users belonging to role IEL

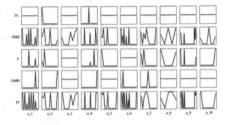

Fig. 3. (right) Privacy leaking trajectory of the 10 most active users belonging to role EL

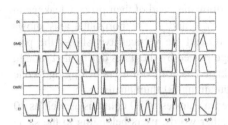

Fig. 4. (left) Privacy leaking trajectory of the 10 most active users belonging to role MIEL

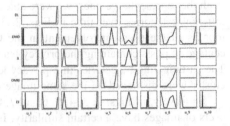

Fig. 5. (right) Privacy leaking trajectory of the 10 most active users belonging to role MIL

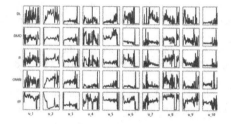

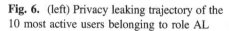

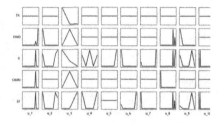

Fig. 6. (left) Privacy leaking trajectory of the 10 most active users belonging to role AL

Fig. 7. (right) Privacy leaking trajectory of the 10 most active users belonging to role IIL

5 Discussion and Conclusion

In this study, we collected and analyzed 4.3 million posts over 11 years from an OHC of breast cancer, identifying the privacy leakage and revealing the dynamics of users' behavior change. Using supervised machine learning techniques, we categorized posts into different categories of privacy leakage and found that emotional feelings are the most common way of users to expose themselves on the selected OHCs. Using an unsupervised clustering algorithm, we identified 6 different user roles in leaking privacy. After verifying the roles change over time, we drew the privacy leaking trajectory of active user samples from different clusters. The findings indicate that most users reduced the expression of emotional feelings gradually. On the contrary, the leakage of personal sensitive information about medical and identity were relatively increased over time.

This research helps to better understand the privacy leaking behavior of network users and has an important practical significance for platform management and users' privacy protection in OHCs. For example, OHCs can periodically prompt users who have been active for a long time to focus on protecting personal privacy and avoid unnecessary expressions about sensitive personal information when communicating with others. In conclusion, the outcome of the paper provides directions of protecting users in the OHCs.

Acknowledgements. Supported by Beijing Natural Science Foundation (9184032) and Program for Innovation Research in Central University of Finance and Economics.

References

1. Wang, X., Zhao, K., Street, N.: Analyzing and predicting user participations in online health communities: a social support perspective. J. Med. Internet Res. **19**(4), e130 (2017)
2. Acquisti, A., Brandimarte, L., Loewenstein, G.: Privacy and human behavior in the age of information. Science **347**(6221), 509–514 (2015)

3. Bol, N., et al.: Understanding the effects of personalization as a privacy calculus: analyzing self-disclosure across health, news, and commerce contexts. J. Comput.-Mediated Commun. **23**(6), 370–388 (2018)

4. Wolak, J., Finkelhor, D., Mitchell, K.J., Ybarra, M.L.: Online 'predators' and their victims: myths, realities, and implications for prevention and treatment. Am. Psychol. **63**(2), 111–128 (2008)

5. Zhang, X., Liu, S., Chen, X., Wang, L., Gao, B., Zhu, Q.: Health information privacy concerns, antecedents, and information disclosure intention in online health communities. Inf. Manag. **55**(4), 482–493 (2018)

6. Kordzadeh, N., Warren, J.: Communicating personal health information in virtual health communities: a theoretical framework. In: 2014 47th Hawaii International Conference on System Sciences, Waikoloa, HI, pp. 636–645 (2014)

7. Li, H., Sarathy, R., Xu, H.: Understanding situational online information disclosure as a privacy calculus. J. Comput. Inf. Syst. **51**(1), 62–71 (2010)

8. Yan, L., Tan, Y.: Feeling blue? Go online: an empirical study of social support among patients. Inf. Syst. Res. **25**(4), 690–709 (2014)

9. Chen, L.: Research on user privacy of network health community. Wirel. Internet Technol. **4**, 19–21 (2017)

10. Mulliner, C.: Privacy leaks in mobile phone internet access. In: 2010 14th International Conference on Intelligence in Next Generation Networks, pp. 1–6 (2010)

11. Ge, J., Peng, J., Chen, Z.: Your privacy information are leaking when you surfing on the social networks: a survey of the degree of online self-disclosure (DOSD). In: 2014 IEEE 13th International Conference on Cognitive Informatics and Cognitive Computing, pp. 329–336 (2014)

12. Michalopoulos, D., Mavridis, I.: Surveying privacy leaks through online social network. In: 2010 14th Panhellenic Conference on Informatics, pp. 184–187 (2010)

13. Irani, D., Webb, S., Li, K., Pu, C.: Modeling unintended personal-information leakage from multiple online social networks. IEEE Internet Comput. **15**(3), 13–19 (2011)

14. Du, S., et al.: Modeling privacy leakage risks in large-scale social networks. IEEE Access **6**, 17653–17665 (2018)

15. Zhao, L., Lu, Y., Gupta, S.: Disclosure intention of location-related information in location-based social network services. Int. J. Electron. Commer. **16**(4), 53–90 (2012)

Detection of Atrial Fibrillation from Short ECG Signals Using a Hybrid Deep Learning Model

Xiaodan Wu[1], Zeyu Sui[1], Chao-Hsien Chu[2(✉)], and Guanjie Huang[2]

[1] Hebei University of Technology, Tianjin 300130, People's Republic of China
xwu@hebut.edu.cn, szyaptx@163.com
[2] The Pennsylvania State University, University Park, PA 16802, USA
{chu, gzh8}@ist.psu.edu

Abstract. Atrial fibrillation (AF) is one of the most common arrhythmic complications. The diagnosis of AF usually requires long-term monitoring on the patient's electrocardiogram (ECG) and then either having a domain expert examine the results, or extracting key features and then using a heuristic rule or data mining method to detect. Recently, researchers have attempted to use deep learning models, such as convolution neural networks (CNN) and/or Long Short-Term Memory (LSTM) neural networks to skip the feature extraction process and achieve good classification results. In this paper we propose a hybrid CNN-LSTM model which uses the short ECG signal from the PhysioNet/CinC Challenges 2017 dataset to explore and evaluate the relative performance of four data mining algorithms and three deep learning architectures, CNN, LSTM and CNN-LSTM. Our results show that all deep learning architectures except LSTM performed much better than machine learning algorithms without needing complicated feature extraction. CNN-LSTM is the best performer, achieving 97.08% accuracy, 95.52% sensitivity, 98.57% specificity, 98.46% precision, 0.99 AUC (Area under the ROC curve) value and 0.97 F1 score. With proper design of configuration, deep learning can be effective for automatic AF detection while data mining methods require domain knowledge and an extensive feature extraction and selection process to get satisfactory results.

Keywords: Atrial fibrillation · Convolution Neural Network · Long Short-term Memory Neural Networks · Short ECG signals · Feature engineering · Data mining

1 Introduction

Atrial fibrillation (AF) is one of the most common arrhythmic complications. Patients with AF usually have symptoms such as palpitation, shortness of breath and weakness [1]. Studies have shown that patients with AF not only have a five-fold increased risk of stroke, but the sequelae caused by the stroke were more difficult to treat. No matter from the complications associated with AF, or the increasing morbidity year by year, there is no doubt that it has brought serious threat to human life, health and social life [2].

© Springer Nature Switzerland AG 2019
H. Chen et al. (Eds.): ICSH 2019, LNCS 11924, pp. 269–282, 2019.
https://doi.org/10.1007/978-3-030-34482-5_24

If a patient is suspected to have AF, the common approach for detecting AF is to deploy a 12 lead ECG monitoring in hospital, from which signals are captured and tested by a medical expert or key features are extracted and then use a heuristic rule or data mining method to detect AF. Many of the current studies used long-term ECG data from the MIT-BIH database [3] for AF detection. Moreover, the use of long-term ECG signals for AF detection will greatly increase the patient's medical expenses and time costs [2]. A number of researchers have conducted in-depth research on AF detection using short ECG signals, but these studies are dependent on the extraction of signal features (see Sect. 2 for details). However, because feature extraction is difficult and extremely susceptible to interference from noise, also requires the professional knowledge of a domain expert, and a large amount of time to adjust the extraction results. Although these algorithms have achieved satisfactory results in terms of the detection accuracy, the inefficiency and complication of feature extraction and selection is a major drawback.

Recently, researchers have attempted to use deep learning models to skip the feature extraction process while still achieving good classification results. The purposes and contributions of this study are three-fold: (1) examining how different options of deep learning architectures can be configured for automatic detection of AF; (2) evaluating the relative performance of different machine learning algorithms and deep learning architectures; and (3) exploring the difficulty and effect of using short ECG signals for AF detection. We used the dataset from the PhysioNet/CinC Challenges 2017 database [4] for training and testing. This data set has shorter recording time and less information. Deep neural network architectures examined including convolutional neural networks (CNN), Long Short-Term Memory networks (LSTM) and their combination, CNN-LSTM. These models need properly design and configure to obtain efficient and effective detection performance. To validate the relative performance of these models we used a 10-fold cross-validation experiment.

2   Related Works

Researchers have conducted extensive and in-depth research on automatic detection of AF from three aspects, statistical models, machine learning methods and deep learning methods. Some of the popular classifiers used include K-Nearest Neighbor (KNN), Decision Trees (ID 3), Support Vector Machine (SVM) and Random Forest (RF). Table 1 summarizes the characteristics and results of selected studies. Because the database, data processing and slitting methods used in these studies varied, the performance results as shown are for reference only may not be able to use for direct benchmark.

In order to relieve the difficulty in feature extraction of traditional statistical and machine learning methods, Hinton [5] used neural networks to learn features automatically from large-scale data. Compared to handmade features, features learned by neural networks have higher levels of feature abstraction, richer content and stronger expression ability. Therefore, some researchers have begun to use deep learning to detect AF.

Table 1. Summary of selected existing studies

Ref.	Data set used	Feature considered	Solutions methods	Se	Sp	Acc
[6]	MIT-BIH AF (partial)	Average P wave amplitude, variance, skewness and kurtosis, etc.	Statistical models	98.09%	91.66%	NA
[7]	MIT-BIH Arrhythmia (partial)	P-wave mode components, variance and standard deviation, etc.	EMD	96.00%	93.51%	NA
[8]	University of Virginia	Sample entropy of RR interval	Heuristic	91.00%	98.00%	NA
[9]	MIT-BIH AF	Variance of the RR interval	Heuristic	NA	NA	84.70%
[10]	MIT-BIH AF	Shannon entropy difference of the RR interval	ANN	85.31%	84.82%	85.39%
[11]	MIT-BIH AF (partial)	Short-term Fourier transform and Static wavelet Transform	DCNN	98.34%	98.24%	98.63%
[12]	PhysioNet/CiC Challenges 2017	Not necessary	CNN	NA	NA	85.99%
[13]	PhysioNet/CiC Challenges 2017 (partial)	Not necessary	MS-CNN	93.77%	98.77%	98.13%
[14]	MIT-BIH AF; MIT-BIH Arrhythmia; MIT-BIH NSR	1-beat segments of RRI	CNN-BiLSTM	98.98%	96.95%	NA

Note: Se: Sensitivity; Sp: Specificity; Acc: Accuracy; NA: Not available; EMD: Empirical Mode Decomposition; SVM: Support Vector Machine; ANN: Artificial Neural Network; CNN: Convolutional Neural Networks; DCNN: Deep CNN; MS-CNN: multi-scaled fusion of deep CNN; CNN-BiLSTM: Convolutional and Bi-directional Long Short-Term Memory Neural Networks; RRI: RR Intervals.

Afdala et al. [10] used the Shannon entropy difference of the RR interval to detect AF. Principal component analysis was used to determine the correlation of the features of each segment of the signal after segmentation of the ECG signal, and classification by ANN. The MIT-BIH AF database was used for experimental verification. Xia et al. [11] used short time Fourier transform (STFT) and static wavelet transform (SWT) to analyze ECG signal segments, and developed two DCNN models for evaluation. They validated the proposed algorithms using ECG data from the MIT-BIH AF database. Kamaleswaran et al. [12] proposed a 13-layer CNN model which was trained on 8528 short single-lead ECG recordings and evaluated on a test dataset of 3658 recordings.

Fan et al. [13] proposed a multi-scaled fusion of DCNN to screen out AF recordings from single-lead short ECG recordings. Andersen et al. [14] proposed a model combining the CNN and RNN to extract high level features from 1-beat segments of RR intervals in order to classify them as AF or normal sinus rhythm.

As can be seen from the previous research, deep learning algorithms have achieved good results in the detection of AF. However, [10, 11] still reply on feature extraction and have not fully exploited the advantages of deep learning algorithms in automatically learning data features. [12] have applied the deep learning algorithms, but only used simple neural network algorithms for applications. Only [13, 14] have improved and innovated the models. This paper proposes a more efficient hybrid deep neural network model to automatic AF detection.

3   Technical Background and Methodology

3.1   Convolutional Neural Network (CNN) Model

CNN is one of the most widely used deep learning models in the field of image recognition [15]. The model structure has been constantly optimized and has also played an outstanding role in the field of signal analysis. A CNN mainly consists of an input layer, convolutional layers, pooling layer, full connection layer and output layer. Data enters the neural network through the input layer. The CNN fully mines the features contained in the data by combining local perception area, sharing weight, and spatial or temporal down-samples, thereby improving the expression ability of the features and optimizing the network structure. The convolutional layer can be formulated as:

$$X_j^l = f\left(\sum_{i \in M_j} X_i^{l-1} * k_{ij}^l + b_j^l\right) \tag{1}$$

Where, X_j^l is the feature map of layer l, $*$ represents the convolution operation, M_j is the set of feature regions to be processed, k_{ij}^l is the convolution kernel, b_j^l is the bias term, and $f(*)$ represents activation function. The specific form of activation function is:

$$f(x) = max(0, x) \tag{2}$$

3.2   Long Short-Term Memory (LSTM) Networks

LSTM is an improved model of the recurrent neural network (RNN), which inherits most of the characteristics of RNN model and solves the problem of gradient disappearance due to gradual reduction in the process of gradient back propagation [16]. In addition, LSTM can acquire and store effective time series information through memory cells composed of input, output and forget gates. Therefore, it can achieve excellent performance in dealing with time series related problems. At time t, the process between the input and output of an LSTM unit is formulated as:

$$i_t = \sigma(W_{it}x_t + W_{hi}h_{t-1} + W_{ci}c_{t-1} + b_i) \tag{3}$$

$$f_t = \sigma(W_{xf}x_t + W_{hf}h_{t-1} + W_{cf}c_{t-1} + b_f) \tag{4}$$

$$c_t = f_t * c_{t-1} + i_t * tanh(W_{xc}x_t + W_{hc}h_{t-1} + b_c) \tag{5}$$

$$o_t = \sigma(W_{xo}x_t + W_{ho}h_{t-1} + W_{co}c_t + b_o) \tag{6}$$

$$h_t = o_t * tanh(c_t) \tag{7}$$

Where, σ represents the sigmoid function, * represents the multiplication between elements, and i, f, o, and c are input gate, forget gate, output gate, and memory cells respectively.

3.3   CNN-LSTM Model

Compared with the normal rhythm, the atrial fibrillation rhythm has structural differences such as the disappearance of the P wave and temporal differences such as arrhythmia. See Fig. 1. The CNN has shown good performance in learning structural features and the LSTM model can fully learn the temporal features of the data [15]. In order to make full use of the advantages of both neural network models to mine the hidden information in the data, this paper proposes a hybrid CNN-LSTM model that combines the strengths of two models. The structure is shown in Fig. 2. First, the ECG signal is randomly down-sampled to balance the amount of data between the AF and the normal signals. Then the model is initialized, and the results can be optimally obtained by automatically updating the parameters of the model after iterative training processes. After many experiments, we arrive at the optimal model structure.

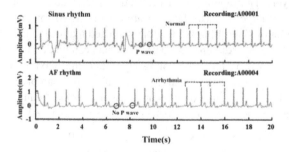

Fig. 1. Comparison of Sinus ECG signal and AF ECG signal

Input Layer. ECG records are digital signals whose shape vary with time and data forms. For deep learning models, the format of the input layer is a one-dimensional matrix form with variable length to facilitate input ECG signals with different lengths for training. As shown in Fig. 1. of digital signals in ECG records, the heart of a healthy person is regularly contracted and diastolic, and the rhythm is maintained at 60–100 times per minute, which is called the sinus rhythm. During AF, various parts of the heart exhibit a rapid and disorderly electrical activity, which is much faster than normal sinus rhythm, and the rhythm is irregular.

Convolutional Units. The convolutional layer makes full use of the local features of the data itself through local connection and weight sharing, thus reducing the number of parameters to be learned in the network. The convolution kernel in the convolutional layer works repeatedly in the whole field of perception, and the feature graph of the input signal is obtained through combining the bias and the activation function, thereby, extracting the local features of the signal. Since the information contained in the short-term ECG signals is relatively small, it is more difficult to learn the characteristics of these ECG signals compared with that of long-term ECG signals.

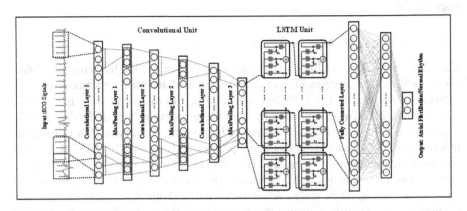

Fig. 2. Schematic diagram of CNN-LSTM structure

Maxpooling Layer. The dimension of the feature vector obtained after the convolution process is very large. If these features are directly used for classification, it will lead to long calculation time. Before using the extracted features to train the classifier, it is necessary to reduce their dimensions. The input data can be divided into several non-overlapping sub-regions by the maxpooling layer, and the maximum values of these sub-regions can be used to represent the features after downsampling. The size of the pool is set to 5 * 1. The computational complexity of the model can be greatly reduced and the robustness of the model to displacement can be enhanced.

Long Short-Term Memory Units. As a variant of the RNN, the LSTM neural network can effectively overcome the problems of gradient explosion or disappearance in the learning process mentioned above. The key rationale of the LSTM model is that it introduces a set of memory cells as hidden layer nodes of the network. The input and output of this unit are controlled by three structures: input gate, output gate and forget gate.

Fully Connected Layer. In order to enhance the nonlinear mapping ability and limit the size of the model, the model will be connected to a full connection layer after the features are extracted by the convolutional layer. The full connection layer can perceive global information and aggregate local features learned by the convolutional layer to form global features for the final classification task. Each neuron in this layer is interconnected with all the neurons in the previous layer, while the neurons in the same layer are not connected to each other. L2 Regularization is used to prevent overfitting and improve the generalization ability and computational efficiency of the model.

Output Layer. After the ECG signal is processed by the full connection layer, the Softmax function is used as the activation of the output layer to calculate the probability value of different categories, and the maximum probability value is output as the category of the ECG signal.

Dropout Strategy. The dropout strategy adopted in each layer of this study include maximum pooling and L2 regularization. They were used to prevent over-fitting, accelerate the training time and increase stability. We set the dropout rate as 0.5 according to pilot test, through the training effect of the model is not necessarily optimal.

4   Performance Evaluation

4.1   Dataset Used

We use the short electrocardiogram (ECG) signal contained in the PhysioNet/CinC Challenges 2017 database to evaluate the relative performance of the selected machine and deep learning models. The data set contains 5076 sinus rhythm (SR) ECG signals and 758 atrial fibrillation (AF) ECG signals. This is the latest data on short time single-lead ECG for AF. The duration of each ECG record in the database ranges from 9 s to 60 s. The average length of the AF signal is 31.6 s/strips, the average length of the sinus rhythm is 31.9 s/strips. The sampling frequency of the ECG signal is 300 Hz. They were collected and band pass filtered by the AliveCor device. Compared with the long-term ECG data in the commonly used MIT-BIH AF database, the ECG data used in this paper has shorter recording time, less information, and the signal features are not obvious, so the recognition is more difficult.

4.2   Data Splitting

In order to avoid the impact of extreme imbalance in the proportion of sinus ECG signals and AF ECG signals in the database on the experimental results, the random undersampling method was used to randomly select 760 signals from the SR data and conduct experimental verification together with 758 AF signals. The data distribution is shown in Fig. 3. We avoid reusing the training set for the validation and test sets to reduce overfitting. Due to the small amount of data we have, this paper adopts the 10-fold cross-validation method to divide the data into 10 samples on average, among which one-fold is selected as the test set and the remaining nine folds as the training set.

We repeated training 10 times to ensure that each piece of data can be tested as a test set, effectively avoiding over-fitting and under-learning, and thereby achieving a more convincing result.

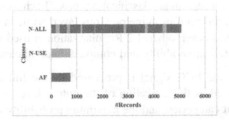

Fig. 3. Schematic diagram of data distribution and data quantity

4.3   Performance Metrics Used

In classification problems, an instance may be judged to be one of the following four types in a confusion matrix: True Positive (Positive sample predicted positive by the model), False Positive (Negative sample predicted positive by the model), False Negative (Positive sample predicted negative by the model) and True Negative (Negative sample predicted negative by the model).

From the confusion matrix, common performance metrics such as sensitivity (also known as recall), specificity, precision, accuracy and F1 score can be calculated to evaluate the classification results of the model. In addition, the ROC curve can be plotted as an aggregated indicator reflecting the sensitivity and specificity of continuous variables. The larger the area under the curve, the higher the accuracy of classification. For quantified purposes, the area under the ROC line, AUC value, is calculated to illustrate the classification results.

4.4   The Implementation Environment

The deep learning models were deployed in Keras and TensorFlow. In order to avoid the disappearance of the gradient and speed up the update of the weight, the cross entropy function is selected as the loss function, and the Adam function is selected as the optimization function [5]. The reason for using the Adam optimizer is that it is robust to the selection of hyperparameters to some extent [17] and it is usually very effective in previous experience. According to previous research experience [18] and our preliminary tests, good results can be obtained when the learning rate was set as 0.00001, $\beta_1 = 0.9$, $\beta_2 = 0.999$. We intend to further optimize these hyper-parameters in future studies. Machine learning algorithms are deployed in the Scikit-learn module which is a fast and efficient machine learning tool. We used a PC with 2.50 GHz i3-3120 M CPU and 16G RAM to perform the tests.

5 Results and Analyses

5.1 Hyperparameter Setting of the Proposed Models

To ensure that the proposed model can obtain the best classification results, the hyperparameter preference experiment was carried out to identify the activation function used and the optimal model structure. The specific hyperparameter settings are shown in Table 2.

Activation Function. Activation function is used to activate neurons and then learn signal features and reflect them to simulate human brain function and solve nonlinear problems. There are several functions commonly used, such as Sigmoid, Tanh and ReLU. Among them, the gradient of the sigmoid function will become very small when its input is far from the origin of coordinates, so the weight cannot be quickly corrected in the process of back propagation of the neural network, which leads to the problem of gradient disappearance. Moreover, the output of the sigmoid function is not zero-centered. This characteristic will cause the model to fluctuate during gradient descent operation and increase the training time. Although the effect of the Tanh function is better than the sigmoid function, it still has the problem of gradient disappearance. The computational complexity of the ReLU function is low, as no exponential operation is required, thus, the gradient disappearance problem is avoided, and its generalization effect and convergence speed are better than either the sigmoid function or the Tanh function. When selecting the activation function of the model, the activation function of the LSTM layer was first set as the default value, and different activation functions were tried in the convolution layer.

Table 2. Configuration of the deep learning models

Unit name	Hyperparameter name	Adjustment range
CNN unit	No. of convolution layers	1, 2, 3, 4, 5
	No. of filters	64, 128, 256, 512
	Kernel size	10, 20, 30, 40, 50, 60, 70, 80, 90, 100
	Activation function	Sigmoid, Tanh, ReLu
LSTM unit	No. of layers	1, 2, 3
	Output dimension	64, 128, 256, 512
	Activation function	Sigmoid, Tanh, ReLu
Full connection layer	No. of layers	1, 2, 3
	Output dimension	64, 128, 256, 512
	Activation function	Sigmoid, Tanh, ReLu

Optimal Model Structure. Through experimentation, we obtained the optimal structure of the deep learning models shown in Table 3.

Table 3. Detailed configuration of the proposed CNN-LSTM model

Layers	Layer types	Activation function	Kernel size	No. of filters	Output shape	No. of trainable parameters
0	Input: ECG signals	–	–	–	–	–
1	Convolution layer	ReLU	70 * 1	256	(None, 8931, 256)	18176
2	Maxpooling	–	8 * 1	256	(None, 2231, 256)	0
3	Convolution layer	ReLU	20 * 1	256	(None, 2212, 256)	1310976
4	Maxpooling	–	5 * 1	256	(None, 442, 256)	0
5	Convolution layer	ReLU	5 * 1	256	(None, 438, 256)	327936
6	Maxpooling	–	2 * 1	256	(None, 219, 256)	0
7	LSTM	tanh	–	–	(None, 219, 256)	525312
8	LSTM	tanh	–	–	(None, 219, 256)	525312
9	Global average pooling	–	–	–	(None, 256)	0
10	Fully-connected layer	ReLU	–	–	(None, 256)	65792
11	Fully-connected layer	ReLU	–	–	(None, 64)	16448
12	Fully-connected layer	ReLU	–	–	(None, 2)	130

5.2 Experimental Results, Analyses and Discussion

Overall Performance. The computational results are summarized in Table 4. As shown, most deep learning models except the LSTM model perform significantly better than machine learning models. Overall, the CNN-LSTM model has the best performance, achieving classification accuracy of 97.08%, and sensitivity, AUC and F1 of 95.52%, 0.99 and 0.97, respectively. In terms of running time, although the training time of CNN-LSTM model is the longest, it skips the time required for feature selection, and only takes 0.13 s to detect an AF signal, which considers as acceptable for practical applications.

Table 4. Summary of computational results

Types	Algorithm	Acc	Se (Recall)	Sp	Pre	AUC	F1	Computational time		
								Feature extraction	Train	Test
Machine learning	K-NN	67.22%	60.08%	100%	100%	0.80	0.75	26.43 s	0.14 s	0.03 s
	ID3	83.11%	79.52%	87.5%	88.59%	0.84	0.84	26.43 s	0.03 s	0.01 s
	SVM	77.48%	95.51%	69.95%	57.05%	0.83	0.71	26.43 s	0.83 s	0.03 s
	RF	90.39%	88.46%	92.47%	92.62%	0.90	0.90	26.43 s	0.98 s	0.02 s
Deep learning	CNN	91.24%	92.58%	90.46%	89.96%	0.96	0.91	No	8.52 h	5.38 s
	LSTM	61.72%	67.39%	60.28%	59.32%	0.75	0.63	No	23.61 h	19.97 s
	CNN-LSTM	**97.08%**	**95.52%**	**98.57%**	**98.46%**	**0.99**	**0.97**	**No**	**18.11 h**	**19.23 s**

Note: Acc: Accuracy; Se: Sensitivity; Sp: Specificity; Pre: Precision; s: seconds; m: minutes; h: hours

As can be seen from Fig. 4 that the deep learning model proposed in this paper reach a stationary state when iterating about 10 times, and the stability is extremely high. The loss function curve and the accuracy curve of the training set are basically coincident with the verification set, which proves that there is no over-fitting. In addition, the accuracy difference between the model testing and training is very small, which indicates that the model proposed in this paper has good generalization ability.

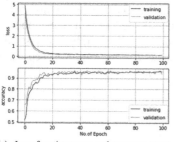
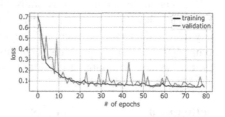

(a) Loss function curve and accuracy curve of CNN-LSTM model

(b) Loss function curve of CNN-LSTM model proposed by Andersen et al. [14]

Fig. 4. Loss function and accuracy curve

Although Fan et al. [13] and Andersen et al. [14] have also applied CNN to AF detection but they need to extract features first. Instead, we directly adopt the original ECG signal without any data segmentation or other processing methods. This reflects the efficiency and simplicity of our model. In addition, our models use variable length input, which is consistent with the actual situation. This can also be seen from Fig. 4 that the model proposed by Andersen et al. [14] is not as stable as the models proposed in this paper. The loss function curve of our models decreases smoothly during training. This is because we have adopted more preventive over-fitting methods than [14], and also adopted dropout strategy to make the model more stable.

Relative Performance of Machine Learning Algorithms. In order to examine the relative performance of the proposed deep learning algorithms, we select the popular data mining algorithms such as KNN, ID3, SVM and RF for comparison. In these experiments, RR interval of AF signal was extracted before ML classification was performed. This is one of the most common features used to detect AF. As shown in Table 4, the sensitivity of SVM is 95.51%, but F1 score is very low, which meant very unreliable in clinical applications. Through the RF achieved high and balanced accuracy and sensitivity, the results were still far lower than that of CNN-LSTM. The reason for this is that there are other features that appear in signals. Although random forests do more calculations through different trees, its classification accuracy is still inferior to the results of CNN-LSTM. This proves the efficiency and accuracy of the proposed deep learning algorithm in the detection of AF.

Relative Performance of Deep Learning Algorithms. The accuracy of the CNN model and LSTM model is only 91.24% and 61.72%, which is much lower than that of the hybrid CNN-LSTM model. Moreover, the LSTM model takes a very long time, more than 23 h to train. This is mainly because the CNN model is more suitable for learning structural features of signals, and the LSTM model is suitable for learning temporal features. However, AF signal has both the structural features of absolutely irregular RR interval and a typical continuous time series signal. Therefore, using either model alone will inevitably lose some features and lead to worse final detection effect. The CNN-LSTM model proposed in this paper can comprehensively learn the structural features and temporal features of ECG signals, so as to achieve a better classification effect. On the other hand, this study also shows that when using the deep learning model for classification tasks, we cannot simply use a certain single model, nor can we only rely on deepening the depth of the model to improve accuracy. Instead, we should comprehensively analyze the data features and combine multiple deep learning architectures to achieve the optimal classification results.

6   Conclusion and Future Works

AF is one of the most common arrhythmic disorders in the clinic with the prevalence rate of AF increasing significantly with age. Therefore, the research on early detection and auxiliary diagnosis of AF has important clinical and social significance for choosing patients' treatment strategies and improving the quality of treatment, reducing the incidence of critical illness and mortality.

In previous studies, machine learning algorithms have been adapted for automatic AF detection, but their results often depend on the proper extraction and selection of signal features. Although certain good results have been achieved, the inefficiency and complication of feature extraction and selection is still a major bottleneck.

In this study, the original ECG signal was directly used as input data, and then the CNN-LSTM model was proposed to detect AF automatically. Using 10-fold cross-validation, the sensitivity, specificity, precision, accuracy, AUC and F1 score of the experimental results reached 98.68%, 94.74%, 94.94%, 96.71%, 0.99 and 0.97 respectively, which are much better than those of the existing studies which used the same data set.

Heart disease has one of the highest morbidities and mortality rates in the world today. AF is one of the diseases, including coronary heart disease, stroke and many other diseases. Hence, we plan to collect more data on other types of heart disease in future research while taking full advantage of the autonomous learning features of the deep learning model, combined with many other methods, such as machine learning, to realize the automatic detection of more types of heart disease.

Since the single-lead short-term ECG signal used in this paper can be easily captured with the newer version of wearable devices such as the Apple smart watch series 4 and others, our next research direction will look at how the proposed deep learning algorithm can be adopted for mobile apps so that smartphones, such as Android or iOS phones, can be more conveniently used for real-time AF detection. In addition, ECG signals, especially heart rate variability, have been initially used to detect sleep apnea (with 90% accuracy), hypertension (with 82% accuracy), falls and diabetes (with 85% accuracy) [19], we will extend our deep learning approach to these potential applications as well.

Acknowledgement. This project was partially supported by the National Social Science Foundation of China (No. 17BGL087). Our deepest gratitude goes to the anonymous reviewers for their careful review, comments and suggestions that have helped improve this paper.

References

1. Rho, R.W., Page, R.L.: Asymptomatic atrial fibrillation. Prog. Cardiovasc. Dis. **48**(2), 79–87 (2005)
2. Jean-Yves, L.H., et al.: Cost of care distribution in atrial fibrillation patients: the COCAF study. Acc. Curr. J. Rev. **147**(1), 121–126 (2004)
3. Moody, G.B., Mark, R.G.: New method for detecting atrial fibrillation using R-R intervals. Comput. Cardiol. **10**, 227–230 (1983)
4. PhysioNet/CinC Challenges Database (2017). http://physionet.org/challenge/2017
5. Lecun, Y., Bengio, Y., Hinton, G.: Deep learning. Nature **521**(7553), 436 (2015)
6. Ladavich, S., Ghoraani, B.: Rate-independent detection of atrial fibrillation by statistical modeling of atrial activity. Biomed. Sig. Process. Control **18**, 274–281 (2015)
7. Maji, U., Mitra, M., Pal, S.: Automatic detection of atrial fibrillation using empirical mode decomposition and statistical approach. Procedia Technol. **10**(1), 45–52 (2013)
8. Lake, D.E., Moorman, J.R.: Accurate estimation of entropy in very short physiological time series: the problem of atrial fibrillation detection in implanted ventricular devices. Am. J. Physiol. Heart Circulatory Physiol. **300**(1), H319–H325 (2011)
9. Nuryani, N., et al.: RR-interval variance of electrocardiogram for atrial fibrillation detection. J. Phys.: Conf. Ser. **776**(1), 012105 (2016)
10. Afdala, A., Nuryani, N., Nugroho, A.S.: Automatic detection of atrial fibrillation using basic shannon entropy of RR interval feature. J. Phys. Conf. Ser. **795**(1), 012038 (2017)
11. Xia, Y., et al.: Detecting atrial fibrillation by deep convolutional neural networks. Comput. Biol. Med. **93**, 84–92 (2017)
12. Kamaleswaran, R., Mahajan, R., Akbilgic, O.: A robust deep convolutional neural network for the classification of abnormal cardiac rhythm using varying length single lead electrocardiogram. Physiol. Measur. **39**(3), 035006 (2018)

13. Fan, X., et al.: Multi-scaled fusion of deep convolutional neural networks for screening atrial fibrillation from single lead short ECG recordings. IEEE J. Biomed. Health Inform. **1**(1), 1744–1753 (2018)
14. Andersen, R.S., Peimankar, A., Puthusserypady, S.: A deep learning approach for real-time detection of atrial fibrillation. Expert Syst. Appl. **115**, 465–473 (2018)
15. Sermanet, P., Chintala, S., Lecun, Y.: Convolutional neural networks applied to house numbers digit classification. In: International Conference on Pattern Recognition (2013)
16. Gers, F.A., Schmidhuber, J., Cummins, F.: Learning to forget: continual prediction with LSTM. Neural Comput. **12**(10), 2451–2471 (2000)
17. Kingma, D., Ba, J.: Adam: a method for stochastic optimization. In: 3rd International Conference on Learning Representations (2015)
18. Ha, R., et al.: Axillary lymph node evaluation utilizing convolutional neural networks using MRI dataset. J. Digital Imaging **31**(1), 1–6 (2018)
19. Ballinger, B., et al.: DeepHeart: semi-supervised sequence learning for cardiovascular risk prediction. In: Proceedings of the Thirty-Second AAAI Conference on Artificial Intelligence (AAAI-18) (2018)

Gradient Boosting Based Prediction Method for Patient Death in Hospital Treatment

Yingxue Ma and Mingxin Gan[✉]

Donlinks School of Economics and Management, University of Science
and Technology Beijing, Beijing 100083, China
ganmx@ustb.edu.cn

Abstract. Patient death in hospital is a concerned topic that is vital for both patients and hospital. The prediction of patient death in hospital is a classification process with extreme label imbalance problem which seriously affects the prediction effect of general classification model. In this paper, we use an ensemble learning method to predict patient death, the coordination of base classifiers in ensemble model can alleviate this imbalance. Patient measurement data, disease data and treatment data are used as inputs of the model, and whether the patient is died in hospital is estimated. From several comparison experiments, we evaluated several machine learning methods for patient mortality, Gradient Boosting based ensemble method outperforms other methods in AUC and other evaluation criteria, the highest AUC achieved by Gradient Boosting Classifier is 0.846. Finally, we proposed several future work based on our research.

Keywords: Machine learning · Patient death · Mortality · Ensemble learning

1 Introduction

Patient death is a serious phenomenon in hospital, especially death during hospital treatment. High patient mortality indicates the poor service provided by hospital which has a negative impact on both patient's family and hospitals. Therefore, it is necessary to accurately predict the occurrence of patient death in hospital, which gives a warning signal to patients and their families and help patients understand their physical condition and disease development, and help hospital to develop personalized treatment plans for high risk patient and make preparations for patient death. In recent years, many in-hospital mortality prediction models have been generated based on various patient data [1, 2]. Overall, such models are based on a variety of medical data during patient's treatment to calculate the probability of patient death.

Generally, the researches about mortality prediction use medical information that reflect patient current condition [3], including patient demographic information (age, gender, marriage, insurance, etc.), treatment information (equipment, examinations and surgery), measurement information (temperature, heart rate, blood pressure, protein, etc.), disease information (historical disease and current disease) [4]. Some detailed information that reflect patient's condition such as disease severity and nursing

© Springer Nature Switzerland AG 2019
H. Chen et al. (Eds.): ICSH 2019, LNCS 11924, pp. 283–293, 2019.
https://doi.org/10.1007/978-3-030-34482-5_25

intensity during treatment also used in modeling process, for example, the sequence of heart rate, medical note generated by medical staff [5, 6].

General medical scoring system that estimate patient mortality include APACHE [7], SOFA [8], SAPS [9]. The prediction of patient death is always regarded as a binary classification problem in which patient death is represented by a label "1" which means patient died during hospital treatment, then label "0" means patient surviving until successfully discharge from hospital.

Simpler models, such as logistic regression, identify some factors as inputs that closely related to patient death, assuming a linear or non-linear relationship between these factors and the occurrence of patient death, then obtain a mapping from input to output [10]. However, this model have been proved by many deep studies that the hypothesis is unreasonable, and it tends to use semi-parametric or non-parametric models to predict mortality [10]. The requirement of models used in mortality prediction got satisfied due to the use of machine learning and deep learning methods. Machine learning methods used in patient death prediction including some classical classification methods such as support vector machine [10], bayesian classifier [10], decision tree [3], etc. and some ensemble learning methods such as random forest. Some deep learning methods are developed based on more detailed data such as sequential measurement data (heart rate, blood pressure, etc.), medical note generated from medical staff [11, 12].

Therefore, the patients are divided into two groups, the "death" patients and the "survival" patients. In fact, it is important to identify a patient whether he is in "death" group or in "survival" group. The ability of model to identify died patients is defined as sensitivity and the ability of model to identify survived patients is defined as specificity. An outstanding model should have both high sensitivity and specificity, the commonly used evaluation criteria is Area Under Roc (AUC) which combines both sensitivity and specificity.

In this paper, we use patient measurement data, disease data and treatment data as inputs to build a Gradient Boosting based ensemble learning model to prediction patient death in hospital and achieve better performance. This paper is organized as the following parts. In Sect. 2, we described the prediction problem and difficulties in prediction, and introduced the method used in death prediction. In Sect. 3, we provided the detail of our experiment process and result analysis. Section 4 contains several conclusions and future works of our research.

2   Problem Description and Method

2.1   Problem Definition and Challenge

The occurrence of death in ICU is a very rare medical accident in real world with tiny probability and patients are divided into two groups "alive" and "death", the occurrence of patient death is marked as "1", and "0" means not occur. Generally, the records number with label "1" is much smaller than label "0". This means there is a serious imbalance problem in ICU mortality prediction, this phenomenon also exists in our experiment dataset.

Therefore, the prediction of patient death in hospital is a binary classification problem with extreme imbalance in class labels. Patient information related to his hospitalization is often used as input to and obtain a possible outcome via a classification model (Fig. 1). In fact, the number of died patients is much smaller than the number of survived patients, which seriously affects the prediction effect of general classification model and is a challenge must to be solved in modeling process.

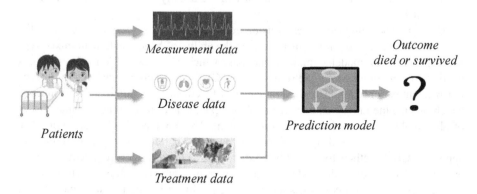

Fig. 1. Problem definition and prediction process for death prediction

2.2 Gradient Boosting Based Ensemble Learning Method for Death Prediction

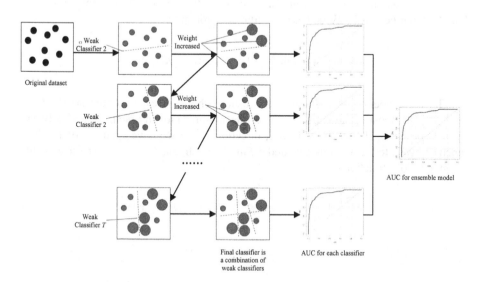

Fig. 2. Gradient boosting based ensemble learning model

Boosting is an enhanced learning model that contains M base learners Fm, each learner is trying to enhance the overall effect as shown in Fig. 2. The training of each base classifier is based on the error of previous. Gradient Boosting Classifier (GBC) considers additive models of the following form [13]:

$$F(x) = \sum_{m=1}^{M} \gamma_m h_m(x) \tag{1}$$

Where hm(x) are the basis functions which are usually called weak learners in the context of boosting.

Gradient Boosting (Tree) uses decision trees with fix size as weak learners. Usually, decision trees is valuable for boosting due to the ability of handle data with mixed type and the ability of model complex functions, which is suitable for model complex relationship and predict multiple source inputs. GBC constructs a decision tree for each independent patient sample, and minimize error by considering different decision trees, which include the unique characteristic of each patient and the common characteristics of all samples for mortality prediction problem. This enables GBC is specialized in solving the impact caused by the incline of dataset. Therefore, this paper attempts to apply the GBC method to mortality prediction to achieve a more efficient mortality prediction. GBC builds the additive model according greedy fashion, each model in Gradient Boosting is a compensation for the error made by the previous model. The training set of the latter model is the error generated by the previous classifiers.

$$F_m(x) = F_{m-1}(x) + \gamma_m h_m(x) \tag{2}$$

Where each the last added tree hm tries to minimize the loss L, which is a function of the actual output and the current prediction result given by the previous ensemble Fm−1, L can be flexibility defined for different problems.

$$h_m = \arg\min_{h} \sum_{i=1}^{n} L(y_i, F_{m-1}(x_i) + h(x_i)) \tag{3}$$

The initial model F0 is problem specific usually chooses the mean of the target values.

Gradient Boosting attempts to solve this minimization problem numerically via steepest descent: The steepest descent direction is the negative gradient of the loss function evaluated at the current model Fm−1 which can be calculated for any differentiable loss function:

$$F_m(x) = F_{m-1}(x) - \gamma_m \sum_{i=1}^{n} \nabla_F L(y_i, F_{m-1}(x_i)) \tag{4}$$

Where the step length γm is chosen using line search:

$$\gamma_m = \arg\min_{\gamma} \sum_{i=1}^{n} L\left(y_i, F_{m-1}(x_i) - \gamma \frac{\partial L(y_i, F_{m-1}(x_i))}{\partial F_{m-1}(x_i)}\right) \tag{5}$$

The algorithms for regression and classification only differ in the used concrete loss function.

Gradient Boosting Algorithm:	
1:	Initialize, set the first classifier F_0 for input x
2:	For m from 1 to M:
3:	Calculate negative gradient for each learning process
4:	Using base learner simulate the prediction value and actual value by minimizing the square error
5:	Calculate the loss function L generated by the current learner
6:	Using linear search determine the step length γ_m to minimize L
7:	Calculate current prediction F_m
8:	End for
9:	Obtain the final prediction result $F_m(x)$

3   Experiment and Result

3.1   Dataset

The experiment dataset is selected from eICU Collaborative Research Database (eICU-CRD) [14], input attribute set A = {temperature, respiratory rate, sodium, heartrate, meanbp, ph, hematocrit, creatinine, albumin, pao2, pco2, bun, glucose, bilirubin, fio2, hepatic failure, metastatic cancer, leukemia, immunosuppression, cirrhosis, elective surgery, activetx, ima, ventday1, oobventday1, oobintubday1, ptcawithin24h} (The details of experiment data is shown in https://mimic.physionet.org/mimictables/admissions/). In real medical dataset, not all attributes are measured and recorded, and some times, due to the careless of medical staff there may exist some blurred records, then data missing is an unavoidable problem. When dealing with missing values, we ignore the records with missing values.

3.2   Comparison Methods and Criteria

In order to confirm the improvement of ensemble methods on hospital mortality prediction, we conducted several extend experiment using the following comparison methods.

Extra Trees Classifier (ETC) [10]: In extremely randomized trees, randomness goes one step further in the way splits are computed. As in random forests, a random subset of candidate features is used, but instead of looking for the most discriminative thresholds, thresholds are drawn at random for each candidate feature and the best of these randomly-generated thresholds is picked as the splitting rule.

Bernoulli NB (BNB) [15]: Bernoulli Naive Bayes implements the naive Bayes training and classification algorithms for data that is distributed according to multivariate Bernoulli distributions.

Decision Tree Classifier (DTC) [3]: Decision Tree is a non-parametric supervised learning method used for classification and regression. The goal is to create a model that predicts the value of a target variable by learning simple decision rules inferred from the data features.

MLP Classifier (MLP) [10]: Multi-layer Perceptron is a supervised learning algorithm that can learn a non-linear function for either classification or regression.

Linear SVC (LSVC) [10]: Linear Support Vector is similar to SVC with parameter kernel = 'linear', but it has more flexibility in the choice of penalties and loss functions and should scale better to large numbers of samples.

We use 5-fold cross-validation to conduct our method (10-fold cross-validation is generally used, with the tiny number of death samples, in order to ensure that the data used in each experiment is sufficient to show regularity, we choose five-fold cross-validation), experiment data is randomly divided into 5 parts, select 4 parts as the training set and remain part as the test set for each experiment. The average of 5 test results was used to evaluate the classification effect of different methods. We obtain four statistics after each experiment, true positive (tp), false positive (fp), false negative (fn) and true negative (tn). Then we use five criteria related to the above factors to evaluate each method, included: Area Under ROC (AUC), Classification Accuracy (CACC), Precision, Recall and F1-score.

tp: patient died in hospital and the predicted result is died in hospital.
tn: patient survived to discharge and the predicted result is survive.
fp: patient died in hospital while the predicted result is survive.
fn: patient survived to discharge and the predicted result is died in hospital.

CACC represents the correct prediction ability of classifiers, we calculate CACC using the following formula. As shown in Fig. 4(4), GBC gets the highest CACC among all comparison methods, in order to further contrast the prediction accuracy of different methods, we draw ROC curve and calculate AUC for different methods.

$$CACC = \frac{t_p + t_n}{t_p + t_n + f_p + f_n} \tag{6}$$

Receiver Operating Characteristic (ROC) is a criteria to measure the classification sensitivity of a classifier, using above four statistics, we obtain the sensitivity and specificity. Sensitivity is true positive rate (TPR) that indicates the proportion that the actual died patients in the predicted died patients, specificity indicates the proportion that the actual survived patients in the predicted died patients and using false positive rate (FPR) to represent it. The horizontal axis of the ROC curve is FPR and the vertical axis is TPR, therefore, the closer distance of the point on the ROC curve to (0, 1), the higher accuracy of the classifier.

$$TPR = \frac{t_p}{t_p + f_n} \tag{7}$$

$$FPR = \frac{f_p}{f_p + t_n} \tag{8}$$

Precision, recall and F1-score are usually used in classification task while not commonly used in medical event prediction, in order to compare and analyze the advantages and shortcomings of comparison methods we further calculate precision, recall and F1-score for different methods and results are shown in Fig. 4.

$$Precision = \frac{t_p}{t_p + f_p} \tag{9}$$

$$Recall = \frac{t_p}{t_p + f_n} \tag{10}$$

$$F1 - score = \frac{2 * Precision * Recall}{Precision + Recall} \tag{11}$$

3.3   Experiment Results

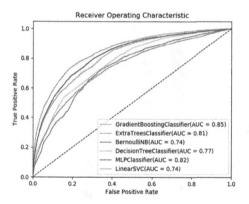

Fig. 3. The curve of area under ROC for different methods

Table 1. AUC of different methods

Methods	AUC (mean $\pm$ std)	Improvement
GBC	**0.846 $\pm$ 0.005**	–
ETC	0.809 $\pm$ 0.005	4.574%
BNB	0.734 $\pm$ 0.004	15.259%
DTC	0.764 $\pm$ 0.007	10.733%
MLP	0.819 $\pm$ 0.004	3.297%
LSVC	0.741 $\pm$ 0.013	14.170%

Experiment results are shown in Table 1 and Fig. 2. GBC achieves the best AUC at 0.846, which gets the best performance in hospital mortality prediction task. GBC uses decision tree as the base classifier, compared with DTC and ETC, GBC gets improvements of 10.733% and 4.574% respectively, the integration of base classifiers dose contribute to higher classification accuracy, which indicates the cooperation of different trees fully considers the classification cost of error prone samples in classification process and achieves higher accuracy when distinguish the dead patients and survived patients. GBC gets 14.170% improvement compared with LSVC, which reflects the non-linear relationship between patient attributes and the occurrence of death in hospital. In Fig. 3, ROC curve of GBC is always at the top of all curves, this means GBC has the highest sensitivity for identify died patients and specificity for identify survived patients followed by MLP, ETC and DTC. For LSVC and BNB, LSVC has higher sensitivity and specificity than BNB when the FPR is lower than 0.23, while BNB outperforms than LSVC when FPR is higher than 0.23, then when the accepted FPR is lower than 0.23, LSVC is more suitable for hospital mortality prediction than BNB.

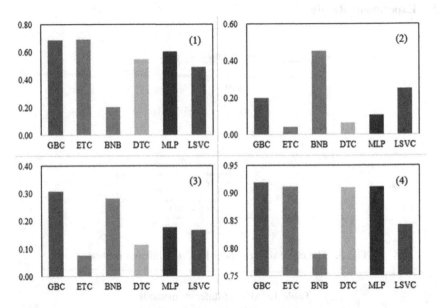

Fig. 4. Prediction performance of comparison methods. (1) Precision. (2) Recall. (3) F1-score. (4) CACC.

Besides AUC, in term of precision in Fig. 4(1), GBC achieves 0.685 close to 0.691 of ETC. the higher the precision, the better the accuracy of prediction. As for recall, the higher the recall the stronger ability of classifier to identify died patients, from Fig. 4(2) we can see BNB gets the highest recall which indicates BNB can be used as the single predictor for high risk patients with high probability of death. F1-score is a combination of accuracy and recall, overall, GBC gets the best comprehensive performance with the highest F1-score of 0.31 followed by BNB, MLP, LSVC, DTC and ETC and CACC of 0.919. The ensemble based methods GBC and ETC are apparently better than other methods which indicates the integration of base classifiers contribute to the imbalance classify process.

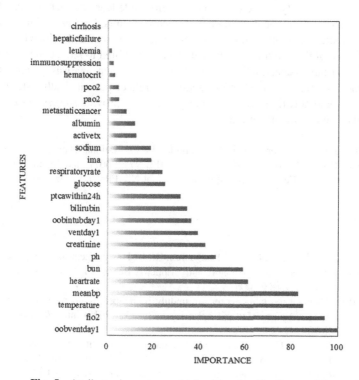

Fig. 5. Attributes importance obtained by classification model.

It is generally believed that the results obtained by a classifier are credible if it obtain an AUC of 0.8 or higher. Then, we use GBC to evaluate the importance of each attribute in input data from the modeling process. The contribution of each attribute to the prediction result is shown in Fig. 5. For easy presentation and understanding, we normalized the importance of each attribute according to maximum normalization. In Fig. 5, oobventday1 contributes the most to prediction and it corresponds to 100% importance in horizontal axis. We can get the descending list of the attributes importance from the bottom to top of the figure. Among them, the top K most important attributes can be used as indicators to monitor the status of patients for doctors and patients.

4 Conclusion

In this paper, we used Gradient Boosting Classifier to predict patient death in hospital. We try to solve the imbalance challenge using the integration of multiple base classifiers, after experiment on real dataset we obtain a better performance in classification sensitivity and specificity. Which indicates the ensemble learning methods can be used in patient death prediction and obtain the acceptable results. Finally, we give a ranking list for the importance of attributes. In the future, many works can be done to enrich our research. Inputs of the classification model can be simplified to reduce the computation cost, while attributes selection is another challenge. When analysis patient death in hospital, the important medical information that reflect patient death risk should be identified and paid attention, which also can be used to provide suggestion for doctors and patients to make treatment plans.

Acknowledgments. This work was partly supported by the National Natural Science Foundation of China (Nos. 71871019, 71471016, 71531013, 71729001), and by the Fundamental Research Funds for the Central Universities under Grant No. FRF-TP-18-013B1.

References

1. Si, Y., Xiao, X., Xiang, S., Liu, J., Mo, Q., Sun, H.: Risk assessment of in-hospital mortality of patients with epilepsy: a large cohort study. Epilepsy Behav. **84**, 44–48 (2018). https://doi.org/10.1016/j.yebeh.2018.04.006
2. Jones, R.P.: Hospital mortality scores are unduly influenced by changes in the number of admissions. Eur. J. Intern. Med. **51**(February), e35–e37 (2018). https://doi.org/10.1016/j.ejim.2018.02.010
3. Rau, C.S., Wu, S.C., Chien, P.C., et al.: Prediction of mortality in patients with isolated traumatic subarachnoid hemorrhage using a decision tree classifier: a retrospective analysis based on a trauma registry system. Int. J. Environ. Res. Public Health **14**(11), 1–10 (2017). https://doi.org/10.3390/ijerph14111420
4. Sadeghi, R., Banerjee, T., Romine, W.: Early hospital mortality prediction using vital signals. Smart Health **9–10**, 265–274 (2018). https://doi.org/10.1016/j.smhl.2018.07.001
5. Jo, Y., Lee, L., Palaskar, S.: Combining LSTM and latent topic modeling for mortality prediction (2017). http://arxiv.org/abs/1709.02842
6. Chettipally, U., Mohamadlou, H., Jay, M., et al.: Using electronic health record collected clinical variables to predict medical intensive care unit mortality. Ann. Med. Surg. **11**, 52–57 (2016). https://doi.org/10.1016/j.amsu.2016.09.002
7. Kho, M.E., McDonald, E., Stratford, P.W., Cook, D.J.: Interrater reliability of APACHE II scores for medical-surgical intensive care patients: a prospective blinded study. Am. J. Crit. Care **16**(4), 378–383 (2007)
8. Lee, J., Cho, Y.J., Kim, S.J., et al.: Who dies after ICU discharge? Retrospective analysis of prognostic factors for in-hospital mortality of ICU survivors. J. Korean Med. Sci. **32**(3), 528–533 (2017). https://doi.org/10.3346/jkms.2017.32.3.528
9. Le Gall, J.-R., Lemeshow, S., Saulnier, F.: A new simplified acute physiology score (SAPS II) based on a European/North American multicenter study. JAMA **270**(24), 2957–2963 (1993). https://doi.org/10.1001/jama.1993.03510240069035

10. Purushotham, S., Meng, C., Che, Z., Liu, Y.: Benchmark of deep learning models on large healthcare MIMIC datasets. ArXiv e-prints (2017). https://doi.org/10.1016/j.jbi.2018.04.007
11. Grnarova, P., Schmidt, F., Hyland, S.L., Eickhoff, C.: Neural document embeddings for intensive care patient mortality prediction (2016). http://arxiv.org/abs/1612.00467
12. Zhang, Y., Jiang, R., Petzold, L.: Survival topic models for predicting outcomes for trauma patients. In: Proceedings - International Conference on Data Engineering, pp. 1497–1504 (2017). https://doi.org/10.1109/icde.2017.219
13. Jain, D.S., Gupte, S.R., Aduri, R.: A data driven model for predicting RNA-protein interactions based on gradient boosting machine. Sci. Rep. **8**(1), 1–10 (2018). https://doi.org/10.1038/s41598-018-27814-2
14. Pollard, T.J., Johnson, A.E.W., Raffa, J.D., Celi, L.A., Mark, R.G., Badawi, O.: The eICU collaborative research database, a freely available multi-center database for critical care research. Sci. Data **5**, 1–13 (2018). https://doi.org/10.1038/sdata.2018.178
15. Zhao, L., Huang, M., Yao, Z., Su, R., Jiang, Y., Zhu, X.: Semi-supervised multinomial naive bayes for text classification by leveraging word-level statistical constraint. In: Proceedings of the 30th Conference on Artificial Intelligence (AAAI 2016), pp. 2877–2883 (2016). http://www.aaai.org/ocs/index.php/AAAI/AAAI16/paper/viewFile/12019/12036

Extracting Medication Nonadherence Reasons with Sentiment-Enriched Deep Learning

Jiaheng Xie[1(✉)], Xiao Liu[2], Daniel Zeng[1], and Xiao Fang[3]

[1] University of Arizona, Tucson, USA
xiej@email.arizona.edu
[2] University of Utah, Salt Lake City, USA
[3] University of Delaware, Newark, USA

Abstract. Medication nonadherence (MNA) refers to the behavior when patients do not take medications as prescribed. Adverse health outcomes of MNA cost the U.S. healthcare systems $290 billion annually. Understanding MNA and preventing harmful outcomes are an urgent goal for researchers, practitioners, and the pharmaceutical industry. Past years have witnessed rising patient engagement in social media, making it a cost-efficient and heterogeneous data source that can complement and deepen the understanding of MNA. Yet, such dataset is untapped in existing MNA studies. We present the first study to identify MNA reasons from health social media. Health social media analytics studies face technical challenges such as varied patient vocabulary and little relevant information. We develop the Sentiment-Enriched DEep Learning (SEDEL) to address these challenges. We evaluate SEDEL on 53,180 reviews about 180 drugs and achieve an F1 score of 90.18%. SEDEL significantly outperforms state-of-the-art baseline models. This study contributes to IS research in two aspects. First, we formally define the MNA reason mining problem and devise a novel deep-learning-based approach; second, our results provide direct implications for healthcare practitioners to understand patient behaviors and design interventions.

Keywords: Deep learning · Text mining · Health analytics · Medication nonadherence

1 Introduction

Medication nonadherence (MNA) is defined as the extent to which patients do not follow the recommendations for prescribed treatments (Hugtenburg et al. 2013). Despite evidence that medical therapy prevents death and improve quality of life, numerous studies have shown that only 50% of patients with chronic diseases adhere to medication regimens as prescribed (Traverso and Langer 2015).

The adverse outcomes of MNA include increased dosage of medications, the risk of adverse effects, physician frustration, misdiagnoses, unnecessary treatment, and exacerbation of disease and fatality (Dunbar et al. 2008). The high morbidity and mortality caused by MNA lead to estimated deaths 125,000 per year and 33% to 69% of medication-related hospital admissions in the United States. MNA accounts for $290

© Springer Nature Switzerland AG 2019
H. Chen et al. (Eds.): ICSH 2019, LNCS 11924, pp. 294–301, 2019.
https://doi.org/10.1007/978-3-030-34482-5_26

billion in preventable annual costs in the United States and 19% of all drug-related emergency room visits (Traverso and Langer 2015).

Understanding the reasons for MNA is the premise for formulating practical and effective strategies to improve medication adherence. In this study, we aim to propose and evaluate an innovative computational approach to understanding MNA reasons for given medications.

Existing studies investigated MNA reasons via surveys. They focus on a single medication or a particular disease class. They are also provider-centered, as direct and timely communications from patients are difficult to obtain. This dominant provider perspective poses a significant barrier to translating these MNA reasons into real-world settings because providers have little control over the actual adoption of daily medication-taking behaviors. A recent survey shows that 61% of adults search online for health information, and 59% of them have participated in health social media platforms (Pew Internet Research 2009). Due to the anonymous nature of health social media discussions, patients are more willing to elaborate their reasons for adhering to or discontinuing medications. This large-scale patient self-reported information creates an unprecedented prospect for studying MNA reasons from patients' decision-making standpoint. To our best knowledge, no social media approach has been taken in MNA studies.

Researchers still face significant challenges to understanding MNA reasons via social media data despite its enormous potential. Patients usually describe diseases and symptoms with a wide range of consumer health vocabulary in social media. Irrelevant discussions in health social media are abundant, far outnumbering those about MNA. Motivated by the critical need for advanced social media analytics techniques to understand MNA reasons, we propose a novel computational method – Sentiment-Enriched DEep Learning (SEDEL) – that addresses patients' varied health vocabulary, scarce MNA-related narratives, and feature sparsity issues.

Our study makes the following contributions to information systems literature and methodology as well as healthcare practice. First, we formally define the MNA reason mining problem, which is generalizable to research questions that aim to detect underlying factors of decisions such as consumer retention, technology adoption, and crowdfunding project investment. Second, we design a Sentiment-Enriched DEep Learning (SEDEL) that could also be generalized to analyze any other opinionated text, such as product reviews, physician reviews, and commentary articles. Third, our empirical findings complement behavioral health science research in medication non-adherence with comprehensive patient experience data. Tailored preventive actions and interventions can be taken accordingly to improve disease management.

2 Literature Review

Prior studies used surveys to investigate reasons for medication nonadherence (MNA). The identified MNA reasons include low health literacy, poor communications between providers and patients, complex medication plan, forgetfulness, cost, severe mental illness, adverse events (Sørensen et al. 2012; Bosworth et al. 2011; Gellad et al. 2009). Investigations on MNA reasons are still limited for the following reasons. First, patients are reluctant to reveal their true adherence status in the surveys or cohorts, and it is time-consuming to obtain research subjects (Krousel-Wood et al. 2009). Second, MNA interventions currently achieve a low success rate, mainly because the interventions are not tailored to address the adherence barriers of individual patients (Gellad et al. 2009).

Health big data from social media platforms addresses the above limitations and makes innovative projects possible. These social media platforms efficiently gather a large volume of timely feedback and opinions from a diverse patient population. To harness the value from social media, we aim to develop advanced and scalable text analytical methods.

Extracting information from health social media is a non-trivial task, as patients use colloquial and diverse expressions about similar medical terms. Deep learning methods have achieved remarkable success in various natural language processing problems. They have also dramatically improved the state-of-the-art in speech recognition (Graves et al. 2013), visual object recognition (LeCun et al. 2015), drug discovery (Chen et al. 2018), and many other domains. We, therefore, develop a deep learning-based method to extract MNA reasons from health social media and address the challenge of patient vocabulary.

3 Research Method

The proposed MNA reason mining approach takes a sentence from social media as the input. The sentiment-enriched word embedding model converts the input sentence to a vector-based embedding sequence. The forward embedding sequence and backward embedding sequence are concatenated and passed to the SEDEL model to identify the MNA reason expressions. Sentiment-enriched word embedding vectors of terms recognized as MNA reason expressions are extracted and analyzed in the reason clustering step. K-means is utilized to cluster those embedding vectors into the meaningful categories of MNA reasons.

The sentiment-enriched word embedding represents each word's sentiment along with the likelihood of co-occurrence of common words. Let S be a training sequence $[w_1, w_2,...,w_T]$. Variable w_i denotes word i in the sequence. The training objective is to maximize the objective function L_s in Eq. 1. Parameter T denotes the number of training words. Parameter c is the window size (the words that appear within distance of c words). Variables w_{t+j} are the words surrounding w_t. Parameter $senti_t$ is the sentiment score of w_t ($senti_t \in [-1, 1]$). Negative score refers to negative sentiment, while positive score refers to positive sentiment.

$$L_s = \frac{1}{T} \sum_{t=1}^{T} \frac{1}{e^{senti_t}} \sum_{-c \leq j \leq c, j \neq 0} \log p\left(w_{t+j}|w_t\right) \tag{1}$$

Different from the standard word embedding, our objective function integrates the sentiment score of words, as contained in the decreasing function $\frac{1}{e^{senti_t}}$. As MNA reasons are associated with negative sentiment, words with negative sentiment have a higher probability of indicating MNA reasons. The decreasing function $\frac{1}{e^{senti_t}}$ could amplify the effect of negative words on the objective function. The new objective function L_s computes the likelihood of the neighboring words that appear together while prioritizing the negative words. This new objective function effectively distinguishes MNA reasons from other words in similar contexts.

To effectively extract sparse MNA-related information, we utilize a bidirectional-LSTM deep learning architecture. Iour model, we devise an element-wise multiplier β to modify the standard LSTM unit. This multiplier allows the weight on each dimension of the embedding vector to adjust according to its relevance to MNA reasons. The multiplier in the LSTM unit addresses the challenge to extract sparse MNA relevant terms by strengthening useful information and degrading irrelevant information in the learning process. The LSTM unit takes the sentiment-enriched word embedding as the input. The computational process in the LSTM unit with the sentiment-enriched word embedding is summarized in Eqs. 2–7.

Sentiment-enriched word embedding:

$$\boldsymbol{\beta} \odot \boldsymbol{x}^{(t)} = \left[\beta_1 x_1^{(t)}, \beta_2 x_2^{(t)}, \ldots \ldots, \beta_{300} x_{300}^{(t)} \right]^T; \tag{2}$$

Sentiment-enriched input gate:

$$i_s^{(t)} = sigm\left(\boldsymbol{W}_i \boldsymbol{\beta} \odot \boldsymbol{x}^{(t)} + \boldsymbol{U}_i \boldsymbol{h}_s^{(t-1)} + \boldsymbol{b}_i \right); \tag{3}$$

Sentiment-enriched forget gate:

$$f_s^{(t)} = sigm\left(\boldsymbol{W}_f \boldsymbol{\beta} \odot \boldsymbol{x}^{(t)} + \boldsymbol{U}_f \boldsymbol{h}_s^{(t-1)} + \boldsymbol{b}_f \right); \tag{4}$$

Sentiment-enriched output gate:

$$o_s^{(t)} = sigm\left(\boldsymbol{W}_o \boldsymbol{\beta} \odot \boldsymbol{x}^{(t)} + \boldsymbol{U}_o \boldsymbol{h}_s^{(t-1)} + \boldsymbol{b}_o \right); \tag{5}$$

Sentiment-enriched memory cell:

$$c_s^{(t)} = tanh\left(\boldsymbol{W}_u \boldsymbol{\beta} \odot \boldsymbol{x}^{(t)} + \boldsymbol{U}_u \boldsymbol{h}_s^{(t-1)} + \boldsymbol{b}_u \right); \tag{6}$$

Sentiment-enriched hidden state:

$$h_s^{(t)} = o_s^{(t)} \odot tanh\left(i_s^{(t)} \odot c_s^{(t)} + f_s^{(t)} \odot c_s^{(t-1)} \right). \tag{7}$$

Variable $\boldsymbol{x}^{(t)}$ is the current input, and $\boldsymbol{h}^{(t-1)}$ is the previous hidden state. Parameters $\boldsymbol{W}$, $\boldsymbol{U}$, and $\boldsymbol{b}$ are weight parameters with values between 0 and 1.

The β parameter is learned through the training process in the LSTM unit. The β parameter assigns different weights to different dimensions in the input embedding vector according to its relevance to the learning objective. Parameters W, U, and b assign different weights to different word embedding inputs. Such a difference is facilitated by using different computation: the computation between β and $x^{(t)}$ is element-wise multiplication $\odot$, thus allowing weight adjusting within the input embedding vector $(x_1^{(t)}, x_2^{(t)}, \ldots, x_{300}^{(t)})$. The computation between W and $\beta \odot x^{(t)}$ is matrix multiplication, thus enabling weight adjusting on the word level $(x^{(t)})$.

Since the bidirectional structure has two reversed LSTM layers, the output of this step is the concatenation of the forward hidden state $h_s^{(t)}$ and backward hidden state $h_s^{(t)'}$. Each forward or backward hidden state has 128 dimensions. We condense useful information from the 300 dimensional $x^{(t)}$ to 128 dimensions in the LSTM cell. The learning rate in the gradient descent is 0.1. The dropout rate is 0.2. Finally, a Softmax layer (Eq. 8) is stacked on the top to predict the word type (MNA reason or not). Variable y is the predicted word type. Variable x is the input to the Softmax layer or the output of the sentiment-enriched BLSTM layer. Parameter w is the weight parameter.

$$p(y = j|x) = \frac{e^{x^T w_j}}{\sum_{k=1}^{K} e^{x^T w_k}}. \tag{8}$$

4 Empirical Analyses

Our research testbed comes from a leading health IT platform, WebMD. We collected all the drug reviews from the start of WebMD in January 2005 to October 2016. The dataset encompasses 233,325 sentences from 53,180 reviews about 180 drugs. We randomly selected 4,500 reviews and annotated them for MNA reason extraction model training and evaluation. Five expert annotators with a bioinformatics background independently read the reviews and tagged MNA reasons in five batches. IOB labeling scheme is used to assign tags for each word in the sentence. We use Cohen's kappa for this inter-annotator reliability measurement (Blackman and Koval 2000). The kappa value is 0.98 for the MNA reason annotation, indicating excellent reliability.

We evaluate our models on the annotated dataset, with 4,500 sentences as the training set and 900 sentences as the test set. We repeat the training procedure for each model 50 times and report the average performance in Table 1.

Table 1. Evaluation of SEDEL

Method	Precision	Recall	F1 score
SVM	29.30%	53.60%	37.90%
CRF	**94.00%**	46.30%	62.04%
RNN	77.71%	77.95%	77.69%
LSTM	83.06%	79.06%	80.93%
BLSTM	84.80%	82.36%	83.49%
SEDEL (Ours)	87.29%	**93.27%**	**90.18%**

Our proposed SEDEL model achieves the highest recall (93.27%) and F1 score (90.18%). Our SEDEL model has the most salient advantage in the recall.

The SEDEL model identifies 24,832 MNA reason expressions from the entire research data. These reason expressions are the actual phrases that patients used in health social media. We group similar reason expressions using k-means to interpret the reason expressions comprehensively. Table 2 shows the MNA reason types and their percentages in our results.

Table 2. MNA reason type

MNA reason type	Description	Percentage
Adverse event	The medication has adverse events or leads to complications	56.76%
Drug switching	The patient switches to another medications by his/herself	15.21%
Complex medication plan	The medication regimen is complicated. The patient does not like the complicated procedure or forget to take the medication	13.98%
Social influence	The patient stops the medication because his/her peers/caregivers/friends/professionals encourage the patient to stop	7.67%
Cost prohibitive for patient	The price of the drug is too high, or insurance does not cover. The patient cannot afford	0.93%
Medication ineffectiveness	The medication is ineffective, so the patient stops it	0.09%
Low health literacy	The patient discontinues the medication because of low health literacy	0.04%
Specific population	The patient stops/reduces the medication because the patient is pregnant/is a child/has liver disease and more	0.02%
Others	Others	5.30%

The results shed valuable insights to understanding patients' intentional medication nonadherence behavior. Adverse drug events are the most common type of reason for patients to discontinue medications. Not only have adverse drug events resulted in medical injuries among patients, they also significantly affect patients' adherence decision and indirectly hamper disease management. Healthcare providers and pharmaceutical companies should be aware of the leading adverse drug events associated with nonadherence and provide alternatives timely. In addition, social influence and specific population have not been noted by prior survey studies. These additional findings may be attributed to the unique advantage of social media where social influence is a remarkable impact on patients.

5 Conclusion

Our research objective was to understand why patients do not adhere to their medications. We designed a patient and drug-specific analytical framework to collect relevant data from health social media, extract the medication nonadherence (MNA) reasons, and analyze the types of reasons. Consistent with design science research methodology, we performed a series of empirical analyses to test the components of our framework rigorously and to compare it with the state-of-the-art methods. Evaluation results show that our SEDEL model outperforms all the baseline models in recognizing relevant MNA reasons. We design the sentiment-enriched deep learning approach for patient- and drug-specific MNA reason detection. We are among the first to analyze MNA reasons in a large-scale health social media data. Many of these reasons have not been noted by previous studies. The MNA reasons detected by our framework allow the stakeholders to gain insight from patients' perspective and understand the patients' thoughts about medications. Knowing the precise reasons for individual patients and drugs, proactive measures and early preventions can be applied to avoid harmful outcomes caused by MNA.

References

Blackman, N.J.-M., Koval, J.J.: Interval estimation for Cohen's kappa as a measure of agreement. Stat. Med. **19**(5), 723–741 (2000). https://doi.org/10.1002/(sici)1097-0258 (20000315)19:5%3c723:aid-sim379%3e3.0.co;2-a

Bosworth, H.B., et al.: Medication adherence: a call for action. Am. Heart J. **162**, 412–424 (2011). https://doi.org/10.1016/j.ahj.2011.06.007

Chen, H., Engkvist, O., Wang, Y., Olivecrona, M., Blaschke, T.: The rise of deep learning in drug discovery. Drug Discovery Today **23**(6), 1241–1250 (2018). https://doi.org/10.1016/j.drudis.2018.01.039)

Dunbar, S.B., Clark, P.C., Quinn, C., Gary, R.A., Kaslow, N.J.: Family influences on heart failure self-care and outcomes. J. Cardiovasc. Nurs. **23**(3), 258–265 (2008). https://doi.org/10.1097/01.jcn.0000305093.20012.b8

Gellad, W.F., Grenard, J., Mcglynn, E.A.: A review of barriers to medication adherence: a framework for driving policy options, RAND Corporation, Santa Monica (2009)

Graves, A., Jaitly, N., Mohamed, A.: Hybrid speech recognition with deep bidirectional LSTM, pp. 273–278. University of Toronto, Department of Computer Science, 6 King's College Rd, Toronto, M5S 3G4, Canada (2013)

Hugtenburg, J.G., Timmers, L., Elders, P.J., Vervloet, M., van Dijk, L.: Definitions, variants, and causes of nonadherence with medication: a challenge for tailored interventions. Patient Prefer. Adherence **7**, 675–682 (2013). https://doi.org/10.2147/ppa.s29549

Krousel-Wood, M., Islam, T., Webber, L.S., Re, R.N., Morisky, D.E., Muntner, P.: New medication adherence scale versus pharmacy fill rates in seniors with hypertension. Am. J. Manag. Care **15**(1), 59–66 (2009). http://www.ncbi.nlm.nih.gov/pubmed/19146365

LeCun, Y., Bengio, Y., Hinton, G.: Deep learning. Nature **521**, 436–444 (2015). https://doi.org/10.1038/nature14539

Pew Internet Research: 61% of American adults look online for health information. Pew Research Center (2009). http://www.pewinternet.org/2009/06/11/61-of-american-adults-look-online-for-health-information/. Accessed 8 Sept 2017

Sørensen, K., et al.: Health literacy and public health: a systematic review and integration of definitions and models. BMC Public Health **12**(1), 80 (2012). https://doi.org/10.1186/1471-2458-12-80

Traverso, G., Langer, R.: Perspective special delivery for the gut. Nature **519**(7544), S19–S19 (2015). https://doi.org/10.1038/519s19a

Perceived Usefulness of Online Health Information Sharing: A Text Mining Based Empirical Research

Jiahui Gao[1], Zhenyan Xiao[2], Jingxuan Cai[1], Chengkun Wang[1], and Jiang Wu[1(✉)]

[1] School of Information Management, Center for E-Commerce Research and Development, Wuhan University, Wuhan 430072, Hubei, China
jiangw@whu.edu.cn
[2] International Business School, Jinnan University, Guangzhou 510632, Guangdong, China

Abstract. Due to the concern for time and geological distance, the seeking health information behavior of patients has transferred from offline to online. The online information sharing has become one of the main sources where patients can obtain health information. Thus, the usefulness of online health information sharing is particularly important. This paper collects 9902 articles in health field from Baidu Experience which is the largest experience-sharing platform in China. It adopts the Information Adoption Model to analyze the impact of author's credibility, text attributes, and pictures on the perceived usefulness of health-information-sharing articles. Results show that readers prefer long articles with more detailed health information and negative emotions in articles can affect readers' perception of usefulness. And illustrated articles are easier to receive recognition. On the other hand, authors' motivation in utilitarianism may lead to challenges to quality of the health-information-sharing article and, in return, hinder readers from adopt the information from the article.

Keywords: Information sharing · Online health information · Perceived usefulness · Information adoption · Baidu Experience

1 Introduction

Information sharing refers to the process in which community users voluntarily share the information they have to help other users solve problems [1]. It is a process of information exchange and information sublimation between users to create new knowledge [2], and a process in which information is acquired, understood and reused.

Baidu Experience is one of the key channels for netizens to obtain information. According to *Chinese netizens' demand for popular science search behavior report (first quarter of 2019)* [3] by Baidu Data Research Center and China Research Institute for Science Popularization, health and medical services ranked first among all search topics, accounting for 66.83% of all online information searches with an increase of 35.63% over the same period of last year. Thus, users are in increasingly demand for health information sharing in virtual communities.

© Springer Nature Switzerland AG 2019
H. Chen et al. (Eds.): ICSH 2019, LNCS 11924, pp. 302–308, 2019.
https://doi.org/10.1007/978-3-030-34482-5_27

Existing literatures in information sharing mainly focus on three aspects: the motivation of information providers [4], behavior of information receivers [5], and the information content [6]. Few scholars explore the online health information sharing. Only a few researches have focused on online health community that are for health field specifically. Therefore, this paper takes the health information sharing on Baidu Experience as the research object, and studies the influencing factors of the perceives usefulness of online health information sharing in the comprehensive virtual community.

2 Theoretical Background and Hypothesis

2.1 Information Adoption Model

Sussman et al. come up with the Information Acceptance model (IAM) [7]. According to IAM, information quality and information source credibility will affect the perceived usefulness of information, thus affecting the information adoption behavior.

For health information on virtual information-sharing platform, the attributes of text and pictures would have influences on the perception of information quality. The attributes of information providers, such as identity, reputation, and influence, would affect information seekers' perception from the aspect of information source credibility. Thus, we constructed a model about the influencing factors of the perceived usefulness of online health information sharing from these three aspects, as shown in Fig. 1.

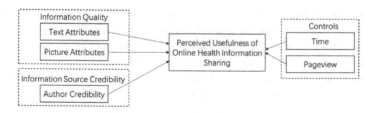

Fig. 1. Theoretical model

2.2 Hypothesis Development

Text Attributes of the Article. Cue Utilization Theory argues that consumers will use all cues they see or hear to assist decision-making. There are two types of cues: task-relevant cues and affection-relevant Cues [8]. In the case of online health information seeking, users with health information needs are equivalent to consumers with consumption needs. They hope to obtain cues that can meet their needs by browsing articles shared by other users in the community of Baidu Experience. Therefore, this theory can be applied in the context of online health information sharing.

Task-relevant Cues refer to the functional features of text that are consistent with information seeker's need. These cues can effectively meet information seekers' needs.

Hypothesis 1. The functional features of the text (H1a: the perception of text; H1b: the cognition of text; H1c: the health characteristics of text; H1d: the social characteristics of text) would impact the perceived usefulness of the health information.

Affection-relevant Cues refer to the emotional characteristics embodied in the text, which will affect the sense of identity of information seekers [9]. Thus, we propose:

Hypothesis 2. The emotional features of the text would impact the perceived usefulness of the health information.

The writing style will significantly affect the reader's experience, and then affect the reader's judgment of information. In the text, different parts of speech, such as verbs and adverbs, take on different tasks, enrich the language and convey more information [10]. Meanwhile, the length of text reflects the amount of information carried by the article, which will affect the information seeker's perception of usefulness.

Hypothesis 3. The writing style (H3a: the use of verb; H3b: the use of adverb; H3c: the length of text) would impact the perceived usefulness of the health information.

Picture Attributes of the Article. Compared to plain text, pictures are more intuitive, which can carry more information and enhance memory. Moreover, pictures can make up for the lack of sensory experience brought by the virtual environment for information seekers, which would exert a positive impact on decision-making by influencing the emotional response of information seekers [11]. Thus, we propose:

Hypothesis 4. The number of pictures would positively impact the perceived usefulness of the health information.

Author Credibility. Health information seekers, in most case, are lack of expertise in this field. It is difficult for them to judge the information reliability directly. They will make decisions through the edge path - information source credibility. Previous studies have proved that information source credibility is an important antecedent variable for knowledge adoption [12], including information providers' identities, reputation, and influence in the virtual community. Thus, we propose:

Hypothesis 5. The credibility of author (H5a: identity; H5b: reputation; H5c: influence) would impact the perceived usefulness of the health information.

3   Research Methodology

3.1   Data Collection

This paper develops a Python program to collect data from Baidu Experience. A total of 12,364 article were collected from 156 tags related to health care on Baidu Experience. After dismissing irrelated records and missing valve, the sample includes 9902 articles. The variable descriptions are presented in Table 1.

Table 1. Definitions and description statistics of variables

Dimension		Variable	Definition
Dependent variable	Perceived information usefulness	*Like*	The number of thumb up obtained by the sharing text
Text attributes	Perception	*Percept*	The proportion of words expressing the perceptual process
	Cognition	*CogMech*	The proportion of words expressing the cognitive process
	Health characteristic	*Body*	The proportion of words expressing something about body
		Health	The proportion of words expressing something about health
		Sexual	The proportion of words expressing something about sexuality
		Ingest	The proportion of words expressing something about ingestion
	Social characteristic	*Social*	The proportion of words expressing social relation
	Affection-relevant cues	*PosEmo*	The proportion of words expressing positive emotion
		NegEmo	The proportion of words expressing negative emotion
	Writing style	*Verb*	The proportion of verbs
		Adverb	The proportion of adverbs
		WordCount	The number of words in the text
Picture attributes	Picture feature	*PicNum*	The number of pictures in the article
		PicSq	The square of the number of images in the article
Author attributes	Identity	*Au_Contracted*	Authors who have signed up with Baidu and get paid for sharing articles
		Au_Prior	Authors who have the privilege that their sharing text can be first reviewed by Baidu
		Au_SelfCommended	Authors who can recommend their sharing articles as quality articles
		Au_Productive	Authors who publishes many sharing articles
	Reputation	*Au_Reputation*	The reputation of the author in the community
		Au_Wealth	The amount of wealth that can be consumed in community
	Influence	*Au_Followers*	The number of the author's followers
Control variable	Time	*Time*	Days after the article being published
	Pageview	*ViewsNum*	The number of views of the article

3.2   Model Specification

To analyze the impact of author's credibility, text attributes, and pictures attributes on the perceived usefulness of information-sharing article, the formula below is applied.

$$\begin{aligned}
Like = \ & \alpha + \beta1Percept + \beta2CogMech + \beta3Body + \beta4Health + \beta5Sexual + \beta6Ingest + \\
& \beta7Social + \beta8PosEmo + \beta9NegEmo + \beta10Verb + \beta11Adverb + \beta12WordCount + \\
& \beta13PicNum + \beta14PicSq + \beta15Au\_Contracted + \beta16Au\_Prior + \\
& \beta17Au\_SelfCommended + \beta18Au\_Productive + \beta19Au\_Reputation + \beta20Au\_Wealth \\
& + \beta21Au\_Followers + \beta22Time + \beta23ViewsNum + \varepsilon
\end{aligned}$$

$$(1)$$

The dependent variable is Like. The perceived information usefulness of the information-sharing article is measured by the number of Like. Since Like is a non-negative integer, and the variance is much larger than the mean value, the negative binomial regression model is adopted for estimation. Independent variables include three dimensions: text attributes, picture attributes, and author attributes. We leveraged the latest version of TextMind to construct measures of text content.

4   Results and Analysis

The estimation results of Negative Binomial Regression Model are shown in Table 2. Through VIF, we can know there is no serious collinearity issues among variables.

Table 2. Model estimation results

	Model 1	Model 2	Model 3	VIF
Percept	−0.050*(0.023)	−0.046*(0.023)	−0.053*(0.023)	1.18
CogMech	0.009 (0.031)	0.002 (0.031)	0.024 (0.030)	1.97
Body	0.030 (0.023)	0.028(0.023)	0.021(0.022)	1.18
Health	0.048*(0.022)	0.042(0.022)	0.049*(0.022)	1.14
Sexual	−0.044*(0.019)	−0.045*(0.019)	−0.051**(0.019)	1.02
Ingest	−0.138***(0.023)	−0.139***(0.023)	−0.118***(0.023)	1.18
Social	0.089**(0.026)	0.084**(0.026)	0.096***(0.026)	1.47
PosEmo	−0.013(0.022)	−0.017(0.022)	−0.026(0.022)	1.13
NegEmo	−0.077***(0.020)	−0.075***(0.020)	−0.070***(0.020)	1.10
Verb	−0.076**(0.026)	−0.079**(0.026)	−0.059*(0.027)	1.68
Adverb	0.069*(0.027)	0.067*(0.027)	0.060*(0.027)	1.67
WordCount	0.089***(0.025)	0.107***(0.026)	0.085**(0.025)	1.14
PicNum		0.177**(0.053)	0.243***(0.054)	6.13
PicSq		−0.230***(0.054)	−0.265***(0.054)	5.87

(*continued*)

Table 2. (*continued*)

	Model 1	Model 2	Model 3	VIF
Au_Contracted			−0.090**(0.028)	2.00
Au_Prior			−1.055***(0.190)	1.66
Au_SelfCommended			1.883***(0.294)	1.38
Au_Productive			0.088**(0.028)	1.58
Au_Reputation			−0.229***(0.033)	2.13
Au_Wealth			−0.253***(0.029)	1.59
Au_Followers			0.572***(0.081)	1.50
Time	−0.012 (0.022)	0.001(0.023)	−0.050*(0.024)	1.34
ViewsNum	0.0002***(0.000)	0.0002***(0.000)	0.0002***(0.000)	1.01
Constant	0.949***(0.024)	0.944***(0.024)	0.922***(0.024)	
observations	9902	9902	9902	
Log likelihood	−20100.412	−20092.016	−19933.859	

*p<0.05, **p<0.01, ***p<0.001

For the core path of information quality, the functional features of the text (H1a: the perception of text; H1c: the health characteristics of text; H1d: the social characteristics of text), the negative emotions behind text and the writing style of the text have significant impact on the perceived usefulness for the information seeker. To the picture attributes, the number of pictures is advantages of the health information sharing articles.

As for the edge path of the information source credibility, the credibility of author has significant impact on the perceived usefulness for the information seekers.

5 Discussion and Conclusion

From this paper we can know that when the information seekers browse the health sharing articles, the more health-related term in the articles, the longer the article is, their seeking task can be easily achieved. The social relations mentioned in the article will arouse a strong feeling of empathy for the information seeker. However, they dislike words related to sex out of privacy issue and full of negative emotions.

Once the information provider signs a contract with the platform, he/she would enjoy special privileges, either obtaining monetary rewards for the sharing behavior or getting priority over the articles review process which makes the information seeker doubt the author's motivation in sharing and the quality of sharing. On the contrary, the author's self-recommendation reflects author's self-confidence. High productivity reflects the author's capability and knowledge level. The number of fans represents the author's influence. All these factors are indirectly cues for information quality. Information seeks prefer to adopt articles published by authors with above characteristics.

This study contributes to the platforms and authors. The results carry guiding importance in improving the perceived usefulness of health information sharing. It can better help information seekers and promote the dissemination of health information.

Acknowledgments. This research is supported by the National Natural Science Foundation of China (No.71573197).

References

1. Yong, S.H., Kim, Y.G.: Why would online gamers share their innovation-conducive knowledge in the online game user community? Integrating individual motivations and social capital perspectives. Comput. Hum. Behav. **27**(2), 956–970 (2011)
2. Hooff, B.V.D., Ridder, J.A.D.: Knowledge sharing in context: the influence of organizational commitment, communication climate and CMC use on knowledge sharing. J. Knowl. Manage. **8**(6), 117–130 (2004)
3. China Association for Science and Technology: Chinese netizens' demand for popular science search behavior report (first quarter of 2019), 26 April 2019/05 September 2019. http://www.cast.org.cn/art/2019/4/26/art_1281_94546.html
4. Kankanhalli, A., Tan, B.C.Y., Wei, K.K.: Contributing knowledge to electronic knowledge repositories: an empirical investigation. MIS Q. **29**(1), 113–143 (2005)
5. Ma, M., Agarwal, R.: Through a glass darkly: information technology design, identity verification, and knowledge contribution in online communities. Inf. Syst. Res. **18**(1), 42–67 (2007)
6. Galunic, D.C., Rodan, S.: Resource recombinations in the firm: knowledge structures and the potential for schumpeterian innovation. Strateg. Manag. J. **19**(12), 1193–1201 (2015)
7. Sussman, S.W., Siegal, W.S.: Informational influence in organizations: an integrated approach to knowledge adoption. Inf. Syst. Res. **14**(1), 47–65 (2003)
8. Parboteeah, D.V., Valacich, J.S., Wells, J.D.: The influence of website characteristics on a consumer's urge to buy impulsively. Inf. Syst. Res. **20**(1), 60–78 (2009)
9. Hwang, K.O., et al.: Social support in an Internet weight loss community. Int. J. Med. Informatics **79**(1), 5–13 (2010)
10. Krishnamoorthy, S.: Linguistic features for review helpfulness prediction. Expert Syst. Appl. **42**(7), 3751–3759 (2015)
11. Yoo, J., Kim, M.: The effects of online product presentation on consumer responses: a mental imagery perspective. J. Bus. Res. **67**(11), 2464–2472 (2014)
12. Allen, W.: The influence of source credibility on communication effectiveness. Audiov. Commun. Rev. **1**(2), 142–143 (1953)

Clinical Informatics and Clinician Engagement

Character-Based Deep Learning Approaches for Clinical Named Entity Recognition: A Comparative Study Using Chinese EHR Texts

Jun Wu[1(✉)] ⓘ, Dan-rui Shao[1] ⓘ, Jia-hang Guo[1] ⓘ, Yao Cheng[1] ⓘ,
and Ge Huang[2] ⓘ

[1] School of Economics and Management, Beijing University
of Posts and Telecommunications, Beijing, China
wujun1127@126.com
[2] School of Software, Beijing University of Posts and Telecommunications,
Beijing, China

Abstract. Previous studies on clinical sequence labeling require large amounts of task specific knowledge in the form of handcrafted features. Using latest development in representation learning, this paper introduces BERT embedding as character based pretrained model and incorporates it with three competing deep learning models (CNN-LSTM, Bi-LSTM and Bi-LSTM-CRF) to extract clinical entities from electronic health records. A comparative evaluation based on CCKS-2017 task 2 benchmark dataset reveals that: (1) BERT embedding not only facilitates improving performance of clinical NER tasks but also acts as good candidate for building end-to-end NER model requiring no feature engineering from Chinese EHR. (2) Bi-LSTM-CRF has the highest performance, i.e., 93% F1 scores when it uses BERT embedding. This paper may enhance our understanding of how to use BERT embedding in clinical NER researches.

Keywords: Clinical NER · BERT embedding · Deep learning · Comparative evaluation

1 Introduction

Fast adoption of the Electronic health record (EHR) systems in China has witnessed the growing magnitudes of clinical information or knowledge entailed in EHR. Although well-organized clinical results may improve the quality of diagnose accuracy, many health records in Chinese EHR systems are in unstructured text format. How to effectively extract clinical information containing the syndrome of the patient, as well as treatment during the hospitalization is a key concern for the academicians and practitioners to facilitate the establishment of smart health information systems.

In natural language processing (NLP) research, named entity recognition (NER) is generally viewed as a relatively mature field since many studies have been performed in the past decades. However, NER application in Chinese EHR environment is still challenging for several reasons: First, different hospitals have different clinical record

© Springer Nature Switzerland AG 2019
H. Chen et al. (Eds.): ICSH 2019, LNCS 11924, pp. 311–322, 2019.
https://doi.org/10.1007/978-3-030-34482-5_28

preferences which hinder the labelling standardization of the named entity extraction. Second, NER technologies developed for English text may not suitable for Chinese text. Especially, unique language attributes mixed with traditional Chinese and modern Chinese exist when dealing with clinical NER problems.

This study tries to explore NER on Chinese clinical discharge summaries using latest developed approaches. Specifically, our purpose is to conduct several character-based deep learning methods and compare their performances for extracting the terms or units, which are further used in smart healthcare information systems, as the fundamental task in Chinese clinical NLP. The extracted clinical entities vary from patient related healthcare information to clinical related treatment information. Because of the correct identification of clinical entities is important for the maximum utilization of EHR, High accuracy of clinical NER would facilitate the successive NLP works like clinical knowledge graph building, automatic classification of diseases or treatments, etc.

Extant researches focusing on NER from clinical EHR can be categorized into three different approaches: dictionary lookup-based string matching, feature-based supervised learning and neural network-based deep learning. Traditionally, string matching methods have been used for named entities extraction in situations like identification of medical risk factors [1] and adverse drug event [2]. In addition, Conditional random fields (CRF), a probabilistic sequence labeling model has been used to generate the most likely label sequence corresponding to a given word sequence input. Several studies reporting comparison performances reveal that CRF outperforms string matching methods when identifying clinical events from English, Sweden and Korean clinical documents [3–5]. In contrast, Kenneth's research reported that, when large scale dataset available, dictionary-based NER method can be comparable with the supervised learning-based model. One disadvantage of dictionary-based string matching and CRF method lies in that both of them need entity feature. In view of the limitations of relatively complex feature selection, high cost of manual annotation, and great dependence on clinical text structure and standardization, neural network-based deep learning methods have emerged in recent years and exhibited improved accuracy in clinical NER tasks.

In this paper, we compare the performance of character level neural network sequence labeling method with and without language embedding to extract the complex clinical entities from the EHR texts. Specifically, taking Convolution Neural Network (CNN) and Long Short-Term Memory Network (CNN-LSTM), Bi-directional Long Short-Term Memory (Bi-LSTM) and Bi-directional Long Short-Term Memory and Conditional Random Field (Bi-LSTM-CRF) as the competing model, using Bidirectional Encoder Representations from Transformers (BERT) as the pretrained character embedding, comparative performance evaluations are conducted based on CCKS-2017 task 2 benchmark dataset.

Potential contributions of this paper are twofold: First, we demonstrate how to combine BERT embedding with CNN-LSTM, Bi-LSTM and Bi-LSTM-CRF model and apply them in clinical NER field. Second, we assess the comparative performance among three models on the CCKS-2017 task 2 dataset. The computational results suggest that BERT embedding approach performs remarkably well compared to no pretrained embedding models. By incorporating BERT embedding into basic models, an end- to-end data driven approach can be used to improve the accuracy of clinical entities extraction.

The rest of the paper proceeds as follows: Sect. 2 details the character-based deep learning approaches like CNN-LSTM, Bi-LSTM-CRF and BERT embedding. Section 3 presents the analysis and results. In Sect. 4, some noteworthy observations related to performance implications among character-based deep learning approaches are further discussed. Conclusions as well as future directions are drawn in the final section.

2 Related Work

This section first introduces latest representation learning model—BERT and its application in NER domain. We further review recently used state-of-the-art deep learning models like CNN-LSTM and Bi-LSTM-CRF and their potential in clinical NER field.

2.1 Bert

Language representation model pre-training has shown to be effective for improving many successive NLP tasks [6, 7]. Pretrained embeddings varying from word to sentence and paragraph are widely used as features in a downstream model. BERT's model architecture is a multi-layer bidirectional Transformer encoder and uses bidirectional self-attention. For a given token in a single text sentence or a pair of text sentences, BERT's input representation is constructed by summing the corresponding token, segment and position embeddings. This is given in Fig. 1.

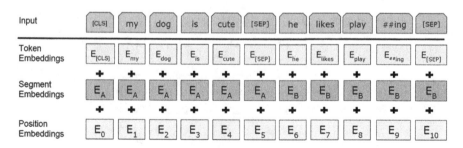

Fig. 1. BERT input representation

Using masked language model to train a deep bidirectional representation and pre-training a binarized next sentence prediction task to understand sentence-pair relationships, the pre-trained model of BERT can be finetuned on token tagging task like NER. Given its excellence performance in English NLP tasks, we can adapt it to Chinese clinical NER domain. Specifically, we can feed the tokenized input word into the final hidden representation layer of the model, i.e., BERT embedding, and use the hidden state corresponding to the sub-token as input to the state-of-the-art NER deep learning model.

2.2   Bi-Directional LSTM and CRF

Traditional high-performance sequence labeling model like Conditional Random Fields (CRF) is a kind of linear statistical model which rely heavily on manually defined features and task specific resources. Since task-specific knowledge is costly to develop [7], this make it difficult for sequence labeling models to adapt to new tasks or new domains.

Deep neural networks, especially recurrent neural networks (RNNs) are theoretically viewed as capable to capturing long-distance dependencies while in practice, they fail due to the gradient vanishing/exploding problems [8, 9]. As variant of RNN, Long Short-Term Memory network (LSTM) is designed to cope with gradient vanishing problems and composed of three multiplicative gates which control the proportions of information to forget and to pass on to the next time step [10]. For sequence labeling tasks, it is beneficial to have access to both past (left) and future (right) contexts. Since the LSTM's hidden state takes information only from past, bi-directional LSTM (Bi-LSTM) is proposed to present each sequence forwards and backwards to two separate hidden states to capture past and future information and the two hidden states are then concatenated to form the final output [11].

For sequence labeling tasks, it is beneficial to consider the correlations between labels in neighborhoods and jointly decode the best chain of labels for a given input sentence [12]. Therefore, the bi-directional LSTM is further advanced to a bi-directional LSTM-CRF to capture the dependency between nodes in the output layer. The Bi-LSTM-CRF model architecture is presented in Fig. 2.

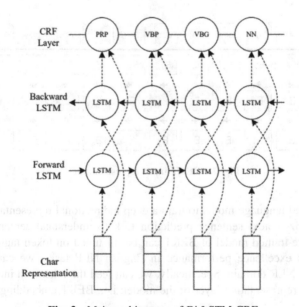

Fig. 2. Main architecture of Bi-LSTM-CRF

2.3   Cnn-Lstm

CNN-LSTM stands for Convolutional Neural Network (CNN) and Long Short-Term Memory network (LSTM) [13]. The CNN-LSTM architecture uses CNN as a front-end function to extract input data and then combine LSTM for sequence prediction [14, 15]. Prior studies have shown that, as a feedforward neural network, CNN can effectively extract morphologically valid information from characters of words and encode it into neural representations.

CNN-LSTM model (Fig. 3) combination consists of an initial convolution layer which will receive word embeddings as input. Its output will then be pooled to a smaller dimension which is then fed into an LSTM layer [16, 17]. The intuition behind this model is that the convolution layer will extract local features and the LSTM layer will then be able to use the ordering of said features to learn about the input's text ordering [18].

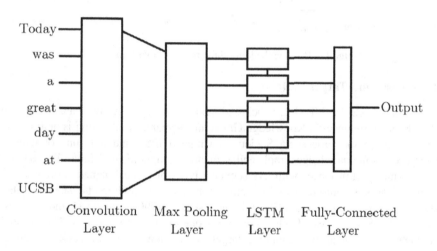

Fig. 3. CNN-LSTM model

3   Methods

In this section we will propose three approaches for our Chinese clinical NER tasks and evaluate their performance when using or not using pre-trained BERT embedding. In addition, we also introduce our benchmark dataset and target entity.

3.1   End-to-End Deep Learning Model for Clinical NER

Our evaluation model (Fig. 3) combination consists of an initial BERT embedding over each tokenized EHR text data input. The output of the hidden representation layer is then fed into three competing model, i.e., CNN-LSTM, Bi-LSTM and Bi-LSTM-CRF which we expect will extract local features. Finally, the output of the model will be BIO sequence label. After training the model, we can predict the clinical NER based on the test dataset (Fig. 4).

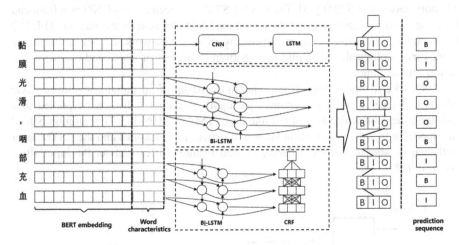

Fig. 4. BERT embedding three neural network model

3.2   Dataset and Target Entity

We use the CCKS-2017 Task 2 benchmark dataset[1] to conduct our evaluations. The 2017 China Conference on Knowledge Graph and Semantic Computing is held by the Chinese Information Processing Society of China (CIPS), and it is one of famous conference about knowledge graph and semantic computing in China. The dataset contains annotated instances with five semantic types of clinical named entities which include diseases, symptoms, examinations, treatments, and body parts. The annotated instances are partitioned into 1198 training instances (7906 sentences) and 398 test instances (2118 sentences). Each instance has one or several sentences. The original text content as well as representative target entities are shown in Tables 1 and 2, respectively.

Table 1. Examples of original clinical EHR texts

Original text (in Chinese)	Annotated text with target entities		
	Entities	Start	End	Notations
1.入院后完善相关检验检查，给予神经外科护理常规，Ⅱ级护理，普食，自动体位2.查血尿常规，各项生化检查3.给予外伤创口间断换药，2-3天换一次4.静点营养脑神经药物及软组织药物抗生素口服药物对症治疗。	血尿常规	40	43	Examination
	生化	47	48	Examination
	营养脑神经药物	75	81	treatment
	软组织药物	83	87	treatment
	抗生素口服药物	88	94	treatment

---

[1] Dataset available at http://www.ccks2017.com/en/index.php/sharedtask/.

Table 2. Semantic types of the target entities

Notations	Representative entities (in Chinese)
Treatment	健骨药物、抗生素、石蜡油、抗炎、抗凝、消炎药、前列腺激光汽化术
Body	腰骶部、左足背、右下肢、双膝关节、胸膜、双肺、肝、心脏、双肾区
Sign	腹胀、咳嗽、骨折、畸形、疼痛、静脉曲张、肿块、隆起、水肿、抽搐
Examination	查体、叩清音、呼吸音、触痛、血常规、心率、呼吸音、肠鸣音、压痛
Disease	前列腺增生、贫血、高血压、糖尿病、腰间盘突出症、支气管肺炎

The annotated text comprised single words and phrase-like expressions. Using standard BIO annotation standard, an entity, therefore, could include the headword for health information as well as a body part, direction, or degree of severity. Specifically, B-X is the tag for the first character of X type entity, I-X is the tag for the consecutive parts in X type and O represents for characters out of target entity. By using BIO scheme, the extracted information would maintain the original meaning of the source data. Detailed statistics are provided in the next section.

3.3   EHR Text Preprocessing

Sequence labeling models view a text as a sequence of tokens, each of which serves as the basis for random variables in the model. Since we use BERT embedding, a character embedding as the input layer, we just split the EHR text data into character and don't need to conduct traditional sophisticated tokenization method. In this regard, using BERT embedding as the pretrained layer and feeding to the successive neural network layer may help us built an end-to-end model relying on no task-specific resources and feature engineering.

4   Analysis and Results

4.1   Data Statistics and Experiment Settings

1198 pieces of data involves the case information of 300 patients, including general items, characteristics of medical history, diagnosis &treatment process, and discharge status. The data set is divided into training set and validate set in a ratio of 7:3. Therefore, there are 838 pieces of data in the training set and 360 pieces of data in the validate set. Table 3 shows the distribution of the five entities in the training set and validate set.

Table 3. Annotation statistics

Dataset	Treatment	Body	Sign	Examination	Disease
Train	696	6428	4424	5911	569
Validate	352	4291	3407	3635	153
Total	1048	10719	7831	9546	722

Given the intensive computational requirement for the BERT based model training, a GPU container cloud service provided by OpenBayes AI lab[2] was introduced and the environment configuration is shown in Table 4.

Table 4. Cloud container environment configuration of model training

Environment	Setting
CPU	2 cores
GPU	NVIDIA T4(16G)
Memory	30G
Python	3.6
TensorFlow	1.12.0
Keras	2.2.4

We randomly select 20% data from the training sets to learn the optimized parameter settings which are shown in Table 5. To obtain the highest F1 score performance, we conduct iterative training. If the F1 score does not increase further, it can be considered that the training is converged and need to be terminated. Once the highest F1 score is obtained, we can set these parameters for the whole training sets and further evaluate its performance on the validate sets.

Table 5. Configuration of neural network parameters

Model	Setting description	# of Parameters
CNN-LSTM	conv_layer: filters = 64; max_pool_layer: pool_size = 2; lstm_layer: units = 256	486266
Bi-LSTM	lstm_layer: units=256; dropout_layer: rate = 0.4	873018
Bi-LSTM-CRF	lstm_layer: units = 256; dense_layer: units = 64	933530

4.2 Results and Discussions

Using pretrained BERT embedding for Chinese Simplified and Traditional (12-layer, 768-hidden, 12-heads, 110 M parameters) which was released on Nov 3rd, 2018[3], three state-of-the-art deep learning models in NER (CNN-LSTM, Bi-LSTM and Bi-LSTM-CRF) are used to identify the entities in the validate sets. Evaluation is a necessary task for Natural Language Processing (NLP), information retrieval (IR) and other fields, and the evaluation indexes are usually as follows: Precision, Recall and F1.

---

[2] Accessed at https://openbayes.com/.

[3] BERT-Base, Chinese is available at https://github.com/google-research/bert.

Table 6 details the statistics of the evaluation results of the five entities identified by the above three models.

Table 6. Three deep learning models for clinical NER and their results

Semantic type	Model	Precision	Recall	F1
Treatment	BERT+CNN-LSTM	0.7078	0.8024	0.7521
	BERT+Bi-LSTM	0.8247	0.8723	**0.8479**
	BERT+ Bi-LSTM-CRF	0.8251	0.8602	0.8423
Body	BERT+CNN-LSTM	0.7885	0.8863	0.8346
	BERT+Bi-LSTM	0.8726	0.9051	0.8886
	BERT+ Bi-LSTM-CRF	0.8726	0.9175	**0.8945**
Sign	BERT+CNN-LSTM	0.9496	0.9573	0.9534
	BERT+Bi-LSTM	0.9504	0.9795	0.9647
	BERT-Bi-LSTM-CRF	0.9649	0.9799	**0.9723**
Examination	BERT+CNN-LSTM	0.9060	0.9533	0.9290
	BERT+Bi-LSTM	0.9380	0.9667	0.9521
	BERT+Bi-LSTM-CRF	0.9435	0.9694	**0.9563**
Disease	BERT+CNN-LSTM	0.6350	0.6641	0.6493
	BERT+Bi-LSTM	0.8116	0.8550	**0.8327**
	BERT+Bi-LSTM-CRF	0.7447	0.8015	0.7721

Note: set BERT sequence length = 256, and 60 epochs for the training

In the evaluation process, entities in the text are identified according to the algorithm, and the prediction is considered to be accurate only when the starting and ending positions of the prediction and the prediction of the entity type are both correct. As can be seen from the Table 6, BERT+ Bi-LSTM-CRF model is superior to the other two models in the recognition results of Body, Sign and Examination entities. Another interesting observation is that BERT+ Bi-LSTM outperforms other two models when identifying Treatment and Disease entities. In addition, the precision of entity recognition of Sign and Examination by BERT+ Bi-LSTM-CRF model is more than 95%, especially the precision of entity identification of Sign is up to 97.23%. In contrast, BERT+CNN-LSTM Model has the lowest precision, recall and F1 scores. By exploring the reasons, we find that BERT+CNN-LSTM model has certain requirements on the length of corpus. Since the length of corpus we use most is about 21-200 characters, accounting for about 60% of the whole corpus. In other words, the length of text we use is limited. Therefore, the recognition effect of BERT+CNN-LSTM Model is not significant. The character length distribution of the corpus is shown in Table 7.

Table 7. Character length distribution in corpus

The length of the range	Frequency	The length of the range	Sign
(0,20]	47	(500,600]	63
(21,50]	117	(600,700]	52
(51,100]	327	(700,800]	18
(100,200]	258	(800,900]	5
(200,300]	111	(900,1000]	3
(300,400]	111	(1000,1200]	2
(400,500]	84	average	218.578

In addition, we also compared three model based on their validating results of using BERT-embedding and no BERT-embedding. Comparative results are shown in Table 8. It can be seen from the table that BERT embedding has significantly contribute to the F1 lift when it is used in three competing models. This further illustrates the great potential for BERT application in clinical sequence labelling field.

Table 8. Comparative results of three deep learning models with and without BERT embedding

	Approaches	Precision	Recall	F1	Increasing
No pretrained embedding	CNN-LSTM (base model)	0.8356	0.8823	0.8534	/
	Bi-LSTM	0.8576	0.8887	0.8719	+1.85%
	Bi-LSTM-CRF	0.8674	0.8737	0.8705	+1.71%
BERT-embedding	BERT+CNN-LSTM	0.8664	0.9196	0.8917	+3.83%
	BERT+ Bi-LSTM	0.9120	0.9433	0.9274	+7.40%
	BERT+ Bi-LSTM-CRF	**0.9173**	**0.9471**	**0.9319**	+7.85%

Note: set BERT sequence length = 256, and 60 epochs for the training

5 Conclusion

Clinical NER is an important and early step in the processing of biomedical information. In this work, we propose BERT embedding as character-based tokenization and Bi-LSTM-CRF as sequence labelling neural architecture so as to build an end-to-end model relying on limited annotation features. We achieved best performance when comparing BERT+ Bi-LSTM-CRF with BERT+ CNN-LSTM and BERT+ Bi-LSTM based on clinical benchmark datasets. In addition, using BERT embedding as pre-trained layer, three popular deep learning models in sequence labelling both achieved higher performance than the no pretrained counterparts. This indicates that BERT embedding can be applied to clinical NER and exert much more role than other traditional approaches.

Potential directions for the future work can be extended in several ways: First, our proposed BERT embedding+ Bi-LSTM-CRF model can be further evaluated by exploring more EHR data, especially for Chinese traditional medicine source corpus, to validate the precision and recall advantages of the model. Since our model does not require any domain or task specific knowledge, it might be useful to extract clinical entities from these domain corpora and enhance our understanding of the approaches. Secondly, the prediction outputs of BERT+ Bi-LSTM-CRF Model can be further applied to the downstream tasks such as construction of clinical terminology library and establishment of clinical knowledge map as shown in Fig. 5.

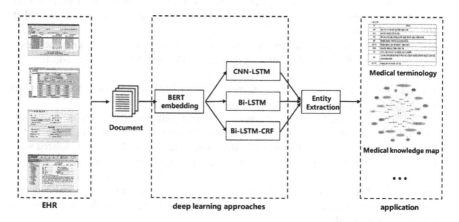

Fig. 5. Downstream application scenarios of the clinical NER

Another interesting direction is to evaluate our model with other emergent competing neural network models, like BGRU and BGRU-CRF so as to improve the accuracy and speed of the entity's extraction.

References

1. Stubbs, A., Kotfila, C., Xu, H., Uzuner, Ö.: Identifying risk factors for heart disease over time: overview of 2014 i2b2/UTHealth shared task Track 2. J. Biomed. Inf. **58**, S67–S77 (2015)
2. Jung, K., LePendu, P., Iyer, S., Bauer-Mehren, A., Percha, B., Shah, N.H.: Functional evaluation of out-of-the-box text-mining tools for data-mining tasks. J. Am. Med. Inf. Assoc. **22**, 121–131 (2015)
3. Ben Abacha, A., Zweigenbaum, P.: Medical entity recognition: a comparison of semantic and statistical methods. In: Proceedings BioNLP 2011 Work, pp. 56–64(2011)
4. Skeppstedt, M., Kvist, M., Nilsson, G.H., Dalianis, H.: Automatic recognition of disorders, an annotation and machine learning study findings, pharmaceuticals and body structures from clinical text. J. Biomed. Inf. **49**, 148–158 (2014)
5. Chen, Y.K., Lasko, T.A., Mei, Q.Z., Denny, J.C., Xu, H.: A study of active learning methods for named entity recognition. J. Biomed. Inform. **58**, 11–18 (2016)
6. Erik, F., Sang, T.K., Meulder, F.D.: Introduction to the conll-2003 shared task: language-independent named entity recognition. In: Proceedings of the Seventh Conference on Natural Language Learning at HLT-NAACL 2003, vol. 4, pp. 142–147. Association for Computational Linguistics (2003)

7. Ma, X., Xia, F.: Unsupervised dependency parsing with transferring distribution via parallel guidance and entropy regularization. In: Proceedings of ACL-2014, pp. 1337–1348, Baltimore, June 2014
8. Bengio, Y., Simard, P., Frasconi, P.: Learning long-term dependencies with gradient descent is difficult. IEEE Trans. Neural Networks **5**(2), 157–166 (1994)
9. Passos, A., Kumar, V., McCallum, A.: Lexicon infused phrase embeddings for named entity resolution. In: Proceedings of CoNLL-2014, pp. 78–86, Ann Arbor, June 2014
10. Xu, K., Yang, Z., Kang, P., Wang, Q., et al.: Document-level attention-based Bi LSTM-CRF incorporating disease dictionary for disease named entity recognition. Comput. Biol. Med. **108**, 122–132 (2019)
11. Na, S.H., Kim, H., Min, J., et al.: Improving LSTM CRFs using character-based compositions for Korean named entity recognition. Comput. Speech Lang. **54**, 106–121 (2019)
12. Shi, X., Chen, Z., Wang, H., et al.: Convolutional LSTM network: a machine learning approach for precipitation nowcasting (2015)
13. Sainath, T.N., Vinyals, O., Senior, A., et al.: Convolutional, long short-term memory, fully connected deep neural networks. In: International Conference on Acoustics (2015)
14. Unanue, I.J., Borzeshi, E.Z., Piccardi, M.: Recurrent neural networks with specialized word embeddings for health domain named-entity recognition. J. Biomed. Inform. **76**, 102–109 (2017)
15. Donahue, J., Hendricks, L.A., Guadarrama, S.: Long-term recurrent convolutional networks for visual recognition and description. In: AB Into Calculation of the Structures and Properties of Molecules (2015)
16. Vinyals, O., Toshev, A., Bengio, S., et al.: Show and tell: a neural image caption generator (2014)
17. Ruch, P., Baud, R., Geissbuhler, A.: Using lexical disambiguation and named-entity recognition to improve spelling correction in the electronic patient record. Artif. Intell. Med. **29**, 169–184 (2003)
18. Liu, H., Mi, X., Li, Y.: Smart deep learning-based wind speed prediction model using wavelet packet decomposition, convolutional neural network and convolutional long short-term memory network. Energy Convers. Manage. **166**, 120–131 (2018)

Cost Optimization Estimation of Medical Institutions in the Hierarchical Medical System Based on System Dynamics Model

Jiang Wu, Yao Yao, and Xiao Huang[✉]

School of Information Management, Wuhan University, Wuhan 430072, China
xiaoh@whu.edu.cn

Abstract. The grading diagnosis and treatment system in China is to improve the first-time diagnosis rate of patients in primary health care institutions, thereby increasing the proportion of people in primary health care institutions, thus achieving the goal of reducing costs. This study constructs a system dynamics model of the number of primary and upper-level visits—the cost of medical institutions, and simulates the effect of the increase in the proportion of patients attending the primary level on the cost of medical institutions. The study found that with the increase in the number of visits, the cost of primary medical institutions will increase, but the total cost of the entire medical system will be reduced significantly. Moreover, the higher the proportion of the number of people attending the primary level, the lower the total cost. If the proportion of primary care in 2017 increases by 15%, and this trend is maintained until 2021, the total cost saved by medical institutions in 2021 will be as high as 903.32 billion yuan.

Keywords: System dynamics · Grading diagnosis and treatment · Primary medical institutions · Medical institution costs · Simulation · Sensitivity analysis

1 Introduction

The grading diagnosis and treatment system is the focus of Chinese medical reform in recent years. The core of the system is to improve the service level of primary medical institutions, change the proportion of reimbursement for hospitals at different levels, and improve the proportion of patients who go to community hospitals, county hospitals and other primary hospitals, by means of the two-way referral method to implement the functions of acute and chronic disease diagnosis and treatment services of various types of medical institutions, so as to clarify the division of responsibilities of various types of medical and health institutions at all levels, then regulate the medical order. The specific problem addressed by the policy is that Chinese primary medical institutions have failed to meet enough medical needs, resulting in waste of medical resources in higher medical institutions.

The focus of grading diagnosis and treatment is to expand the service level of primary medical institutions. Specific measures include improving the basic measures of primary medical institutions, improving the quality of employees in primary medical

© Springer Nature Switzerland AG 2019
H. Chen et al. (Eds.): ICSH 2019, LNCS 11924, pp. 323–332, 2019.
https://doi.org/10.1007/978-3-030-34482-5_29

institutions, and increasing the difference between the reimbursed proportion of primary medical institutions and higher medical institutions. These measures can attract more patients to the primary medical institutions, allowing more patients with chronic diseases to be referred from higher medical institutions, thereby improving the number of visits to primary medical institutions. In short, this measure will enable primary medical institutions to serve a wider range of patients, and thus reduce the total cost of medical care in China. The reform measures can improve the number of visits to primary health care institutions. However, the details of the economic benefits of the increase in the number of visits to primary health care institutions are not known. This issue needs to be further verified. Scholars in many countries have established many models for medical-related research through system dynamics, with a focus on the evaluation of the effects of medical-related policies [1]. The impact of the increase in the number of visits to primary medical institutions on the cost of medical institutions can also be explored through system dynamics methods.

Therefore, this study will construct a system dynamics model for the number of visits to primary medical institutions, the number of visits to higher medical hospitals, and the cost of hospitals at different levels. Second, validate the validity of the model with real data. Finally, evaluate the impact of the increase in the number of visits to primary medical institutions in 2017–2021 on the total cost of Chinese medical institutions through sensitivity analysis.

2 Literature Review

System dynamics methods are often used in policy evaluations, its medical-related applications are also related to policy. Such research mainly includes two types: (1) Assess the impact of macro policy changes on outcomes such as cost optimization. Ahmad et al. assessed the cost-effectiveness of tobacco intervention control, finding that long-term savings in medical costs can offset the investment in tobacco intervention control, it also increases the life expectancy of the implementation of this policy area. Yu et al. predicted that adjustment of different health policies in China would affect the proportion of patients who did not seek medical care, the relationship between adjusting the number structure of hospitals and community hospitals, adjusting outpatient prices, and adjusting the level of health insurance to potential medical needs was found [2]. Hungary introduced a new labor law in 2012, which allows informal payments to be accepted. Márta Somogyvári evaluated the impact of this policy on the country's health care industry and found that the policy created mistrust between doctors and patients and increased the total cost of social and health insurance funds [3]. Ahmad, S. assesses the policy that California hopes to implement—increasing the legal minimum purchase cigarette age to 21—the cost-effectiveness of this policy, and found that after 50 years of implementation, the youth (14–17 years old) smoking rate 13.3% fell to 2.4% (82% reduction), actually saving the country and residents 24 billion US dollars [4]. (2) Assess the impact of different disease interventions. Edelstein et al. compared the potential outcomes of nine different preventive interventions for early childhood caries [5]. Because overuse of opioid analgesics is prone to death, Wakeland et al. evaluated the impact of three different drug education interventions on the number of overuse deaths during the 2008–2015 evaluation period [6].

In addition, the system dynamics method is widely used in the assessment of medical resources supply and demand, mainly including the supply and demand of medical resources such as the supply and demand of doctors, the inventory of medical resources, and the simulation evaluation of the allocation of relevant resources in the crisis. Researchers from different countries have used the system dynamics method to simulate the number of doctors and supply and demand in the country. From Japan [7, 8], Spain [9], Canada [10] have found their country or a certain region within the country, they have found that the number of doctors will be in short supply at certain times. Wang et al. established a new hospital inventory demand-driven replenishment model that determines the optimal replenishment time and the total inventory cost [11]. The model developed by Senese et al. predicts the evolution of the supply of Italian medical experts and combines demographics, service utilization and hospital beds to measure the potential effective allocation of medical allocations [12]. Diaz et al. demonstrates the utility of the system dynamics approach to model and simulate US demand for ambulatory health care service both for the general population and for specific cohort subpopulations over the 5-year period, from 2003 to 2008. A system dynamics approach that is shown to meaningfully project demand for services has implications for health resource planning and for generating knowledge that is critical to assessing interventions [13]. Decision-making simulations in times of crisis are also the focus of researchers. Khanmohammadi et al. proposed a system dynamics simulation model that describes the dynamic characteristics of the hospital's post-earthquake recovery process, which enables managers to gain insight into how their decisions about available resource use before and after the earthquake affect hospital function, and Assist administrators in assessing the impact of various readiness policies on their hospital resilience [14]. Wenya et al. used the system dynamics method to establish a system dynamics model of mass casualties. The model, based on Shanghai, China, found that adjusting the efficiency of rescue ambulances and the allocation of emergency medical personnel to the efficiency of organization and command [15].

3 Model Building

3.1 The Logic of Model Building

The services of the primary medical institutions are significantly different from those of the second-tier and third-tier hospitals. For example, most of people choose inpatient services in higher-level hospitals, which leads to the tightness of beds in second-tier and third-tier hospitals, but not in primary hospitals. According to the relevant literature, news, and consulting experts in relevant fields, this study sorts out the relationship between the number of medical institutions and the cost of medical services at different levels, and completes the model construction with the system dynamics modeling tool Vensim, as shown in Fig. 1.

As shown in Fig. 1, our model consists of two subsystems, which are the primary medical institution's medical treatment-cost subsystem and the higher medical

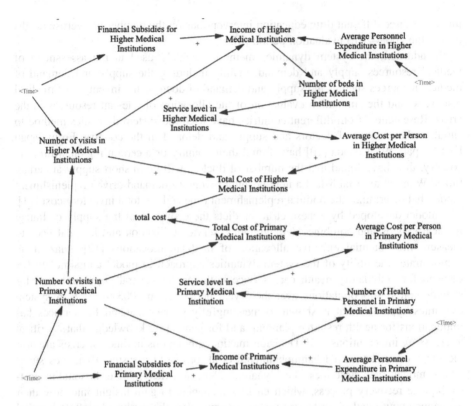

Fig. 1. Model of relationship between medical visits and medical costs at different levels of medical institutions

institution's medical treatment-cost subsystem, in which the number of visits to higher-level medical institutions will be reduced due to the diversion effect of primary medical institutions. In the subsystem of the higher medical institutions, the amount of medical treatment of the higher medical institutions and the per capita expenditure of the higher medical institutions jointly affect the income of the higher medical institutions. This part of the income together with the government financial subsidies constitutes the total income of the higher medical institutions; the accumulation of total annual income will have a positive impact on the number of beds in higher medical institutions in the next year; thus, the service level of higher medical institutions will be improved, that is, the amount of medical care for the next year will be increased; the promotion has caused an increase in the per capita cost of the higher medical institutions; the per capita cost and the amount of medical treatment of the superior medical institutions jointly affect the total cost of the higher medical institutions. In the subsystems of primary medical institutions, there are similar relationships between variables, and ultimately caused changes in the total cost of primary medical institutions. In addition, since the per capita expenditure for medical treatment in primary medical institutions is lower than the per capita expenditure in higher medical institutions, as the flow of people from the higher medical institutions to the primary medical institutions, the total medical costs will be reduced, thereby increasing the utilization rate of medical resources.

3.2   Model Parameter Relationship Determination

This study obtains various types of data of the above model from the 2014–2017 China Health Statistical Yearbook and the 2018 China Health and Wellness Statistical Yearbook, and combined with relevant demographic data and economic data, the parameter relationships in the above models are clarified. The parameters in the above model are divided into three categories:

The number of visits, per capita expenditure, and financial subsidy income are parameters that exhibit a linear relationship at the same time. This type of parameter has a significant linear relationship with time, and the relationship between the data and time is found by data from different years.

(2) The cost of primary medical institutions, the cost of higher medical institutions and the total cost. These parameters are directly calculated from the data in the model. Total Cost of Primary Medical Institutions = Average Cost per Person in Primary Medical Institutions * Number of visits in Primary Medical Institutions; Total Cost of Higher Medical Institutions = Average Cost per Person in Higher Medical Institutions * Number of visits in Higher Medical Institutions; Total cost = Total Cost of Higher Medical Institutions + Total Cost of Primary Medical Institutions.

(3) Other various types of parameter relationships. In this study, the parameter relationship between the remaining parameters is clarified by least squares method, curve fitting and consulting the corresponding literature. For example, it is generally believed that the number of beds in a medical facility and the number of medical staffs will affect the number of visits to the medical institution. Therefore, the study initially determined that the service level of the medical institution was significantly correlated with the number of beds and the number of medical staffs, and the relationship between these variables was calculated by the least square method. However, it is found through calculation that the number of visits to higher hospitals is only significantly related to the number of beds, while the level of service of primary care institutions is only significantly related to the number of medical staffs. The most stressful resource in the upper hospital is the bed. Patients who are unwilling to see a doctor at the grassroots level often rely on the distrust of primary care workers and the lack of adequate medical staff at the primary health care facility to complete the consultation of most diseases. Therefore, the above results are consistent with the facts, so the factors related to the service level of different levels of hospitals are also different. It can be known that the service level of the superior medical institutions is significantly related to the number of beds, and the service level of the primary medical institutions is significantly related to the number of hospital personnel. Then, the relationship between these parameters is clarified by curve fitting with real data.

3.3   Model Test

In this study, various system parameter relationships are uploaded to the above model to simulate the total cost of higher medical institutions and the total cost of primary medical institutions in the Chinese medical treatment system from 2013 to 2017. The simulation data is compared with the actual value to calculate the actual value of the higher-level medical institution and the cost of the primary medical institution and the error of the analog value. The results are shown in Table 1.

Table 1. Comparative analysis of medical institution cost simulation results and real results from 2013 to 2017

Year	Higher level of medical institutions (Billions of Yuan)			Primary medical institutions (Billions of Yuan)		
	Actual value	Simulation value	Error (%)	Actual value	Simulation value	Error (%)
2013	1693.65	1731.22	2.22	338.36	337.72	−0.19
2014	1952.42	1962.74	0.53	364.17	378.87	4.04
2015	2212.71	2216.09	0.15	410.00	420.62	2.59
2016	2496.78	2492.48	−0.17	458.02	462.96	1.08
2017	2790.13	2793.11	0.11	521.84	505.91	−3.05

As shown in Table 1, except for 2.2% in 2013, the cost error of higher-level medical institutions in other years is less than 1%; although the cost error of primary medical institutions in 2014 is 4.04%, the overall error is within the acceptable range. Using the cost of different levels of medical system in 2013–2017 to verify the authenticity of the model, the overall error rate of the model is small, which indicates that the simulation model we have established is practical.

4   Simulation Analysis

Graded diagnosis and treatment will increase the proportion of visits to primary care institutions, affect the cost of primary care institutions and higher-level medical institutions, and ultimately affect the total cost of medical institutions. This study assumes that the proportion of primary care clinics per year will increase by 5%, 10%, and 15% from 2017 to 2021. Based on this, the cost and total cost of the medical institutions at different levels in the five-year increase ratio are calculated. At the same time, these values are compared with the original values (real and simulated values) to assess the impact of the increase in the number of primary consultations on total cost optimization.

First, calculate the cost of the primary medical institutions in different years and make a fold line, as shown in Fig. 2.

Figure 2 shows that the increase in the proportion of people attending the primary level will lead to an increase in the cost of primary care. Moreover, the higher the proportion of people attending the primary level, the higher the cost of primary care. According to calculations, when the proportion increases by 5%, the cost of primary medical institutions will increase by 3.74%, 7.02%, 7.03%, 7.04%, and 7.05% from 2017 to 2021 respectively. When the proportion increases by 10%, the cost of medical

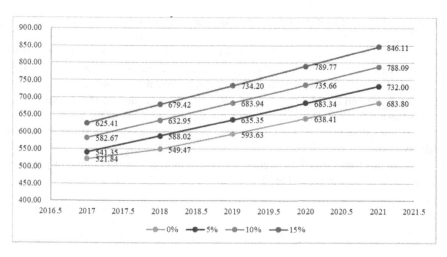

Fig. 2. Sensitivity analysis of the cost of primary care institutions (Billions of Yuan)

institutions increased by 11.66%, 15.19%, 15.21%, 15.23%, and 15.25%, respectively. When the proportion increased by 15%, the cost increased by 19.85%, 23.65%, 23.68%, 23.71%, and 23.74%, respectively. It can be seen that, except for 2017, the increase in the cost of other years is relatively stable.

Calculate the cost of the higher-level medical institutions in different years and make a fold line, as shown in Fig. 3.

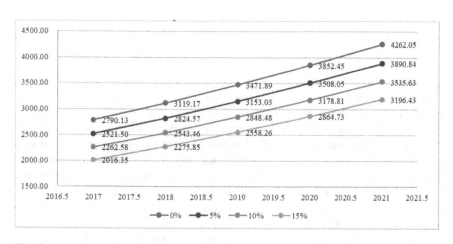

Fig. 3. Sensitivity analysis of the cost of superior medical institutions (Billions of Yuan)

Figure 3 shows that the increase in the proportion of patients attending the primary level will lead to a decline in the cost of higher-level medical institutions. Moreover, the higher the proportion of the number of people attending the primary level, the lower the cost of the higher-level medical institutions. According to the calculation, when the proportion of the number of people attending the primary level increased by 5%, the cost of the higher-level medical institutions decreased by 9.63%, 9.44%, 9.18%, 8.94%, and 8.71% from 2017 to 2021; when the proportion increased by 10%, In the past five years, the cost of higher-level medical institutions decreased by 23.32%, 18.46%, 17.96%, 17.49%, and 17.04%, respectively. When the proportion increased by 15%, they decreased by 27.73%, 27.04%, 26.32%, 25.64%, and 25.00%, respectively. It can be seen that when the proportion of the number of visits to the primary level is increased, the proportion of the cost of the higher-level medical institutions is also relatively stable.

Calculate the total cost of the higher-level medical institutions in different years and make a polyline, as shown in Fig. 4.

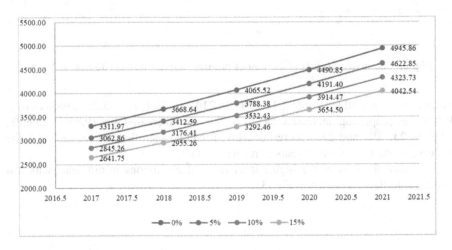

Fig. 4. Sensitivity analysis of total cost of medical institutions (Billions of Yuan)

At the same time, calculate the amount and percentage of total cost reductions of medical institutions in different situations, as shown in Table 2.

Figure 4 shows that when the proportion of primary consultations increased by 5%, 10%, and 15%, the total cost of medical institutions was lower than the original value, and the higher the proportion, the lower the total cost. It can be seen from the Table 2 that when the proportion of the number of visits to the primary level is increased by 5%, the total cost of medical institutions in 2017–2021 is about 7% lower than the original value, and the average annual reduction is 280 billion yuan. When the proportion increases by 10%, the total cost of medical institutions in 2017–2021 is about 13% lower than the original value, with an average annual reduction of 540 billion yuan. When the proportion increases by 15%, the total cost of medical institutions in 2017–2021 is about 19% lower than the original value, with an average annual reduction of 780 billion yuan. In 2021, the decline was the biggest, reaching 903.32 billion yuan.

Through sensitivity analysis, the cost of primary care institutions in 2017–2021 will increase due to the increase in the number of people attending the primary level in

Table 2. The amount and percentage of total cost reduction of medical institutions in different situations

		5%	10%	15%
2017	Amount (Billions of Yuan)	249.11	466.71	670.22
	Rate (%)	7.52	14.09	20.24
2018	Amount (Billions of Yuan)	256.05	492.23	713.38
	Rate (%)	6.98	13.42	19.45
2019	Amount (Billions of Yuan)	277.14	533.09	773.06
	Rate (%)	6.82	13.11	19.02
2020	Amount (Billions of Yuan)	299.45	576.38	836.35
	Rate (%)	6.67	12.83	18.62
2021	Amount (Billions of Yuan)	323.01	622.13	903.32
	Rate (%)	6.53	12.58	18.26

2017–2021, and the proportion of cost increase is relatively stable. Similarly, an increase in the number of visits to the primary level will result in a steady decline in the cost of higher medical institutions during the period 2017–2021. Moreover, due to the large gap between the cost per capita of the upper hospital and the primary medical institution, the cost of the medical institution is much lower than that of the primary medical institution, which leads to a decline in the total cost of medical care. And the higher the proportion of the number of visits to the primary level, the more the total cost of medical care is saved. If the trend of increasing the number of people attending the primary level remains unchanged over time, it will be able to bring about a significant reduction in the total cost of Chinese medical institutions. If the annual 15% increase is maintained until 2021, the total cost savings for Chinese medical institutions will reach 903.32 billion yuan.

5   Conclusion

The purpose of graded diagnosis and treatment is to increase the rate of primary consultation at the grassroots level, and the increase in the proportion of people attending the primary level can reduce the total cost of medical institutions. On this basis, this study constructs a system dynamics model of the relationship between the number of visits to medical institutions at all levels and its cost, and verifies the validity of the model by comparing the actual data with the simulated data from 2013 to 2017.

Secondly, the sensitivity analysis of the ratio of cost to grassroots visits in 2017–2021 is made. The results of the analysis show that although the cost of primary medical institutions will increase due to the increase in the number of visits, the cost of higher-level medical institutions will be significantly reduced, resulting in a reduction in the total cost of the entire medical system. Moreover, the higher the proportion of the number of people attending the primary level, the lower the total cost reduction. If the proportion of primary care in 2017 increases by 15%, and this trend is maintained until 2021, the total cost saved by medical institutions in 2021 will be as high as 903.32 billion yuan.

Acknowledgments. This research is supported by the National Natural Science Foundation of China (No. 71573197).

References

1. Sturmberg, J.P., Martin, C.M., Katerndahl, D.A.: Systems and complexity thinking in the general practice literature: an integrative, historical narrative review. Ann. Fam. Med. **12**(1), 66–74 (2014)
2. Yu, W., Li, M., Ge, Y., et al.: Transformation of potential medical demand in China: a system dynamics simulation model. J. Biomed. Inform. **57**, 399–414 (2015)
3. Somogyvári, M.: The costs of organisational injustice in the Hungarian health care system. J. Bus. Ethics **118**(3), 543–560 (2013)
4. Ahmad, S.: The cost-effectiveness of raising the legal smoking age in California. Med. Decis. Making **25**(3), 330–340 (2005)
5. Edelstein, B.L., Hirsch, G., Frosh, M., et al.: Reducing early childhood caries in a Medicaid population. J. Am. Dent. Assoc. **146**(4), 224–232 (2015)
6. Wakeland, W., Nielsen, A., Schmidt, T.D., et al.: Modeling the impact of simulated educational interventions on the use and abuse of pharmaceutical opioids in the United States: a report on initial efforts. Health Educ. Behav. **40**(1 Suppl), 74S–86S (2013)
7. Ishikawa, T., Fujiwara, K., Ohba, H., et al.: Forecasting the regional distribution and sufficiency of physicians in Japan with a coupled system dynamics—geographic information system model. Hum. Resour. Health **15**(1), 64 (2017)
8. Ishikawa, T., Ohba, H., Yokooka, Y., et al.: Forecasting the absolute and relative shortage of physicians in Japan using a system dynamics model approach. Hum. Resour. Health **11**(1), 41 (2013)
9. Barber, P., López-Valcárcel, B.G.: Forecasting the need for medical specialists in Spain: application of a system dynamics model. Hum. Resour. Health **8**(1), 24 (2010)
10. Vanderby, S.A., Carter, M.W., Latham, T., et al.: Modeling the cardiac surgery workforce in Canada. Ann. Thorac. Surg. **90**(2), 467–473 (2010)
11. Wang, L.C., Cheng, C.Y., Tseng, Y.T., et al.: Demand-pull replenishment model for hospital inventory management: a dynamic buffer-adjustment approach. Int. J. Prod. Res. **53**(24), 14 (2015)
12. Senese, F., Tubertini, P., Mazzocchetti, A., et al.: Forecasting future needs and optimal allocation of medical residency positions: the Emilia-Romagna Region case study. Hum. Resour. Health **13**(1), 7 (2015)
13. Diaz, R., Behr, J.G., Tulpule, M.: A system dynamics model for simulating ambulatory health care demands. Simul. Healthc. **7**(4), 243–250 (2012)
14. Khanmohammadi, S., Farahmand, H., Kashani, H.: A system dynamics approach to the seismic resilience enhancement of hospitals. Int. J. Disaster Risk Reduction **31**, 220–233 (2018)
15. Wenya, Y., Yipeng, L., Chaoqun, H., et al.: Research of an emergency medical system for mass casualty incidents in Shanghai, China: a system dynamics model. Patient Prefer. Adherence **12**, 207–222 (2018)

Knowledge Base Construction Based on Knowledge Fusion Process Model

Hao Fan$^{(\boxtimes)}$ ⓘ and Jianping He ⓘ

School of Information Management, Wuhan University, Wuhan, China
hfan@whu.edu.cn, jianpinghe@qq.com

Abstract. A Personal Health Record (PHR) records health data and relevant information about a healthcare patient. It is necessary to build a knowledge base to make the best of PHRs because of their rich value. Through literature review, this paper clarifies two problems in the field of PHR knowledge base construction, the lack of universal knowledge fusion framework and less consideration of fusion between of different types knowledge. For the problems, this paper proposes a knowledge fusion process model which can be used across fields. It consists of concept fusion, relation fusion, attribute fusion, domain fusion and instance fusion. Based on this theoretical model, this paper constructs hypertension PHR knowledge base through the design of conceptual model, knowledge extraction and knowledge fusion. In the process of knowledge fusion, both fusion of health knowledge from different sources and fusion of different types health knowledge are considered. Further more, this paper implements the application of the hypertension PHR knowledge base.

Keywords: Personal Health Record · Knowledge base · Knowledge fusion

1 Introduction

The National Alliance for Health Information Technology report defines a PHR as an electronic record of health-related information on an individual that conforms to nationally recognized interoperability standards, and can be drawn from multiple sources while being managed, shared and controlled by the individual [1]. Nowadays PHRs are extended to collect, track and share the past and current health information about common people rather than patients, which have characteristics of continuous high speed growth and rich value, and are the prerequisite and foundation for implementing an intelligent healthcare service, personal medicine, remote treatment, disease prevention and prediction, etc.

In order to make the best of PHRs, researchers begin to focus on the construction of PHR knowledge bases. Due to the wide range of knowledge sources in the construction of PHR knowledge base, there are problems such as the quality of knowledge, the

This research is part of the MOE Project of Key Research Institute of Humanities and Social Sciences at Universities "Research on mining and service of big data resources for medical and health _elds" (No: 17JJD870002).

repetition of knowledge from different data sources, and the lack of clear correlation between knowledge. Therefore, knowledge fusion must be carried out. Knowledge fusion (KF) enables different sources to perform heterogeneous data integration, disambiguation, processing, reasoning verification, and updating under a same framework specification, to achieve the integration of data, information, methods, experience, and human thoughts, and to form a high quality knowledge base.

Many scholars use the theory and method of knowledge fusion to construct the PHR knowledge base, which leads to abundant achievements. However, there are still two problems to be solved:

(1) Previous research has proposed and used many knowledge fusion frameworks in the construction of knowledge base, but there is no one-size-fits-all theoretical model.
(2) Health knowledge is divided into two categories, general health knowledge and special health knowledge. Previous studies have mostly focused on the fusion of knowledge from different sources and less on the integration of different types of health knowledge.

To solve problem 1, this paper proposes a knowledge fusion process model which can be used across fields. Based on that model, this paper constructs hypertension PHR knowledge base through the design of conceptual model, knowledge extraction and knowledge fusion. Both fusion of knowledge from different sources and fusion of different types of health knowledge are considered, which solves problem 2. Furthermore, this paper implements the application of the hypertension PHR base.

2 Related Work

Health records can provide reliable information for individuals and departments participating in patient care and they are the key of solving problems related to quality of care, clinical decision support. More and more scholars focus on the study of health records. In order to make drug information exchangeable among electronic health record systems, Wang et al. in [2] build a Normalized Chinese Clinical Drug (NCCD) knowledge base by applying the RxNorm model to Chinese clinical drugs. El-Sappagh et al. formulates a newly constructed knowledge base, Diabetes Mellitus Treatment Ontology (DMTO), which provides the highest coverage and the most complete picture of coded knowledge about T2DM patients [3]. El-Sappagh et al. in [4] propose a standard relational data model for diabetes diagnosis based on HL7 REVI, EHR and SNOMED CT, which works as an operational data store constructing a case-base that providing knowledge for a diabetes diagnosis CBR system. Besides, based on the ontology, they propose a decision support system for diabetes diagnosis which implements a new semantically interpretable fuzzy rule-based systems (FRBS) framework [5]. Nithya et al. in [6] realize a knowledge base of scientific evidences containing associations between two domains of medical and oral health, which has committed to the problem of fragmented healthcare delivery. Sherimon et al. in [7] have developed an ontology based clinical decision support system (CDSS) to assess the risk factors and provide appropriate treatment suggestions for diabetic patients.

Shemeikka et al. in [8] develop and verify proofs of CDSS concepts to support prescriptions of pharmaceutical drugs in patients with reduced renal function. By using crowdsourcing approaches previously developed, Mccoy et al. in [9] generate a knowledge base of problem-medication pairs in a large, non-university health care system with widely used and commercially available electronic health records. Jing et al. in [10] integrates an OWL-DL knowledge base with a standards-based EHR prototype, and provides customized information via the EHR interface, which has the advantage of expanding and maintaining knowledge base of any scale, with the goal of assisting clinicians and other EHR users in making better informed health care decisions. Rao et al. in [11] integrate patient health data from various sources and provide a comprehensive view of patient health status, by modelling data requirements, designing a Public Health Ontology to represent domain knowledge, and mapping relational health data into instances of the ontology to form the health record knowledge base.

Many studies focusing on the construction of health record knowledge base have considered data heterogeneity between health records from different sources and tried to solve the problem. However, there is less discussion about the integration of different types of health knowledge and there is no unified knowledge fusion framework to be used.

3 The KF Process Model

In the previous work [12], we define a knowledge ontology as the form of five-tuple, consisting of concepts, attributes, relations, domains and instances, upon which we classify five KF patterns composing the KF process model. All knowledge bases are composed of these five basic knowledge elements, so the KF process model based on the five basic elements is universal. The KF process model are as follows.

1. **Instance Fusion** is removing redundancy, deducing noise, correcting error and merging content for entity objects and producing a new set, in which knowledge sources usually have the same modeling structure, or can be converted into the same one. After instance fusion, the modeling structure of source knowledge is totally or partly inherited into the fused target in accordance with user definitions and requirements, where the pertinence, consistency and correctness of knowledge entities are improved. There is a substantial overlap between instance fusion and traditional information fusion, so that the former can be implemented by using the latter fusing methods as references. Instance fusion is concerned mainly having four activities: *Named Entity Recognition, Alignment, Disambiguation* and *Linking*, in terms of extracting named entities, finding the same real world entity belonging to heterogeneous knowledge sources, and solving the name ambiguity problem by linking ambiguous entity reference items to a given knowledge base.

2. **Domain Fusion** is applying set operations like UNION, INTERSECT, MINUS and EXCEPT on attribute fields or value ranges of source knowledge entities, resulting in attribute definitions of fused knowledge entities. When Instance Fusion is applied, knowledge sources might be in the same modeling structure but different domains, which is required to redefine the attribute domain of fused knowledge.

Domain fusion remains the modeling structure of source knowledge, but change its attribute fields or value ranges, which is an extension and expansion of Instance Fusion.

3. **Attribute Fusion** is comparing, analysing, transforming and merging attributes of knowledge concepts, in terms of classifying, selecting and reorganising the object features according to users requirements. In attribute fusion, there are usually differences between modelling structures of knowledge sources, especially including complementary, contradiction and homograph differences in attribute definitions. Fusion strategies vary according to different situations. After attribute fusion, new attributes appear in fused knowledge and new relations are also required to correspond with them. Thus, attribute and relation fusion are two complementary and alternately iterative processes, both are important parts of knowledge discovery processes.

4. **Relation Fusion** is merging relations in source knowledge by removing redundancy and combining structures, as well as applying inductive and deductive reasoning over relations for inferring and mining a new one. Relations in knowledge ontology include interactions between concepts, affiliations between concepts and attributes, functions defining particular mappings, and axioms representing true assertions. Relation fusion explores and derives new relations according to original ones in the source, in which modelling structures might be different from either each other, or the fused one where the new knowledge is generated. After fusing relations, the fused knowledge structure will be different from the source, as well as knowledge instances, which includes new knowledge that is produced during the inference process.

5. **Concept Fusion** is constructing new knowledge concepts, which might bring about new attributes and relations as well. Therefore, it is not possible to individually produce concept fusion separately from the other KF patterns, which have to be based on instance fusion, iteratively and incrementally applying domain, relation and attribute fusions to achieve a whole fusion process.

Different KF patterns meet different requirements and produce different fusion results. Figure 1 gives a KF process mode to illustrate relationships among the five KF patterns. Concept fusion is considered as the high level of the KF hierarchy, where domain, relation and attribute fusion are middle levels between the low level instance fusion and the high level one.

The requirement of domain fusion is generated on the basis of instance fusion. In different knowledge sources, value ranges of concepts might vary from each other, which is required to be adjusted, merged and redefined, i.e. producing domain fusion, to meet the demand of instance fusion. After changes of concept domains, relations between the concepts may also need to change so as to affect the inferring results of relation fusion. E.g. the increase or decrease of a concept value ranges is likely to affect the establishment of equal relationships between the concepts. At the same time, relation and attribute fusion are also two interactive and complementary processes. The production of new attributes might lead to the generation of new relations, and vice versa.

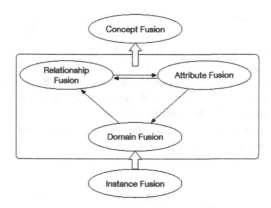

Fig. 1. Knowledge fusion process model

Therefore, the three KF patterns, i.e. Domain Fusion, Relationship Fusion and Attribute Fusion, are performing in a way of loop iterations. In order to eventually achieve Concept Fusion, each iteration makes a further step in the progress of generating new knowledge. Thus, KF processes could not be completed only by a single fusion pattern, nor by a stepwise linear procedure. Fusion patterns need to be comprehensively considered, KF is realized in a way of loop iteration, incremental progression and spiral development.

4   The Design of PHR Knowledge Base Conceptual Model

Knowledge in the health field is divided into general health knowledge and special health knowledge. General health knowledge refers to some public medical and healthcare knowledge, such as doctor information, hospital information, drug prices, and certain disease characteristics. Special health knowledge is usually related to personal privacy, and is generally individual experiences, such as medical records, painful treatment experiences, and personal health status.

These two types of knowledge are indispensable in a high-quality PHR knowledge base, which should be considered in the design of conceptual model. The final conceptual model consists of four categories: **individual profile, medical service, patient** and **disease**, as shown in Fig. 2.

The category **individual profile** covers basic information of patients, including **demographics**, e.g. *dob, sex, height, weight, pregnancy status*; **family history** e.g. *genetic genes, susceptible diseases*; **geographical environment**, e.g. *country, district*.

The category **medical service** encompasses information might be recorded at any point during a disease management process, and consists of two subcategories, **historical record** and **care plan**. The category **historical record** represents medical behaviours that have happened to the individual in the past, which has subclasses **observation** and **action**. Instances of class **observation** contain records of any phenomenon or state related to an individual, and it corresponds to **measurement**, **symptom expression** and **lifestyle** information that occur during the individual's daily life. Instances of class **action** are intervention activities that happened to an individual. The category **care plan** contains subclasses **assessment** and **instruction**, which are used to describe the evaluation statements and suggestions for personal health. The class **assessment** is used to assess the risk of disease and the class **instruction** is used to specify the observation and action requests according to the requirements of medical workers, which enables both simple and complex specifications to be expressed, including **investigation** and **intervention request**.

The **disease** category describes **definition**, **etiology**, **treatment**, **epidemiology** and **clinical manifestation** information of the disease.

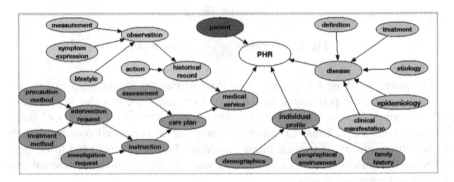

Fig. 2. The structure of conceptual model for PHR knowledge base

5   Constructing the Hypertension PHR Knowledge Base

Based on the PHR conceptual model designed above, we construct hypertension PHR knowledge base through knowledge extraction and knowledge fusion. Data sources consists of web articles, the eighth edition textbooks *Internal Medicine* [13] and *Obstetrics and Gynecology* [14], the structured knowledge base *Disease Ontology* [15].

5.1   Knowledge Extraction

Knowledge extraction is extracting knowledge elements from raw data (unstructured, semi-structured, structured data) by a set of automatic or semi-automatic techniques.

Based on the definition of the knowledge ontology [12], knowledge extraction in this paper can be divided into **concept**, **relation**, **attribute**, **domain**, and **instance** extractions.

(1) Materialize the Conceptual Model

The specific conceptual model of the hypertension PHR knowledge base contains more comprehensive information than the general one. The model categories need to be further refined, such as the **measurement** class is divided into three subcategories: **basic item**, **recommended project** and **select project**. The final conceptual model of hypertension PHR knowledge base consists of 4 top, 10 secondary and 38 low level classes. This step is completed by medical experts.

(2) Instance Extraction

We recruit graduate students with medical backgrounds to extract seven types of meaningful medical entities, i.e. **body**, **disease**, **symptom**, **sign**, **surgery**, **drug**, **laboratory examination**. The medical entities are added to the knowledge base as instances. For example, the concept (class) **drug therapy** has instances **amiloride**, **amlodipine**, **atenolol**, **benazepril**, **betaxolol**, **bisoprolol**, **candesartan**, **captopril**, **carvedilol**, **cilazapril**, etc.

(3) Relation Extraction

Hierarchical and association relations exist between classes simultaneously. At the same time that the conceptual model is created, the hierarchical relationship exists. The relation here is defaulted as association relations. According to medical experts, we defines four relations that exist between medical entities. As shown in Fig. 3, based on the named entity recognition in the previous section, we implement the process of relation extraction. We believe that the co-occurence of different types of medical entities in the same sentence represents a relation between them. The type of relation depends on the type of medical entity. However, we only consider the four types of relations mentioned above. For example, disease **essential hypertension** and drug **amiloride** are in the same sentence. We can draw a conclusion that **amiloride therapy essential hypertension**.

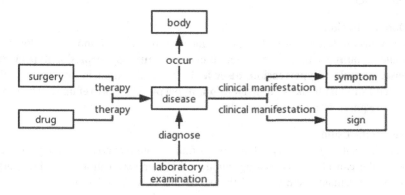

Fig. 3. Relations between medical entities

(4) Attribute Extraction

An attribute is the characteristic of a class itself, which can be inherited by its subclasses and owned by all instances of the class. Attributes also need to be further constructed through domain analysis and expert evaluation. This article defines several attributes for each class according to characteristics of hypertension. For instance, the class **drug treatment** contains four attributes, i.e. **DTdrug name**, **DTbegin time**, **DTend time**, and **DT time of duration**. The attributes indicate the specific drug name, the begin time of the drug treatment, the end time of the drug treatment and the period of drug treatment. We also define data type of each attribute which is determined by specific data contents.

(5) Domain Determination

A domain set refers to the value range of a relation or attribute. We determine **definition** domains and **value** domains separately for relations defined above. For example, the definition domain of relation **suffer from** is **patient** and the value domain is **disease**.

5.2   Fusion of Knowledge from Different Sources

As mentioned above, there are three data sources for hypertension PHR knowledge base construction. The KF process model is necessary as theoretical guidance for the fusion of knowledge from different sources.

(1) Instance Fusion

Instance fusion is normally considered at the first step. Using DO as a reference standard, there are two possible outcomes for the entities extracted from other sources. On the one hand, there are equivalent entities in DO. What we need to do is find its equivalent entity and link it to DO. On the other hand, there are no equivalent entities in DO. What we need to do is classify it and add it to the DO. For example, the entity **secondary hypertension** extracted from the textbook has equivalent entity **secondary hypertension** in DO and can be linked to each other directly. However, the entity **elderly hypertensive** has no equivalent entity in DO. It needs to be classified and added to DO.

(2) Domain Fusion

Domain fusion follows the step of instance fusion. For example, the domain of attribute **Synonyms** in DO is {**High blood pressure**, **hyperpiesia**, **hypertensive disease**, **vascular hypertension disorder**}, while the domain of same attribute extracted from text book is {**hypertension**, **hyperpiesia**, **wind vertigo**}. The domain sets are required to be merged together.

(3) Relation Fusion

The key in relation fusion is to clarify two similar relation expression. They can be the same or the can be one containing another. For our verification, it is necessary to compute the semantic similarity of the words that describe relations.

(4) Attribute Fusion

For example, in DO, the attribute of entity **hypertension** is {**DOID**, **Definition**, **Name**, **Synoyms**, **Xrefs**}, and the attribute of same entity extracted from textbooks includes {**definition**, **diagnosis**, **treatment**, . . .}. Usually, text similarity calculation and semantic similarity calculation are required to clarify two similar attribute. After that these attributes can be merged.

(5) Concept Fusion

Concept fusion is considered to be a process of generating new concepts. For example, the concept **hypertension** in DO refers to {**primary hypertension**, **malignant hypertension**, **pre-eclampsia**, **pulmonary hypertension**, **secondary hypertension**}. However, the same concept **hypertension** extracted from the textbooks refers to {**primary hypertension, secondary hypertension, elderly hypertension, resistant hypertension**}. We should incorporate the knowledge elements from different sources to generate new concept **hypertension**.

5.3   Fusion of General and Special Health Knowledge

In order to realize the fusion of general and special health knowledge, we defines nine association relations according to the principle that general health knowledge can influence the occurence and personal health states, and further influence special health knowledge. As shown in Fig. 4, the different colored lines represent different relations, i.e., **influence, therapy, prevent, manifest, suffer from, direct, has property, had the experience** and **plan to experience**. They exist between different categories. For example, The relation of **influence** connects **geographical environment, lifestyle**, and **family history** with the **disease** concept, representing effects of etiologies on the disease.

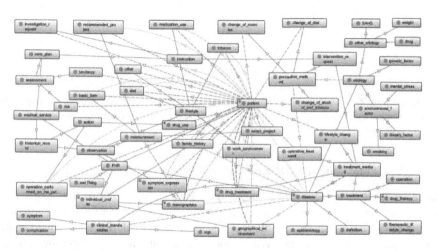

Fig. 4. Relations in the hypertension PHR knowledge base

After the process of knowledge extraction, the general health knowledge and special health knowledge exists as knowledge elements. Based on these nine types of relations, the elements from two types of knowledge can be connected like a network structure. Figure 5 illustrate an example.

There is a piece of special health knowledge text "the patient suffers from essential hypertension, lives in Liaoning province and is 30 years old, who had headache and had the medicine hydrochlorothiazide for seven years from year 2010 to 2017. The recommend drug therapy plan is to take propranolol two times a day, 15 mg for each time." and a piece of general health knowledge text "Symptoms of essential hypertension have headache, dizziness etc. It can be treated with drug hydrochlorothiazide, propranolol etc." They are translated the logical structure shown in Fig. 5. Three knowledge elements which exist in two pieces of text at the same time are reused, i.e. headache, propranolol and hydrochlorothiazide.

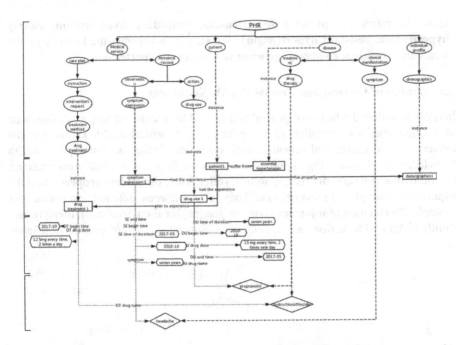

Fig. 5. Fusion of general and special health knowledge (The circles represent concepts, the rectangles represent instances, and the hexagons represent attributes. Rhombuses represent the reused knowledge elements.)

5.4   The Application of PHR Knowledge Base

Based on the hypertension PHR knowledge base mentioned above, this paper constructs a knowledge service platform, illustrated in Fig. 6. The platform can be divided into five modules according to different functions, the module for conceptual navigation, the module for linked data visualization, the module for explaining the concept, the module for displaying related concept and the module for knowledge seeking. It is worth mentioning that four modules are connected organically. When one module changes, other modules changes accordingly.

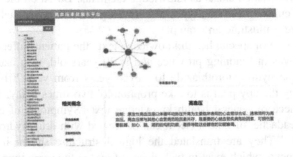

Fig. 6. The platform for knowledge service (Chinese edition)

6 Discussion

The contributions of this paper are as follows:

(1) We proposes a knowledge fusion process model, which is universal.
(2) In the process of knowledge fusion in hypertension PHR knowledge base construction, two dimensions of knowledge fusion are considered. It can provide researchers with new research ideas.
(3) This paper constructs a hypertension PHR knowledge base and implements its application. It is conducive for the better management of healthy big data in the field of chronic diseases, which is the foundation of improving public health, conquering medical problems, and improving health policies.

However, there are also some limitations in our research. We are committed to making improvements in the future.

(1) The method used in the process of construction is semi-automatic, which leads to low efficiency. In the future, the method will be transformed to automated ways.
(2) The scale of the hypertension PHR knowledge base is small. In the future, we will build a complete chronic disease PHR knowledge base.
(3) The functions of knowledge service platform is less. In the future, we will add more functions to the platform, such as natural language queries and decision support services.

References

1. Ed-informatics.   http://ed-informatics.org/healthcare-it-in-a-nutshell-2/emr-vs-ehr-vs-phr/. Accessed 21 May 2019
2. Wang, L., et al.: Toward a normalized clinical drug knowledge base in China—applying the RxNorm model to Chinese clinical drugs. J. Am. Med. Inf. Assoc. **25**(7), 809–818 (2018)
3. El-Sappagh, S., Kwak, D., Ali, F., Kwak, K.S.: DMTO: a realistic ontology for standard diabetes mellitus treatment. J. Biomed. Semant. **9**(1), 8 (2018)
4. El-Sappagh, S., El Mogy, M., Riad, A.M.: A standard fragment of EHR relational data model for diabetes mellitus diagnosis. In: 9th International Conference on Informatics and Systems, pp. DEKM-1. IEEE (2014)
5. El-Sappagh, S., Alonso, J.M., Ali, F., Ali, A., Jang, J.H., Kwak, K.S.: An ontology-based interpretable fuzzy decision support system for diabetes diagnosis. IEEE Access **6**, 37371–37394 (2018)
6. Nithya, G., Shabu, S.L.: A novel framework in reusing the ontological health record. Res. J. Pharm. Bio. Chem. Sci. **7**(3), 215–220 (2016)
7. Sherimon, P.C., Vinu, P.V., Krishnan, R.: Using concept based OWL2 rules in risk assessment of diabetic patients. In: IEEE Information Technology, Networking, Electronic and Automation Control Conference, pp. 270–274. IEEE (2016)
8. Shemeikka, T., et al.: A health record integrated clinical decision support system to support prescriptions of pharmaceutical drugs in patients with reduced renal function: design, development and proof of concept. Int. J. Med. Inf. **84**(6), 387–395 (2015)

9. McCoy, A.B., Wright, A., Krousel-Wood, M., Thomas, E.J., McCoy, J.A., Sittig, D.F.: Validation of a crowdsourcing methodology for developing a knowledge base of related problem-medication pairs. Appl. Clin. Inf. **6**(02), 334–344 (2015)

10. Jing, X., Kay, S., Marley, T., Hardiker, N.R.: Integration of an OWL-DL knowledge base with an EHR prototype and providing customized information. J. Med. Syst. **38**(9), 75 (2014)

11. Rao, R.R., Makkithaya, K., Gupta, N.: Ontology based semantic representation for public health data integration. In: International Conference on Contemporary Computing and Informatics (IC3I), pp. 357–362. IEEE (2014)

12. Fan, H., Wang, F., Zheng, M.: Research on knowledge fusion connotation and process model. In: Chen, H., Ji, H., Sun, L., Wang, H., Qian, T., Ruan, T. (eds.) CCKS 2016. CCIS, vol. 650, pp. 184–195. Springer, Singapore (2016). https://doi.org/10.1007/978-981-10-3168-7_18

13. Author, F., Author, S., Author, T.: Book title. 2nd edn. Publisher, Location (1999)

14. Ge, J., Xu, Y.: Internal Medicine, 8th edn. People's Medical Publishing House, Beijing (2013)

15. Xie, X., Gou, W.: Obstetrics and Gynecology, 8th edn. People's Medical Publishing House, Beijing (2013)

16. Disease Ontology. www.disease-ontology.org. Accessed 21 May 2019

CrowdMed: A Blockchain-Based Approach to Consent Management for Health Data Sharing

Mira Shah, Chao Li, Ming Sheng, Yong Zhang$^{(\boxtimes)}$,
and Chunxiao Xing

Research Institute of Information Technology, Beijing National Research Center
for Information Science and Technology, Department of Computer Science
and Technology, Institute of Internet Industry, Tsinghua University,
Beijing 100084, China
wuml18@mails.tsinghua.edu.cn, {li-chao, shengming,
zhangyong05, xingcx}@tsinghua.edu.cn

Abstract. The need for greater health data sharing is widely acknowledged in the healthcare industry. The provision of healthcare services and attempts to harness Big Data analytics are adversely affected by the fragmentation of medical data across healthcare providers. However, attempts to encourage greater data sharing have been unsuccessful due to privacy concerns and lack of motivation for patients to share their data. We propose CrowdMed, a medical data management framework to facilitate greater data sharing, empowering patients with full control over access to their medical data. The framework is fully transparent, ensuring that patients have full knowledge over how who has access to their data, and how their data is being used. Using blockchain as the foundation for consent management, patients can trust that only parties with permission can view their data. Permissions are also finely specified, and can be revoked or modified according to the patient's wishes. Following these permissions, data is transferred automatically between parties, conveniently and efficiently alleviating the problem of data fragmentation. CrowdMed also addresses the lack of motivation for data sharing, incentivising patients to share more of their data for research purposes through reward tokens and an innovative pricing mechanism. The framework integrates fully with existing data storage architecture, aiding in its widespread adoption.

Keywords: Blockchain · Health data · Privacy · Data sharing

1 Introduction

The problem of medical fragmentation has been well known and studied. As people move from place to place, they leave fragments of their medical history in various medical organisations [8]. Patients are thus unable to obtain a holistic, complete view of their medical history, and are unable to provide accurate information to doctors. This adversely affects the quality of medical care patients receive. They might have to repeat tests unnecessarily, or a portion of their medical history may simply be missing.

© Springer Nature Switzerland AG 2019
H. Chen et al. (Eds.): ICSH 2019, LNCS 11924, pp. 345–356, 2019.
https://doi.org/10.1007/978-3-030-34482-5_31

With more complete information, doctors can make more accurate diagnoses. Additionally, ensuring that complete medical records are available would unlock the potential of big data analytics in the healthcare industry and greatly benefit medical researchers [7]. Hence, the need for a framework to facilitate medical data sharing is real and urgent.

Given the sensitive nature of medical data, protecting patient's rights must be the highest priority when designing such a framework [2]. The framework should provide transparency and auditability, and ensure patients are aware of who can access their data and for what purpose. In fact, patients should have the ability to control who can access their data and what exactly they choose to share. In this way, ownership over medical data is restored to the patients themselves. Thus, a system supporting medical data sharing should empower patients with knowledge and control over their medical data records.

When it comes to sharing medical data for research, patients lack the motivation to do so. Patients may be hesitant to share their data with medical researchers despite the benefits to society at large from medical research due to privacy concerns. Patients also do not receive immediate benefits and thus are unlikely to participate in medical data sharing. Hence, a system that provides patients with direct benefits from sharing their data would facilitate the creation of an ecosystem where patients are incentivised to share their data, and the community as a whole benefits from improved research outcomes.

A blockchain-based system has the potential to meet these requirements. A blockchain is an immutable, append-only chain of records that are stored in multiple machines. Using public-key cryptography, it maintains a consistent record of transactions in the absence of a trusted third party [10]. Since a copy of the blockchain is stored in every machine, the contents of the blockchain are available to all members, providing for auditability and accountability. Using a consensus algorithm, the blockchain is extended by mining nodes that compete for the rights to append a block of transactions to the chain, according to the specific configuration of the blockchain. The popular Bitcoin network uses the Proof of Work consensus protocol, where miners compete by solving a computationally-intensive puzzle. The mining activities in a blockchain open the possibility of incentivising and rewarding certain behaviours [3].

In this paper, we propose CrowdMed, a novel blockchain-based approach to managing patient consent and sharing medical data. CrowdMed addresses the challenges to data sharing outlined above: lack of interoperability, privacy concerns and lack of motivation. CrowdMed is a framework that enables convenient and secure data transfers between users, places the patient at the center of control over data access, and provides incentives and rewards for data sharing for research purposes. It can be integrated into existing data management infrastructure, facilitating easy adoption [4].

The paper is organised as follows. In Sect. 2, we discuss related work. In Sect. 3, we describe the architecture and stakeholders of the framework. In Sect. 4, we elaborate on the incentives for data sharing. In Sect. 5, we describe the usage of CrowdMed to illustrate its functionality. In Sect. 6, we discuss the added value of the framework and address some caveats. Finally, we conclude the paper and discuss the future direction of this research in Sect. 7.

2 Related Work

In this section we give an overview of research that has been done in medical data sharing. First, we review some proposed systems for integrating heterogeneous health data sources using traditional database management technologies. Next, we explore privacy concerns related to health data sharing, and the implications it has on the design of CrowdMed. Last, we describe some blockchain-based systems that others have proposed.

Using traditional database storage systems, Khennou et al. [7] propose using the mobile agent paradigm to transfer medical data between multiple databases from clinics, as well as to a centralised database. The system ensures hospitals have access to a patient's complete medical history, and the pooling of data in a centralised database enables data analytics. Gui et al. [6] propose an architecture for healthcare big data management and analysis, focusing on pre-processing and transforming data for analytics. Stream analytics is incorporated for real-time monitoring and analysis. Similar to the previous system, medical records are acquired from clinics and stored in a centralised database. Data governance, including data life-cycle management, is mentioned but not considered in detail. These systems involve the storage of data in an external database, which involves a third-party that stores and manages medical data. Due to the privacy and security issues involved in this, CrowdMed does not take the same approach, and uses a distributed storage system using the existing databases in hospitals. These systems also do not consider patient authority and privacy, which is the focus of CrowdMed.

Asghar et al. [2] conduct a thorough review of privacy and consent management in healthcare, emphasising the need for patient control over their medical records. The authors assert that patients should be empowered with the ability to finely specify access permissions to their data, such as how long the data should be accessible, and what specifics parts of the data are accessible. Along with creating these permission protocols, patients should also be able to freely modify or revoke consent. Patient identifiers and anonymity are also addressed. The requirements Asghar et al. describe form the basis for how privacy and access control is built into CrowdMed. In particular, the complexity of consent management relates to the ability to execute smart contracts in blockchains, and opens up the potential of incorporating blockchain in medical data management systems for patient consent management.

Kumar et al. [8] gives an overview of the potential applications of blockchain in healthcare, including for data sharing, data access control and maintaining medical history. They also stress the importance of interoperability, security and transparency in the design of blockchain-based medical data management systems, and highlight the use of smart contracts. These strengths of blockchain are highlighted in the design of CrowdMed, but some challenges mentioned such as scalability and data standardisation are outside the scope of this paper and will not be addressed. The authors of [1, 5, 9, 11] and [3] propose blockchain-based systems for securely sharing and transferring medical data, using smart contracts and permissions contracts to protect patients' privacy and data access control. However, [11] does not address data sharing across hospitals for maintaining patients' medical history. [1] and [9] utilise a centralised database for data storage which is difficult to implement in reality due to legal regulations. The upload of data to a third-party is also an obstacle to widespread adoption. [9] utilises a unique approach to the creation of medical records that we adapt in CrowdMed, emphasising patients' ownership over their data. [3] highlights the possibility of incentivising data sharing through mining activities. However, the authors propose using patient data as mining rewards, which is a clear violation of patient control. CrowdMed improves on the ideas proposed, proposing an innovative approach to this, while protecting patients' privacy and authority.

3 General Architecture and Stakeholders

In this section, we first present the general architecture of CrowdMed and describe the components. We then describe the various stakeholders in the framework.

3.1 General Architecture

Figure 1 presents the general architecture of the CrowdMed framework. It is divided into 3 layers: the data storage layer, the central management layer and the user layer. The data involved in the function of CrowdMed can be categorised into two types: medical data and the sharing log. Medical data is stored in the databases in the data storage layer, while the sharing log is stored in the blockchain in the central management layer.

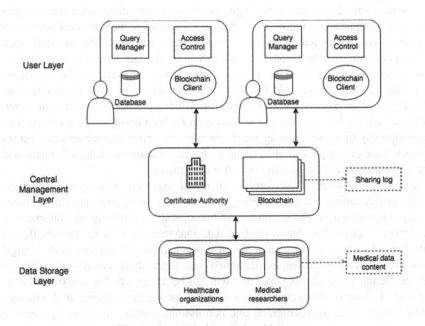

Fig. 1. CrowdMed general architecture

User Layer. Each user can be a patient, doctor/hospital or researcher. Each user node consists of a local database, a query manager, an access control manager and the blockchain client.

The query manager executes queries on medical data and returns results from the user's local database, or retrieves data from the data storage layer. If the user is a doctor or researcher, their local database is part of the data storage layer i.e. query managers can access their database. For patients, the access control manager provides an interface through which they generate permission contracts. These are forwarded to the blockchain client that appends it to the blockchain. The blockchain client executes all actions related to the blockchain.

For the purposes of this paper, we take doctors and hospitals to be interchangeable. We assume doctors act in a larger organisation, and when a hospital joins CrowdMed, all doctors that work in the hospital also join. However, patients form relationships with individual doctors.

Central Management Layer. The central management layer comprises the central query manager and the distributed ledger (i.e. the blockchain) itself.

The certificate authority (CA) is responsible for adding new users to the framework. The CA verifies the new user's identity and links their real-world identity to a unique virtual ID. This is the signature used by the user in transactions on the blockchain. This helps to de-link patient data from their real-world identities in the event of a data leak. The ID can also be periodically changed to prevent data leaks from detecting similarities in transactions. When adding new hospitals/researchers, the CA also ensures that the organisation is legitimate. Hence, when patients receive requests for their data from these organisations, they can trust that it is an actual doctor/researcher who is accessing their data.

The blockchain stores patients' permissions contracts and records actions performed on data (such as creation of data entries or transferral of data to different parties). The permissions contracts are the specification of a patient's consent to sharing their data with another user in the framework. One permissions contract is created per patient-doctor relationship, and provide the patient with fine-grained options, such as how much data to share and how long the doctor should be able to access their data. Additionally, each patient also creates one special permissions contract detailing their willingness to share their data for research purposes. This is elaborated on in Sects. 5.3 and 5.4.

Data Storage Layer. CrowdMed uses a distributed storage system, where healthcare providers and medical researchers maintain their own, pre-existing databases. The framework then connects with these databases and executes queries on them. This approach facilitates adoption of CrowdMed as the framework can be built on top of the existing infrastructure. Moreover, this circumvents security and legal issues that may surround uploading medical data to a third party storage system (such as cloud storage provided by a commercial entity).

We assume that the medical data stored takes the form of an Electronic Medical Record (EMR) with additional data attached to it. The EMR is identified by an identification number and linked to the patient using the patient's ID, but the patient's personal information is not stored in the EMR itself. Additional data such as medical images, lab test results, comments etc. are linked to the EMR by the EMR's ID.

3.2 Stakeholders

Table 1 summarises the role, functionality and benefits of each stakeholder involved in CrowdMed. Notably, patients are the only party able to create permissions contract. Thus, patients remain in full control of access to their medical data. Additionally, the doctor is considered to be responsible for storing medical data. When data is shared within the framework, the doctors' databases are always the source. There is thus 'one true source' of medical data.

Table 1. Stakeholders in CrowdMed framework.

Stakeholder	Role	Functions	Benefits
Patient	Owner of medical data	Create permissions contracts with doctors and researchers	Improved medical care
Doctor	Creator and primary storage of medical data	Create new medical records, request and receive patients' existing data	Improved decision making from more complete information
Medical researcher	Blockchain mining node	Request and receive patients' data	Improved research outcomes from more sources of health data

The framework can be extended as needed to add new stakeholders. The framework considers data creators and receivers. New stakeholders would be afforded certain functions depending on which of these they are. For example, a physical examination center that is external to a hospital would be a data creator, and would be able to create new medical records that are accessible to other users. As patients are able to add permission contracts for sharing medical records with doctors, they will be able to add contracts for sharing the results of physical examinations. Other stakeholders that may be added to the framework include medical insurance companies, as data receivers.

4 Incentives for Data Sharing

In this section, we describe the incentives in mining the blockchain and in sharing data with researchers. We envision that CrowdMed will be self-sustaining, and encourages patients to share data for research purposes.

Research institutions are the mining nodes on the blockchain and receive tokens as a reward. When a patient shares their data with the researcher, the researcher transfers these tokens to the patient. The patient can then exchange the tokens for actual rewards according to the regulations of that country. This reward might be cash rewards, discounts when they purchase medical services among others. Another possible reward that is more novel could be the findings of the research institution's work that was made possible using the patient's data. Carrying from the earlier example of a diabetes researcher, the patient might be informed of drugs that might be more effective for their disease.

The price attached to a patient's data is proportional to the amount of data they share (such as the number of EMRs) and the value of the data (e.g. textual EMRs vs imaging results), and the uniqueness of the data. For example, patient A who chooses to disclose their exact date of birth may receive a greater reward than patient B who does not as patient A's data is more specific and useful to the researcher. This pricing mechanism incentivises patients to share a greater amount of data, as well as improves the quality and usefulness of data shared with researchers.

5   Use Case Scenarios

We describe several use case scenarios below to illustrate the various functions of CrowdMed, and show how patient privacy and control is carefully considered and protected in the framework.

5.1   Registering a New User

A Certificate Authority (CA) is charged with adding new users to the framework.

5.2   Adding New Medical Records

Figure 2 describes the process of adding a new EMR.

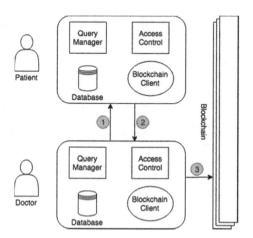

Fig. 2. Adding a new EMR

1. Doctor creates and signs the EMR and sends it to the patient.
2. Patient signs the EMR and returns it to the doctor (the patient can optionally choose to save the EMR to his own database as well).
3. Doctor saves the EMR in his database and appends a transaction to the blockchain.

The doctor's signature provides for accountability, in that an EMR can be traced back to a specific source, since the EMR may reside in various databases and be transferred between various parties. The patient's signature signifies their ownership over the EMR, and also represents the patient's acknowledgement and approval of the creation of the new EMR. After signing the EMR, the patient may optionally save it to their own local database. Doing so ensures the availability of their data, but the patient may choose not to do so due to resource constraints. The EMR is saved in the doctor's database, and a new transaction is added to the blockchain, representing the creation of a new EMR and ensuring that its location can be found by other parties.

If an existing EMR is modified, the above process is repeated as though the EMR is new. However, in step 3, an additional transaction is appended to the blockchain nullifying the previous transaction related to this EMR.

5.3 Visiting a New Doctor

Figure 3 describes the process of sharing data with a doctor that a patient has not visited before. This process transfers the patient's complete medical history to the doctor.

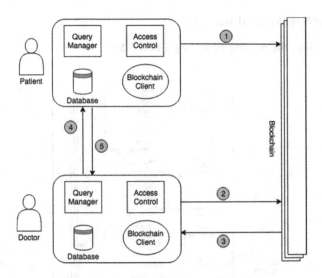

Fig. 3. Sharing medical history with a doctor

1. Patient creates a new permissions contract (PC), giving the doctor permission to access their data.
2. Doctor searches the blockchain for the indices of the patient's medical records.

3. After verifying with the PC, the blockchain returns the indices of the EMRs. A new transaction is added to the blockchain showing the transfer of data to the doctor.
4. The doctor sends a request for the EMRs to the appropriate database, with the indices.
5. The database manager verifies the PC, and returns the data to the doctor.

The process is initiated when a doctor sends a query to his local database requesting a patient's data. If this data does not exist on his database, he searches the blockchain for the indices of the required data. Before returning the indices, the blockchain client checks that there is a permissions contract authorising the doctor to access this patient's data. If none exists, the doctor sends a request to the patient for access. The patient can approve this request and add a permissions contract to the blockchain, or reject it by not taking action. If/when the doctors request is approved, he can search the blockchain for the required indices. The required indices are returned, and a new transaction is added to the blockchain showing the transfer of data. The doctor then sends a request to the appropriate database with the indices of the data. The database manager verifies via the blockchain that there is a permissions contract authorising the doctor to access the data, and returns the data to the doctor.

In some situations, the patient may wish to share their data with a doctor/researcher that is not a member of the framework. Then, the process described above is not possible as the third-party does not have access to the central query manager and blockchain. For example, a patient in an emergency situation may be sent to a hospital that he has never visited before and is not a registered user of CrowdMed. The framework must consider such exceptional life-or-death cases and allow the patient to send data from their own local database to the third-party directly. However, as the identity of the third-party has not been verified by the CA, the patient shares his data in this manner at his own risk. We envision that this will only occur in highly exceptional cases.

5.4 Sharing Data with Researchers

Sharing data with researchers using CrowdMed is similar to the previous scenario in terms of data flow, but with a different initiation process. The priority in this process is ensuring that patients are not personally identifiable using the data they share with researchers.

On registering for CrowdMed, patients enter their preferences on the type of data they are willing to share with researchers, as well as what personal information they share about themselves (henceforth referred to as identifiers). These are stored in a special permissions contract specifically for sharing data with researchers, and appended to the blockchain. Modifications can be made to this permissions contract, and the blockchain will be updated accordingly. The settings patients store with respect to identifiers concerns obscuring their identities. For example, instead of sharing their exact date of birth with researchers, patients can share only the month and year of birth, or even only the year. This helps to ensure that the data they share with researchers cannot be linked to them.

When requesting data from patients, a researcher could search for the data of patients relevant to their research goals. For example, a researcher interested in studying diabetes could search for patients with diabetes, who are between the ages of 50 to 70. The data shared with the researchers is drawn from the pool of patients who are willing to share their data and have these characteristics. From there, the data is transferred to the researchers in a process similar to that explained before. The incentives and exchange of tokens related to sharing data with researchers is explained in Sect. 4.

5.5   Reviewing EMRs

As time progresses, patients/doctors may wish to review their previous EMRs and add notes on the diagnoses and treatments received. For example, a patient may add a comment describing the adverse side-effects of a drug prescribed to him, or on the particular efficacy of a certain drug. Recognising the value of this to doctors, researchers and to patients themselves, CrowdMed provides a mechanism for both patients and doctors to add comments and notes to previous EMRs. These are additional blocks of data that contain a link to the parent EMR. They are stored in the databases and added to the blockchain in the same way EMRs are added.

6   Discussion

CrowdMed empowers patients with access and knowledge of their own medical history, enabling them to make better decisions with regards to their health. Additionally, patients are truly in control of their data, increasing trust between patients, doctors and researchers. Quality of medical care also significantly improves as doctors have more information to base their decisions on. Accountability and transparency are also encouraged. Lastly, the medical research community benefits from the sharing of medical data.

CrowdMed integrates with existing data storage infrastructure, aiding in the widespread adoption of the framework. Due to the distributed storage system, duplication of data in patient and doctor's databases, and distributed nature of blockchain, there is no central target for attackers, reducing the likelihood of massive data breaches.

The novel way CrowdMed handles patient data and data sharing rests on the transparency and accountability provided by the blockchain. However, Bitcoin is known for its issues with scalability and efficiency. Hence, the viability of CrowdMed is dependent on the improvements in blockchain. Research in this field has been progressing at a rapid pace, and many new consensus algorithms have been proposed that may address the current shortcomings in blockchain. The specifics of the blockchain can be configured separately from the rest of our proposed design, and can be easily changed as the technology develops.

CrowdMed also does not fully address the security issues arising from targeted attacks on hospital's databases. Even using our architecture, individual databases may be hacked into, resulting in data leaks. However, CrowdMed takes steps to de-link patient real-world identities from their IDs in the framework. While this does not solve the problem completely, some of the risk is alleviated.

7   Conclusion and Future Work

CrowdMed takes an innovative approach to data management in the healthcare sector. We improve on existing systems by giving patient privacy and authority the highest priority at every step of the design. The proposed framework also seeks to encourage patients to share as much of their medical data with researchers as they are comfortable with, benefitting the medical community at large.

In the future, we intend to create a working prototype of the CrowdMed framework. Experiments regarding the performance and scalability of the framework will also be carried out to optimise the underlying data structures for efficient retrieval. Finally, data harmonisation remains an obstacle in previous attempts to integrate heterogeneous sources of medical data. We will explore this topic more, and integrate these processes into CrowdMed to fully realise a future where medical data can be easily shared, and mined for valuable insights.

Acknowledgements. This work was supported by NSFC (91646202), National Key R&D Program of China (2018YFB1404400, 2018YFB1402700).

References

1. Amofa, S., et al.: A blockchain-based architecture framework for secure sharing of personal health data. In: 2018 IEEE 20th International Conference on e-Health Networking, Applications and Services (Healthcom), September 2018, pp. 1–6. https://doi.org/10.1109/HealthCom.2018.8531160
2. Asghar, M.R., Lee, T., Baig, M.M., Ullah, E., Russello, G., Dobbie, G.: A review of privacy and consent management in healthcare: a focus on emerging data sources. In: 13th IEEE International Conference on e-Science, e-Science 2017, Auckland, New Zealand, 24–27 October 2017, pp. 518–522 (2017). https://doi.org/10.1109/eScience.2017.84
3. Azaria, A., Ekblaw, A., Vieira, T., Lippman, A.: MedRec: using blockchain for medical data access and permission management. In: 2nd International Conference on Open and Big Data, OBD 2016, Vienna, Austria, 22–24 August 2016, pp. 25–30 (2016). https://doi.org/10.1109/OBD.2016.11
4. Cohen, S., Zohar, A.: Database perspectives on blockchains. CoRR abs/1803.06015 (2018). http://arxiv.org/abs/1803.06015
5. Fan, K., Wang, S., Ren, Y., Li, H., Yang, Y.: MedBlock: efficient and secure medical data sharing via blockchain. J. Med. Syst. **42**(8), 136 (2018). https://doi.org/10.1007/s10916-018-0993-7
6. Gui, H., Zheng, R., Ma, C., Fan, H., Xu, L.: An architecture for healthcare big data management and analysis. In: Health Information Science - 5th International Conference, HIS 2016, Proceedings, Shanghai, China, 5–7 November 2016, pp. 154–160 (2016). https://doi.org/10.1007/978-3-319-48335-1_17

7. Khennou, F., Khamlichi, Y.I., Chaoui, N.E.H.: Designing a health data management system based hadoop-agent. In: 4th IEEE International Colloquium on Information Science and Technology, CiSt 2016, Tangier, Morocco, 24–26 October 2016, pp. 71–76 (2016). https://doi.org/10.1109/CIST.2016.7804983

8. Kumar, T., Ramani, V., Ahmad, I., Braeken, A., Harjula, E., Ylianttila, M.: Blockchain utilization in healthcare: key requirements and challenges. In: 20th IEEE International Conference on e-Health Networking, Applications and Services, Healthcom 2018, Ostrava, Czech Republic, 17–20 September 2018, pp. 1–7 (2018). https://doi.org/10.1109/HealthCom.2018.8531136

9. Liu, J., Li, X., Ye, L., Zhang, H., Du, X., Guizani, M.: BPDS: a blockchain based privacy-preserving data sharing for electronic medical records. In: 2018 IEEE Global Communications Conference (GLOBECOM), pp. 1–6, December 2018. https://doi.org/10.1109/GLOCOM.2018.8647713

10. Nakamoto, S.: Bitcoin: a peer-to-peer electronic cash system. Cryptography Mailing List (2009). https://metzdowd.com

11. Theodouli, A., Arakliotis, S., Moschou, K., Votis, K., Tzovaras, D.: On the design of a blockchain-based system to facilitate healthcare data sharing. In: 2018 17th IEEE International Conference On Trust, Security And Privacy In Computing and Communications. 12th IEEE International Conference On Big Data Science And Engineering (TrustCom/BigDataSE), pp. 1374–1379, August 2018. https://doi.org/10.1109/TrustCom/BigDataSE.2018.00190

Research on the Construction of Information Service Platform for Autism Based on Knowledge Map

Wang Zhao[1,2](✉)

[1] School of Information Management, Wuhan University, Wuhan, China
199223263@qq.com
[2] Suzhou Zealikon Healthcare Co., Ltd., Suzhou, China

Abstract. With the development of social economy and the aggravation of environmental pressure, autism has been gradually recognized and its incidence has become higher and higher. At present, the research on autism at home and abroad is still in its infancy, and the research methods and tools are relatively few, especially the research on the acquisition and display of autism-related knowledge is relatively scarce. Doctors and various rehabilitation institutions as well as the vast number of autistic patients have an urgent need to acquire knowledge about treatment and rehabilitation of autism. In the information age, the Internet provides people with convenient access to information and knowledge. The purpose of this study is to use Internet technology to collect information and knowledge about autism. The autism database is designed and the autism information service platform based on knowledge map is constructed. Autism information service platform can provide doctors and patients with efficient access to autism information and knowledge, help them to acquire the required knowledge at any time and anywhere, and promote the early diagnosis and treatment of autism.

Keywords: Autism · Knowledge map · Information service platform

1 Introduction

Autism, also known as autism or autism disorders, is a representative disease of generalized developmental disorders. In recent years, the incidence of autistic children has become higher and higher, experiencing a transition from rare diseases to epidemics, and the number of autistic children has exceeded our imagination. But there are few autism related knowledge websites or information platforms. It is difficult for people to acquire autism related knowledge. Rehabilitation treatment of autism is generally effective before the age of 6. How to make the knowledge of autism popularized and easily acquired by the public is the focus of current research. Knowledge maps show the relationship between knowledge in a visual form, which makes knowledge easier to understand. With the efficient communication channel of the Internet, the rapid dissemination of autism information and knowledge is possible.

The purpose of this paper is to study the information and knowledge of autism, build the knowledge map of autism, and establish a visual autism query system. In

© Springer Nature Switzerland AG 2019
H. Chen et al. (Eds.): ICSH 2019, LNCS 11924, pp. 357–368, 2019.
https://doi.org/10.1007/978-3-030-34482-5_32

order to systematize and standardize the knowledge of autism, promote the diagnosis and treatment of autism, and improve the public's awareness of autism, so as to provide an opportunity for patients with autism to seek medical treatment and treatment as soon as possible.

2   Autism and Its History

Autism (autism disorder) is a neurodevelopmental disorder, also known as autism. The diseases are collectively referred to as autism spectrum disorder (ASD) [1]. Since Kanner, an American child psychiatrist, first reported autism in 1943, the incidence of autism has risen rapidly worldwide. In the 1980s, about 3–5 out of every 10,000 people suffered from the disease, while in 2000, 6.7 out of every 1,000 children suffered from the disease [2]. According to the National Center for Health Statistics, the probability of autism among children aged 3-14 in the United States reached 2.76% in 2016 [3]. The incidence of autism has been increasing steadily for more than 40 years.

There is no statistical survey on autistic children in China. However, according to the data of "Report on the Development of Autism Education and Rehabilitation Industry in China II", the number of autism population in China is estimated to exceed 10 million people, of which 2 million are autistic children. At the same time, it is growing at the rate of nearly 200,000 per year [4].

Autism brings serious financial burden to both society and family. Families with autistic children, on the one hand, spend a lot of time caring for children, working hours are reduced, so that work income is reduced. On the other hand, the cost of family rehabilitation treatment for autistic children is huge, which increases the family's financial burden [5]. According to the survey of family financial burden of preschool autistic children, 33% of parents of autistic children reported that the care of autistic children seriously affected their career, their annual income was significantly lower than that of ordinary families, with an average annual income loss of 30,957 yuan. Meanwhile, the average annual cost of autistic children's families for children's education and training is significantly higher than that of ordinary families [6]. Society and government also need to invest a lot of money in rehabilitation education for autistic children. At the same time, autism also brings depression to the patients'families, which has a negative impact on their quality of life [7, 8].

It can be seen that the incidence of autism in children is relatively serious, and the harm to society and family is enormous. However, there is no systematic and standardized knowledge system for medical research on autism. Doctors often rely on personal experience to diagnose and treat autism, so it is worthwhile to build a knowledge map of autism. This can provide comprehensive information and knowledge services to autistic children. It plays an important role in alleviating the economic and mental pressure of families with autistic children.

3   Current Situation of Knowledge Map of Autism

3.1   Knowledge Map and Its Application

Knowledge map is an important part of AI. Knowledge maps originate from semantic networks [9]. On May 16, 2012, Google introduced the concept of knowledge map, which aims to improve the accuracy of search engines and make search engines more intelligent [10]. Knowledge map is essentially a semantic network that reveals the relationship between entities and can formally describe the relationship between things in the real world.

In recent years, knowledge map has been applied to search engines, intelligent question answering systems, e-commerce and many other fields. The application of knowledge map makes these software more intelligent. Knowledge map also plays an important role in the process of medical intellectualization. Using knowledge map technology, medical knowledge can be integrated and expressed more accurately and normatively.

3.2   Current Status of Knowledge Map of Autism

Overseas research on knowledge map of autism is relatively early. Before the concept of knowledge map was put forward, many scholars studied the ontology of autism.

The research on the construction and reasoning of children's autism knowledge map is relatively few in China, and most of them are based on literature research hotspots and visual analysis of research status. There are few studies on the construction of autism knowledge map.

Therefore, building an autism information service platform based on knowledge map has important scientific research and application value.

4   Construction of Information Service Platform for Autism

Autism Information Service Platform includes Autism Knowledge Base, Autism Knowledge Map, Data Import, Association Query, User Interface, etc.

4.1   Construction Principles

The construction of information service platform for autism has several characteristics, such as accuracy, advanced, popular and practical.

- Accuracy: Autism knowledge base is required to be accurate and reliable, in line with hospital and national standards. Current diagnostic criteria for autism include the World Health Organization's International Statistical Classification of Diseased and Related Health Problems (ICD-10) and the American Psychiatric Association's Revised Manual on Diagnosis and Statistics of Mental Abnormalities (DSM-IV-TR, APA, 2000).

- Advanced: The platform can collect timely data for the knowledge base, including the latest autism diagnosis, treatment and rehabilitation knowledge. Information service platform can use the latest technology to meet the knowledge needs of all kinds of users.
- Popularization: The goal of system platform design is to meet the needs of autism patients to acquire knowledge of autism in any area and at any time through network channels, relying on the Internet and mobile Internet.
- Practicality: The design requirement of information service platform is to achieve practical purposes, provide comprehensive and necessary autism knowledge, reduce the workload of doctor diagnosis, and reduce the cost of autism diagnosis and treatment.

4.2 Design Idea

Autism information service platform includes data processing and knowledge visualization display, which includes two main parts: one is the collection of basic data, the other is the analysis and visualization of collected data, including user interface interaction design. The design idea is as follows: The system platform has the function of automatic data acquisition and processing, and can store and visualize the knowledge data collected before. The principles of user interface design are as follows.

- Beautiful Interface: The interface design meets the requirements of conciseness, professionalism and user-friendliness. Each component of the program interface has independent functions, clear classification and comprehensive information display.
- Visual Knowledge Display: The program can realize the display of knowledge association. For example, after searching for "diagnoses", the information display area can display the knowledge map and specific diagnostic methods of autism diagnosis.
- Structured Presentation of Knowledge: By using knowledge map, the structure and relevance of knowledge can be displayed, and the content of knowledge can be displayed comprehensively and abundantly.

4.3 Overall Structure of the Information Service Platform

The information service platform adopts Browser/Server structure, the server part of the system includes knowledge database, and the client part of the system includes program interface. The overall structure of the system is shown in Fig. 1.

The system includes four layers: Collection layer, data layer, function layer and user layer. Each layer depends on each other and gradually forms the whole information service platform. Collection layer is mainly responsible for collecting various information and knowledge of autism, including medical books, medical knowledge base, medical websites. Data layer is the data center of the information service platform, which stores information and knowledge about autism. Function layer includes knowledge retrieval, knowledge map, ontology navigation, knowledge concept display, knowledge content editing, knowledge management and other business functions. User layer is the user interface, including the client page and the server page.

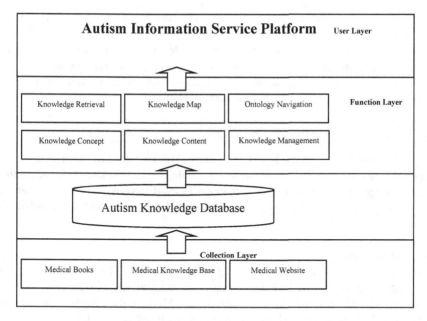

Fig. 1. Overall structure of the information service platform

4.4   Network Topology

According to the network environment and equipment of the information service platform, the network topology can be divided into four levels. The network topology diagram is shown in Fig. 2.

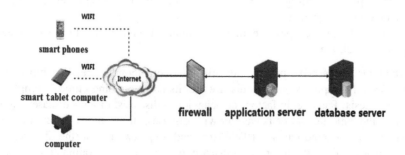

Fig. 2. Network topology diagram

The first layer is the application layer, which consists of users, computers and various smart devices. Smart devices include smart tablet computer, smart phones and other electronic devices. Users access and use the information service platform through computers and various smart devices.

The second layer is the communication layer, mainly based on the Internet network environment, providing access channels for users and systems.

The third layer is the application server layer, which is composed of firewall and application server, and has an ontology display system for autism. The application server manages various business functions, handles various business requests submitted by users, and can access the database server for various data exchange.

The fourth layer is the database server layer, which stores all kinds of data and knowledge resources of the information service platform.

4.5   Design of Knowledge Map of Autism

Autism knowledge map is the key of this study. The key steps of autism knowledge map design include knowledge extraction, knowledge fusion and knowledge reasoning.

Knowledge map are usually stored in graph-based databases, RDF-based databases and relational databases. In this study, relational database is used to complete the storage of knowledge map.

4.5.1   Data Sources

Data is needed to construct the knowledge map of autism. The data sources of the knowledge map of autism include open source medical knowledge map, network resources, scientific research literature and so on. Most of the data such as network resources and scientific research literature are unstructured data, so the construction of knowledge map is mainly based on unstructured data.

4.5.2   Ontology Construction

The ontology construction of knowledge map is the definition of knowledge map structure. The definition of autism knowledge map ontology includes the definition of class and the definition of relationship. Combining various data types and referencing medical knowledge map, this paper defines the following six basic categories: "disease", "symptoms", "drugs", "training and treatment", "examination methods", "pathogenic factors or behavior".

According to the six types of entities, five kinds of semantic relations are created in this paper, which are:

- Symptoms: disease-symptoms, indicating the corresponding relationship between disease and symptoms, namely disease and its corresponding clinical symptoms.
- Pathogenesis: Pathogenic factors or behaviors - diseases, drugs - diseases, used to link pathogenic factors or behaviors with diseases, drugs and diseases, indicating that such pathogenic factors or behaviors and drugs can lead to the disease.
- Examination: Examination mode - disease, used to connect examination mode and disease, indicating that this examination mode can be used to examine and diagnose the disease.
- Treatment: Treatment - disease, treatment - symptoms, used to link treatment and disease, treatment and symptoms, indicating that the treatment is directed at the disease or the treatment is directed at the symptoms.
- Co-occurrence disease: disease-disease, used to connect disease and disease, means that these two diseases can occur in the same patient, that is, the same patient can suffer from both diseases at the same time.

4.5.3   Storage of Knowledge Map

Knowledge map essentially represents entities, their attributes and the relationship between entities and entities in the form of graphs. At present, graph data structure and RDF (Resource Description Framework) structure in Semantic Web framework are widely used to store data in knowledge map.

This paper uses RDF structure database to store data. RDF is a standard data model developed by the World Wide Web Consortium (W3C) to describe real resources on the semantic web, which can be read and understood by computers. In RDF, each resource has its unique URI (Uniform Resource Identifiers). RDF is a set of finite triples (s, p, o). Each triple represents a fact statement sentence, in which s is the subject, P is the predicate and O is the object. Its meaning is that s has the attribute P and its value is o or that there is a relationship p between S and o. For example (autism, symptoms, communication disorder), it means that the symptoms of autism have communication disorder.

4.6   Software Development Tools

- Database: This paper uses MySQL 5.7 and Structured Query Language (SQL) to develop database.
- Programing language: The information service platform is developed by Java, using JavaScript scripting language. Java is an object-oriented language.
- Software development tools: The information service platform uses MyEclipse development tools, and MyEclipse uses visual editors for coding.
- Visualization tools: Using Echarts for visual display, Echarts provides an intuitive and easy-to-use interactive way to mine, extract, modify or integrate the displayed data.

4.7   Database Design

4.7.1   Disease Table

The disease table stores data about autism diseases, including disease id, disease classification, disease name, disease definition, and disease source data. See the Table 1 below.

Table 1. Disease table

Name	Type	Length	Description
id	bigint	10	disease id
Class	bigint	10	disease classification
Name	varchar	20	disease name
Definition	varchar	100	disease description
source	varchar	20	disease source data

4.7.2   Disease Classification Table

The disease classification table stores the classification data of autism diseases, including the disease classification ID and the disease classification name. It is a dictionary table of disease classification. See the Table 2 below.

Table 2. Disease classification table

Name	Type	Length	Description
id	bigint	10	disease id
Name	varchar	20	disease classification

4.7.3   Three Tuple Table

This table stores the classification information of autism diseases, including triple id, subject, predicate and object, which represent the relationship among them. It is a data table used to visualize triples. See the Table 3 below.

Table 3. Three tuple table

Name	Type	Length	Description
id	bigint	10	triple id
Subject	varchar	20	Subject description
Predicate	varchar	20	Predicate description
Object	varchar	20	Object description

4.8   System Interface

4.8.1   Main Interface

The main interface of the Autism Information Service Platform is shown in Fig. 3. The following is the description of each display area.

4.8.2   Search and Tree Display

Users can enter keywords in the search bar, search, and display relevant content in the tree structure. See Fig. 4.

4.8.3   Knowledge Map of Autism

Autism knowledge map supports multi-level knowledge display. Nodes at all levels can be dragged, enlarged and narrowed. Clicking on the node can show details of relevant knowledge. See Fig. 5.

Autism Information Service Platform
Navigation Bar
search
Scale
medicine
behavior
Symptom
Autism
Treatment
Ethology
gene
Analysis
image
Related Concepts
DSM-IV
DSM-IV
ICD-10
Diagnostic scale

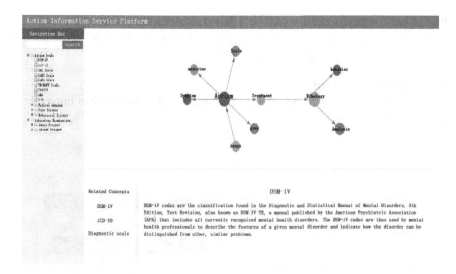

Fig. 3. Main interface

Navigation Bar
search
Autism Scale
DSM-IV
ICD-10
ABC Scale
CABS Scale
CARS Scale
VB-MAPP Scale
TEACCH
ABA
DIR
Medical imaging
Gene Science
Behavioral Science
Laboratory Examination
Basic Project
Select Project

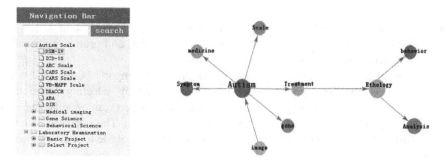

Fig. 4. Search interface

Scale
medicine
behavior
Symptom
Autism
Treatment
Ethology
gene
Analysis
image

Fig. 5. Knowledge map

4.8.4 Relevant Knowledge Display

On the left is the concept of knowledge. Choose any one and the right will show the details of the concept. See Fig. 6 below.

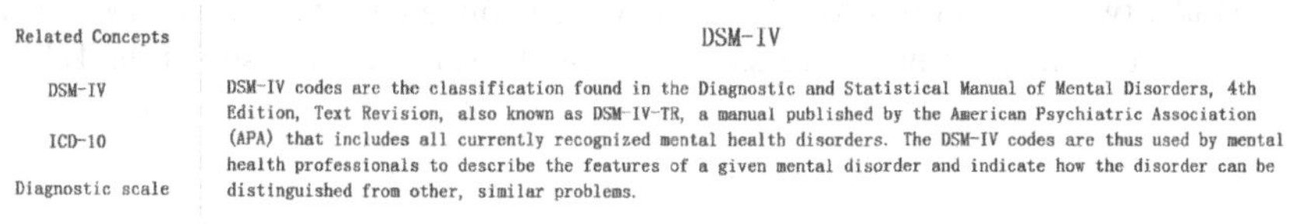

Related Concepts
DSM-IV
ICD-10
Diagnostic scale
DSM-IV
DSM-IV codes are the classification found in the Diagnostic and Statistical Manual of Mental Disorders, 4th Edition, Text Revision, also known as DSM-IV-TR, a manual published by the American Psychiatric Association (APA) that includes all currently recognized mental health disorders. The DSM-IV codes are thus used by mental health professionals to describe the features of a given mental disorder and indicate how the disorder can be distinguished from other, similar problems.

Fig. 6. Relevant knowledge display

4.8.5   User Login

The user enters the correct name and password and clicks the login button to login to the system management page. The Fig. 7 is the login interface.

4.8.6   Data Management

Data management mainly includes basic data import and relational data import functions, as shown in Fig. 8.

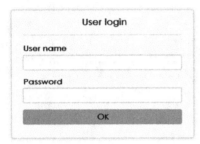

Fig. 7. User login interface

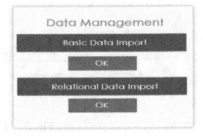

Fig. 8. Data management interface

- Basic Data Import: Click on "Basic Data Import" and a file selection dialog box appears. Users can import data after selecting Excel files, and prompt information will be given after importing.
- Relational Data Import: Click on the "Relational Data Import" button, and a file selection dialog box appears. Users can import data by selecting Excel files. Information will be prompted after importing data. Users can modify the data according to the prompt and then import it into the system. The imported data will be displayed in a relational graph format, the imported Excel file format is shown in Fig. 9.

	A	B	C	D
1	Primary element	Relevant Elements	Relational Direction	Relationship description
2	Autism	Concept	0	include
3	Autism Diagnostic Scale	VB-MAPP Scale	0	include

Fig. 9. Imported Excel file format

4.9   System Testing

In this study, two kinds of mobile phones, personal computers and servers are selected as test environments. The hardware and software environments are shown in Table 4.

Table 4. Testing environment

Testing equipment	Hardware environment	Software environment
OPPO R17 Mobile Phone	CPU: SDM670 RAM: 8 GB	Android
IPhone 8 Mobile Phone	CPU: A11 RAM: 2 GB	iOS
Personal Computer	CPU: Intel i7 RAM: 16 GB	Windows 10
Server	CPU: Intel W2133 RAM: 16 GB	Windows Server 2019

After detailed system testing, the response time of the information platform meets the requirements, the business function is correct, the quality is stable, and it is suitable for applications.

5 Conclusion

The incidence of autism has become more and more high, which has attracted more and more attention from all aspects of society. Using knowledge map and other tools to build an information service platform for autism, to meet the public's understanding of autism and the information needs of the treatment and rehabilitation of autistic patients, has become a research hotspot. This paper initially constructs an autism information service platform based on knowledge map, and achieves the sharing and utilization of autism knowledge. Next, we will study the diagnosis and rehabilitation of autism, expand the business functions of the service platform, promote the sharing of autism knowledge, and improve public awareness and understanding of autism.

Acknowledgements. This research has been possible thanks to the support of projects: National Natural Science Foundation of China (No. 61772375) and Independent Research Project of School of Information Management Wuhan University (No: 413100032).

References

1. Duan, Y., Wu, X., Jin, F.: Advances in etiology and treatment of autism. Chin. Sci. Life Sci. **45**(09), 820–844 (2015)
2. Vismara, L.A., Rogers, S.J.: The early start denver model. J. Early Interv. **31**(1), 91–108 (2008)
3. Zablotsky, B., Black, L.I., Blumberg, S.J.: Estimated prevalence of children with diagnosed developmental disabilities in the United States, 2014–2016. NCHS Data Brief. (291), 1–8 (2017)
4. Academy of Autism of Five Coloured Deer: Report on the Development of Autism Education and Rehabilitation Industry in China 2. Huaxia Publishing House (2017)
5. Wu, X., Chen, S., Jin, F.: Research progress on quality of life and its influencing factors of primary caregivers of autistic children. General Nurs. **16**(18), 2206–2208 (2018)
6. Yang, Y., Wang, M.: Employment and financial burdens of families with preschool-aged children with autism. Chin. J. Clin. Psychol. **22**(2), 295–297, 361 (2014)

7. Singh, P., Ghosh, S., Nandi, S.: Subjective burden and depression in mothers of children with autism spectrum disorder in India: moderating effect of social support. J. Autism Dev. Disord. **47**(10), 3097–3111 (2017)
8. Wang, Y., Xiao, L., Chen, R., et al.: Social impairment of children with autism spectrum disorder affects parental quality of life in different ways. Psychiatry Res. **266**, 168–174 (2018)
9. Sireteanu, A.N.: A survey of web ontology languages and semantic web services. Ann. Alexandru Ioan Cuza Univ. Econ. **60**(1), 42–53 (2013)
10. Amit, S.: Introducing the knowledge graph: things, not strings (2012)

Data-Driven Hospital Surgery Scheduling Optimization

Zhigang Li, Yan Yi$^{(\boxtimes)}$, and Xichen Wu

School of Management Science, Chengdu University of Technology,
Chengdu 610059, China
lizhigang@mail.cdut.edu.cn, 15881281421@163.com,
lemongress93@qq.com

Abstract. With the deepening reform of the medical system, major hospitals have begun to pay attention to the research on the optimization of medical resource allocation, and seek ways to improve patient satisfaction and reduce hospital operating costs. This paper takes data as the center, collects data through on-site investigation, and analyzes the scheduling problem of the current hospital operating room by using surgical scheduling knowledge and business flow chart. Combining the constraints and the actual situation of the hospital, a multi-objective mixed integer programming model with the lowest operating room operating cost and the highest patient satisfaction was established, and the optimal solution was obtained using Lingo software. The optimization results were verified by FlexsimHC simulation software, and the effects before and after the optimization of the surgical scheduling were compared. The research results provided a basis for optimizing the operation schedule, reducing the operating cost of the operating room and improving patient satisfaction, and established an event data-driven analysis paradigm for operating room scheduling optimization.

Keywords: Surgical scheduling · Multi-objective · FlexsimHC simulation software

1 Introduction

According to the data of the 2017 China Health and Safety Business Development Statistics Bulletin, the bed utilization rate of the tertiary hospital is as high as 98.6%, the operating room utilization rate is 95.6%, and the bed utilization rate of the first-level general hospital is only 57.5%, the operating room utilization rate is only 45.8%, The operating room is the most densely populated place in the hospital. Its investment accounts for 10% of the hospital's fiscal expenditure [1], and profits account for 40% of the hospital's total profit [2]. The utilization of surgical resources directly affects the operating costs and economic benefits of the entire hospital. [3, 4].

The research on hospital surgery scheduling can start from four aspects: business scheduling optimization method, multi-objective planning method, hospital surgery scheduling optimization, operating room cost and patient satisfaction. From the business scheduling optimization method, Cardoen et al. used the goal planning theory to

© Springer Nature Switzerland AG 2019
H. Chen et al. (Eds.): ICSH 2019, LNCS 11924, pp. 369–380, 2019.
https://doi.org/10.1007/978-3-030-34482-5_33

optimize the operation scheduling problem [5]. Tan et al. verified the feasibility of heuristic optimization algorithm scheduling [6]. Vincent et al. used the ant colony algorithm to solve the multi-objective flexible job shop scheduling problem, and realized the optimization of the job shop scheduling [7]. Landa et al. developed a hybrid two-stage optimization algorithm to optimize hospital processes [8]. From the perspective of multi-objective planning methods, currently, multi-objective planning is widely used in surgical scheduling [9, 10]. Beliën et al. established a mathematical scheduling model for surgical scheduling based on the use of mixed integer programming theory and heuristic algorithm, based on the patient's needs and capabilities [11]. Lamiri et al. divided the patients into: ordinary patients and emergency patients, and then established a mathematical model of the surgical scheduling [12]. Wang et al. established a mathematical model simulating the arrangement of patient beds to optimize the current patient bed arrangement [13]. Silvaab et al. propose a heuristic method based on integer model and integer programming to maximize the use of the operating room [14]. Ma et al. extended the single-objective mathematical model to multiple goals, a complete study of the hospital operating room short-term Surgical scheduling model [15]. Guido et al. propose a multi-objective integer linear programming model that can effectively plan and manage hospital operating room suites [16]. From the hospital surgery scheduling optimization, Arenas M and others used the goal planning theory to establish a mathematical model of surgical scheduling with the goal of reducing patient waiting time [17]. Guinet et al. used the dual structure heuristic algorithm to target surgical re-source utilization and patient satisfaction, and established a heuristic mathematical model to optimize the surgical schedule [18]. Daiki et al. classify patients into different priorities according to their severity and perform surgical scheduling according to their priorities [19]. Zhao and Li used mixed integer nonlinear programming and constrained programming methods to determine the operating room arrangement and the patient's surgical sequence [20]. Wang et al. established a model with the goal of minimizing the cost of surgery and operation time [21]. Meng and Chen optimized the operating room cost from the aspects of surgical priority and limited doctor resources [22]. Zhou et al. the operating room utilization results, the minimum hospital operating costs and the highest patient satisfaction [23]. From operating room costs and patient satisfaction optimization, Risser defines patient satisfaction as the degree to which a patient experiences differences between ideal conditions and services experienced under real conditions [24]. Angela and Elena constructed a one-week surgical scheduling model using linear programming theory to improve the utilization of the operating room, taking into account the two factors of welfare and patient waiting time [25]. Zhu et al. pointed out the preparation time between the operation groups in the operation, and used the theory of deterioration effect to establish a mathematical model with the goal of minimum surgery completion time [26]. Wang et al. focuses on finding a satisfactory surgery scheduling to patients and efficiently managing scarce medical resources in laminar-flow operating theaters [27]. Heydari and Soudi considered emergency surgery into the entire surgical arrangement and constructed corresponding mathematical models, and proposed a method to solve the problem of maintaining surgical schedule stability [28]. Hao sought the optimal number of operating rooms to reduce the cost of surgery in the surgical scheduling problem, and sought the optimal surgical sequence to reduce the waiting time of patients and the overtime hours of doctors, and established an optimization model for multi-target surgical scheduling problems [29].

In summary, the current research on hospital surgical scheduling mainly focuses on the establishment of theoretical models, ignoring the mining and application of data resources. Therefore, in order to optimize and improve the hospital operating room scheduling process, explore data-driven solutions for hospital operating room operations and management, this paper focuses on the "Site Research - Data Collection - Model Building - Data Simulation - Scheduling Optimization" research technology route, trying to build multi-objective planning and simulation techniques as a tool, data-centric paradigm of event data analysis for hospital operating room scheduling optimization, which makes academic theoretical research results more operational and practical

2 Data Collection and Model Building

2.1 Site Investigation

An orthopedic specialist hospital in Mianyang City is a Grade III B orthopedic hospital. The hospital adheres to the emphasis on both Chinese and Western medicine, focusing on bone injuries and highlighting the development of hospital disciplines with single disease and orthopedic specialty. The hospital's orthopaedic department has 4 operating rooms, 19 surgical teams, 20 surgical assistant nurses, and 300 beds of various types, which can perform various orthopedic surgery. With the continuous increase of the overall strength of the hospital, the artificial surgical scheduling of the operating room has caused problems such as the number of surgical arrangements in each operating room and the imbalance of medical staff workload. In order to balance the utilization rate of each operating room and the working hours of medical staff and improve patient satisfaction, we will combine the actual situation of the hospital and the constraints of medical resources on the surgical schedule to establish a multi-objective mixed integer programming model.

2.2 Model Assumptions and Constraints

Model Assumptions:

(1) The various operating rooms of the four operating rooms of the C hospital can be used normally, and different types of bone injuries can be performed in each operating room.

(2) The normal opening hours of the operating room of the C hospital are 8 h.

(3) C Hospital performed surgical arrangements with T (5 working days in a week) as a scheduling period.

(4) The medical team has been informed about the number of surgical patients and the type of surgery, and all patients have already prepared for surgery before performing surgical scheduling.

(5) In order to reduce unnecessary mistakes during surgery, each auxiliary nurse performs at most one operation per day.

Model Constraints:

(1) The number of nurses assisted with surgery should not exceed the total number of nurses who can participate in the operation during the day.
(2) All patients who have scheduled an operation in a scheduling cycle can be scheduled for surgery.
(3) The operation time of any patient cannot be later than the latest operation time.
(4) In order to prevent the surgeon from causing medical malpractice due to fatigue, the working time of each medical team cannot exceed F_i hours.
(5) The number of operations per day in each operating room cannot exceed four.

2.3   Symbols and Variable Description

In order to facilitate the establishment of mathematical models, combined with the actual situation of C hospital surgery schedule, the symbols and decision variables appearing in the model are defined as follows:

(1) Symbols appearing in mathematical models:
K: a day of a scheduling cycle;
j: the patient number;
r: the operating room number;
b_{kr}: the opening time of the operating room r on day k;
b'_{kr}: the remaining opening time of the operating room r on day k;
b_j: The duration of the patient's operation given by the doctor;
s_1: the unit time loss coefficient of insufficient operating room opening time;
s_2: the remaining unit time loss coefficient of the operating room opening time;
T_j: the duration of surgery of the jth patient;
O_{ij}: the correspondence between patient j and surgical group i;
d_j: represents the latest time when patient j was scheduled for surgery;
A_{ij}: the surgery group i can be scheduled for surgery on day k;
n_j: the number of nurses required to perform surgery on the jth patient;
N_k: the total number of nurses who can participate in surgery on day k;
(2) Decision variables appearing in mathematical models
x_{jrk} is the decision variable indicating whether surgery is performed in the operating room r on the kth day;

$$x_{jrk} = \begin{cases} 1 & \text{Indicates that patient j is undergoing surgery on the kth day in the operating room} \\ 0 & \text{Indicates that patient j did not undergo surgery in the operating room on day k} \end{cases}$$

A_{ik} is the decision variable indicating whether the surgery group i can perform surgery on day k;

$$A_{ik} = \begin{cases} 1 & \text{surgery team i can perform on day K} \\ 0 & \text{surgery group i cannot perform surgery on day k} \end{cases}$$

2.4   Mathematical Model

Based on the multi-objective planning of surgical scheduling optimization, this paper constructs a multi-objective mixed integer programming model with the minimum operating cost of operating room and the highest patient satisfaction. The multi-objective mixed integer programming mathematical model can use the linear weighting method to assign different weights to two different targets into a single-objective mixed integer programming mathematical model, as follows:

$$MinZ = \lambda \sum_{K=1}^{T} \sum_{r=1}^{m} (s_1 b_{kr} + s_2 b'_{kr}) - (1 - \lambda) \sum_{j-1}^{s} m_j$$
$$\cdot \frac{d_j - \sum_{k=1}^{T} \sum_{r=1}^{m} K x_{jrk} + 1}{d_j} \tag{1}$$

$$\left[\sum_{k=1}^{T} \sum_{r=1}^{m} x_{jrk} = 1; (j = 1, 2, ..., S) \quad (2) \right.$$
$$\sum_{j=1}^{S} \sum_{r=1}^{m} x_{jrk} n_j \le N_k; (k = 1, 2, ..., T) \quad (3)$$
$$\sum_{j=1}^{s} x_{jrk} \le M; (k = 1, 2, ..., T; r = 1, 2, ..., m) \quad (4)$$
$$\sum_{j=1}^{s} O_{ij} x_{jrk} b_j < F_i; (i = 1, 2, ..., N; k = 1, 2, ..., T; r = 1, 2, ..., m) \quad (5)$$
$$K x_{jrk} \le d_j; (k = 1, 2, ..., T; j = 1, 2, ..., S; r = 1, 2, ..., m) \quad (6)$$
$$O_{ij} x_{jrk} \le A_{ik}; (i = 1, 2, ..., N; j = 1, 2, ..., S; r = 1, 2, ..., m; k = 1, 2, ..., T) \quad (7)$$
$$A_{ik} = 1 \quad \text{Surgery team } i \text{ can perform surgery on day } K$$
$$A_{ik} = 0 \quad \text{Surgery group } i \text{ cannot perform surgery on day } K$$
$$x_{jrk} = 1 \quad \text{Patient } j \text{ is undergoing surgery on the kth day in the operating room } r$$
$$\left. x_{jrk} = 0 \quad \text{Patient } j \text{ did not undergo surgery on the kth day in the operating room } r \right.$$

The objective function (1) indicates that the operating cost of the operating room is minimized as the objective function $Min = \left\{ \sum_{K=1}^{T} \sum_{r=1}^{m} (s_1 b_{kr} + s_2 b'_{kr}) \right\}$ weight is λ, s_1 is 1.5, s_2 is 1 (Wen et al. 2008). The maximum weight of patient satisfaction is the weight of the objective function $Max = \left\{ \sum_{j=1}^{s} m_j U_j(x) \right\}$ is $1 - \lambda$, where $U_j(x)$ represents the satisfaction function of patient j $U_j(x) = \frac{d_j - \sum_{k=1}^{T} \sum_{r=1}^{m} K x_{jrk} + 1}{d_j}$, $(k = 1, 2, ..., T)$ for the surgical scheduling problem, all patients were satisfied with the earliest scheduled operation, and the patient's satisfaction was directly related to the operation date. Due to the certain difference in the patient's condition, the degree of influence of the operation schedule on the patient's condition is also different. Therefore, patients are divided into different priority levels to represent the severity of the patient's condition. Suppose we divide the patient's priority level into 3 levels, and patient j has a priority of m_j, $m_j \in \{1, 2, 3\}$ $\sum_{r=1}^{m} K x_{jrk} + 1$ indicates the patient's date of surgery, d_j means during the scheduling period, The latest time when patient j was scheduled for surgery. When $d_j = k$, the patient j must have a satisfaction greater than 0 as long as it is determined to perform surgery within one week. When $d_j > k$, the satisfaction of patient j must be greater than zero. When $d_j > k$, the satisfaction of patient j must be less than 0, and the patient is in a state of complete dissatisfaction, and this state should be prevented.

Constraints (2)–(4) are related to minimum operating costs, the constraint (2) indicates that all scheduled surgical patients can be scheduled for surgery in a scheduling cycle, constraint (3) indicates that the number of nurses assisted with surgery cannot exceed the total number of nurses who can participate in the operation during the day, Constraint (4) means that the amount of surgery per operating room per day cannot exceed M, x_{jrk} is a 0–1 variable, M is 4. Constraints (5)–(7) are most relevant to patient satisfaction, the constraint (5) indicates that the working time of any one of the surgery groups cannot exceed F_i, constraint (6) indicates that the surgery time of any one patient cannot be later than the latest operation time, and the constraint (7) indicates that the doctor's surgery date is limited by the outpatient date and the teaching day, A_{ij} and x_{jrk} are 0–1 variables.

3   Model Solving

Lingo software is a software mainly used to solve the optimal solution of linear programming. The software can be connected to some data files to accept data files such as spreadsheets and text files. Lingo software provides a more flexible programming language. It is fast and fast when solving large-scale problems. Therefore, Lingo software is widely used in academia and scientific research.

There are many cases in which the value of λ of a single objective function is determined. The weight of the optimal solution of the model is temporarily undetermined. Therefore, in the same way, different values of λ are substituted into the LINGO software program of the single-objective mixed integer programming model, and the program is run. The optimization results obtained under different weight λ values are given below, as shown in Table 1:

Table 1. Optimal results under different weights.

λ	1 − λ	MinZ
0.1	0.9	−55.755
0.2	0.8	−46.910
0.3	0.7	−38.065
0.4	0.6	−29.220
0.5	0.5	−20.375
0.6	0.4	−11.530
0.7	0.3	−2.685
0.8	0.2	6.160
0.9	0.1	15.005

From Table 1, it can be concluded that when the weights λ are taken as 0.1, 0.2, 0.3, 0.4, 0.5, 0.6, and 0.7, respectively, the results of the single-objective mixed integer programming model are not satisfied with the multi-targets constructed. Mixed integer programming model requirements. When λ is 0.8, the result of the single-objective mixed integer programming model is non-negative 6.16. At the same time, according to the constructed multi-objective programming model and the actual situation of the hospital, when the λ is 0.8, the model achieves the lowest comprehensive operating cost at the same time. And the best state of patient satisfaction. Therefore, in summary, when the weight $\lambda = 0.8$, the solution of the single-objective mixed integer programming model obtained at this time is the optimal solution.

4   FlexsimHC Simulation Results

According to the results of the optimization of the surgical schedule of the C hospital, combined with the actual situation of the C hospital, under the same conditions before the optimization of the surgical schedule, the simulation model was established by using the FlexsimHC simulation software to optimize the 5-day surgical schedule of the C hospital. In order to verify the results of the surgical schedule optimization.

4.1   Comparison of Operating Costs of Operating Rooms Before and After Optimization

After the operation of the simulation model was completed in the C hospital, the working state maps of each operating room were collected. The data collected can be used to obtain the utilization of the four operating rooms within 5 days as shown in Table 2.

As can be seen from Table 2, after the multi-objective mixed integer programming model was used to optimize the surgical schedule of the C hospital, the difference in the utilization rate of each operating room was reduced. Most of the operating room utilization rates in the first two days reached 100%, and patients with a priority level above 1 in the patient's severity were scheduled for the first two days. Because the patients with higher severity had priority in surgery, the first 1, 2 days overtime, the total time for overtime has reached 378 min. On the third and fourth days, the utilization rate of the operating room reached more than 85%, the total time for overtime in the operating room was 6 min, and the operating room was idle for 162 min. On the fifth day, the utilization rate of the second operating room was 60%, the idle time was longer, and the others all achieved 85% utilization. The total idle time of the operating room was 288 min, and no overtime was generated.

Table 2. Utilization of 4 operating rooms in 5 days.

Surgical date	Operating room number	Operating room utilization (%)	Operating room idle rate (%)	Total operating room idle time (minute)	Operating room overtime (minutes)
1	1	100	0	0	180
	2	100	0		
	3	100	0		
	4	100	0		
2	1	100	0	90	198
	2	100	0		
	3	100	0		
	4	81.25	18.75		
3	1	98.75	1.25	78	0
	2	100	0		
	3	86.25	13.75		
	4	98.75	1.25		
4	1	93.75	6.25	84	6
	2	100	0		
	3	97.5	2.5		
	4	91.25	8.75		
5	1	96.25	3.75	288	0
	2	60	40		
	3	95	5		
	4	88.75	11.25		

The comparison of the effects of the 5-day surgical schedule optimization of C hospital is shown in the following table (Table 3):

Table 3. Comparison of effects before and after C hospital optimization.

Index	Before optimization	Optimized
Operating room utilization is greater than 85%	15	18
Total overtime in the operating room (minutes)	414	384
Total operating room idle time (minutes)	810	540
Operating room overall cost	1431	1116

4.2   Comparison of Patient Satisfaction Before and After Optimization

According to the constructed mathematical function of patient satisfaction, the patient satisfaction before and after the optimization of the surgical schedule is compared and analyzed. The specific data comparison is shown in Fig. 1.

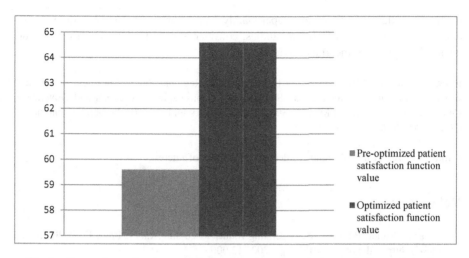

Fig. 1. Comparison of patient satisfaction function values before and after optimization

After optimizing the surgical schedule of the C hospital, patients with a priority of 1 or more were scheduled for the first two days. The patient satisfaction function value of all patients within 5 days increased from 59.6 before optimization to 64.6 after optimization, which greatly improved patient satisfaction. The verification of the simulation results shows that the optimization method of the surgical schedule is feasible.

5 Conclusions

This paper analyzes the current operating room scheduling problem, collects data related to the operation schedule through field investigation, and describes and analyzes existing problems. A multi-objective mixed integer programming model with the lowest operating cost and highest patient satisfaction in the operating room was established. The Lingo software was used to evaluate the optimal solution and compare the effects before and after the operation scheduling optimization. The research results have important reference value for the hospital to solve the surgical scheduling problem, the operation cost problem, and the improvement of the patient's satisfaction. The problems of the use of the operating room in the surgical schedule of C hospital and the lack of reasonable surgical arrangements for the patients have been effectively improved. Because the surgical scheduling optimization model involves many constraints, some problems such as anesthesiologists are not considered in the model construction of this paper, so the research model needs further improvement. In addition, due to the uncertainty and randomness of the hospital emergency department, the data is difficult to collect, this paper mainly focuses on the surgical schedule of non-emergency departments. In future studies, consider how to perform a reasonable surgical schedule in an uncertain environment.

Funding. This work was supported by the Sichuan Regional Public Management Informationization Research Center Project "Study on the Coordination Mechanism and Governance Countermeasures of Shared Medical Stakeholder Network under the Background of Internet +" (No. QGXH18-02).

Conflicts of Interest. The authors declare no conflict of interest.

References

1. Aida, J., Atidel, B., Hadj, A.: Operating rooms scheduling. Int. J. Prod. Econ. **99**, 52–62 (2006). https://doi.org/10.1016/j.ijpe.2004.12.006
2. Bowers, J., Mould, G.: Ambulatory care and orthopaedic capacity planning. Health Care Manage. **8**(1), 41–47 (2005). https://doi.org/10.1007/s10729-005-5215-4
3. Bai, X., Luo, L., Li, R.: Operating room scheduling: research overview and prospect. Manage. Rev. **23**(1), 121–128 (2011). https://doi.org/10.14120/j.cnki.cn11-5057/f.2011.01.001
4. Luo, L., Kang, S.: Theory, method and application of medical service resource scheduling optimization. Science Press, Beijing (2013). ISBN: 9787030396259
5. Cardoen, B., Demeulemeester, E., Beliën, J.: Optimizing a multiple objective surgical case sequencing problem. Int. J. Prod. Econ. **119**(2), 354–366 (2009). https://doi.org/10.1016/j.ijpe.2009.03.009
6. Tan, H., et al.: Simulation of surface segmentation workshop scheduling simulation. Ship Eng. **36**(02), 99–102 (2014). https://doi.org/10.13788/j.cnki.cbgc.2014.0057
7. Vicent, T.: Solving a bicriteria scheduling problem on unrelated paralled machines occurring in the glass bottle industry. Eur. J. Oper. Res. **135**(1), 42–49 (2001). https://doi.org/10.1016/S0377-2217(00)00288-5
8. Landa, P., Aringhieri, R., Soriano, P., Tanfani, E., Testi, A.: A hybrid optimization algorithm for surgeries scheduling. Oper. Res. Health Care **8**, 103–114 (2016). https://doi.org/10.1016/j.orhc.2016.01.001
9. Ozkarahan, I.: Allocation of surgeries to operating rooms by goal programming. J. Med. Syst. **24**(6), 339–378 (2000). https://doi.org/10.1023/A:1005548727003
10. Blake, J.T., Cater, M.W.: A goal programming approach to strategic resource allocation in acute care hospitals. Eur. J. Oper. Res. **140**(3), 541–561 (2002). https://doi.org/10.1016/S0377-2217(01)00219-3
11. Beliën, J., Demeulemeester, E.: Building cyclic master surgery schedules with leveled resulting bed occupancy. Eur. J. Oper. Res. **176**(2), 1185–1204 (2007). https://doi.org/10.1016/j.ejor.2005.06.063

12. Lamiri, M., Xiea, X., Dolgui, A.: A stochastic model for operating room planning with elective and emergency demand for surgery. Eur. J. Oper. Res. **185**(3), 1026–1037 (2008). https://doi.org/10.1016/j.ejor.2006.02.057

13. Wang, K., Zhou, Z., Wang, S.: Application of mathematical model to the allocation of the hospital sickbeds. J. Math. Med. **24**(2), 226–228 (2011). https://doi.org/10.3969/j.issn.1004-4337.2011.02.044

14. Silvaab, T.A.O., de Souzac, M.C., Saldanhad, R.R., Burkee, E.K.: Surgical scheduling with simultaneous employment of specialised human resources. Eur. J. Oper. Res. **245**(3), 719–730 (2015). https://doi.org/10.1016/j.ejor.2015.04.008

15. Ma, C., et al.: The mathematical models of short term operation scheduling optimization problem. Math. Pract. Theory **47**(21), 207–214 (2017). http://www.cnki.com.cn/Article/CJFDTotal-SSJS201721026.htm

16. Guido, R., Conforti, D.: A hybrid genetic approach for solving an integrated multi-objective operating room planning and scheduling problem. Comput. Oper. Res. **87**, 270–282 (2017). https://doi.org/10.1016/j.cor.2016.11.009

17. Arenas, M., et al.: Analysis via goal programming of the minimum achievable stay in surgical waiting lists. J. Oper. Res. Soc. **53**(4), 387–396 (2002). https://doi.org/10.1057/palgrave.jors.2601310

18. Guinet, A., Chaabane, S.: Operating theatre planning. Int. J. Prod. Econ. **85**(1), 69–81 (2003). https://doi.org/10.1016/S0925-5273(03)00087-2

19. Daiki, M., Yuehwern, Y.: An elextive surgery scheduling problem considering patient priority. Comput. Oper. Res. **37**(6), 1091–1099 (2010). https://doi.org/10.1016/j.cor.2009.09.016

20. Zhao, Z., Li, X.: Scheduling elective surgeries with sequence—dependent setup times to multiple operating rooms using constraint programming. Oper. Res.r Health Care **3**(3), 160–167 (2014). https://doi.org/10.1016/j.orhc.2014.05.003

21. Wang, D., Liu, F., Yin, Y., et al.: Prioritized surgery scheduling in face of surgeon tiredness and fixed off-duty period. J. Comb. Optim. **30**(4), 967–981 (2015). https://doi.org/10.1007/s10878-015-9846-1

22. Meng, F., Chen, H.: Consider the elective surgery scheduling constraint planning model under multi-factor conditions. Comput. Appl. Softw. **12,** 83–89 (2018). http://www.cnki.com.cn/Article/CJFDTotal-JYRJ201812016.htm

23. Zhou, B., Yin, M., Zhong, Z.: Lagrangian relaxation-based scheduling algorithm for operating theatres. Syst. Eng. Theory Pract. **36**(1), 224–233 (2016). https://doi.org/10.12011/1000-6788(2016)01-0224-10

24. Risser, N.L.: Development of an instrument to measure patient satisfaction with nurse and nursing care in primary care settings. Nurs. Res. **5**(2), 45–52 (1975). https://doi.org/10.1097/00006199-197501000-00011

25. Angela, T., Elena, T.: Tactical and operational decisions for operating room planning: efficiency and welfare implications. Health Care Manage. Sci. **12**(4), 363–373 (2009). https://doi.org/10.1007/s10729-008-9093-4

26. Zhu, Y., Zhang, Y., Song, Y.: Surgical scheduling considering setup time between surgeries and setup time between surgical teams. J. SE Univ. (Nat. Sci. Ed.) **45**(6), 1218–1222 (2015). https://doi.org/10.3969/j.issn.1001-0505.2015.06.034

27. Wang, Y., Tang, J., Pan, Z., Yan, C.: Particle swarm optimization-based planning and scheduling for a laminar-flow operating room with downstream resources. Soft. Comput. **19**(10), 2913–2926 (2015)

28. Heydari, M., Soudi, A.: Predictive reactive planning and scheduling of a surgical suite with emergency patient arrival. J. Med. Syst. **40**(1), 1–9 (2016). https://doi.org/10.1007/s10916-015-0385-1

29. Hao, Z.: A method of surgical scheduling: improving the satisfaction of doctors and patients while cutting operation costs. Ind. Eng. J. **20**(4), 49–71 (2017). http://www.cnki.com.cn/Article/CJFDTOTAL-GDJX201704007.htm

China's Biomedical Scientific Leadership Flows and the Role of Proximity

Chaocheng He, Xiao Huang, and Jiang Wu[(⊠)]

School of Information Management, Wuhan University, Wuhan 430072, China
jiangw@whu.edu.cn

Abstract. In this paper, we propose the concept of scientific leadership, and examine the effect and evolution of various proximity dimensions (geographical, cognitive, institutional, social and economic) on scientific leadership flows. The data to capture scientific leadership consists of a set of multi-institution papers published between 2013 and 2017 in biomedical field. We filter 244 institutions that have positive scientific leadership every year. The gravity model (Tobit model) sheds light on the role and dynamic evolution of geographical, cognitive, institutional, social and economic proximity in shaping scientific leadership flows. Our findings can provide evidence and support for grant allocation policy to facilitate biomedical scientific research and collaborations.

Keywords: Biomedical · Scientific collaboration · Scientific leadership · Proximity

1 Introduction

Scientific collaboration has become a trend throughout global academia. In biomedical field, scientific collaboration is particularly prevalent. It's common to see a biomedical paper with multiple authors, institutions and countries. Plenty of biomedical literatures explored scientific collaborations from individual, institutional, regional and international level [1]. The rapid increase of scientific collaboration motivate researchers to investigate which measurable factors will promote scientific collaboration. Geographic and social factors are the most common factors to promote scientific collaboration [2]. It's expected that collaboration is greater between closer researchers. Social distance such as friends or previous collaboration relationship is proved to facilitate scientific collaboration [3]. Some researchers also show cognitive factors to influence scientific collaboration [3].

The previous literature about scientific collaboration in biomedical has certain limitations. First, the collaboration relationship is homogeneous among authors for the same article. However, the collaborative relationship with the first author and corresponding author can better reveal scientific collaboration because they often dominate the scientific collaboration. Second, although Boschma [4] identifies five notions of proximity (geographical, cognitive, institutional, social and economic), most studies fail to systematically and comprehensively examined the relationships between these factors and scientific collaboration. Third, few previous studies go deep into the level of institutions. It is institution that have the primary mission of knowledge creation and

H. Chen et al. (Eds.): ICSH 2019, LNCS 11924, pp. 381–387, 2019.
https://doi.org/10.1007/978-3-030-34482-5_34

diffusion. To fill these research gaps, first, we introduce "scientific leadership" and propose its measurement. Second, we examine the effects of five proximity proposed by Boschma [5] on biomedical scientific collaboration. Third, we focus on scientific collaboration on the institution level. Specifically, we study the scientific collaboration between Chinses institutions in biomedical field, because the corresponding authorship is highly valued in China. Research in biomedical fields requires more on complex teamwork, involving tens of and even hundreds of researchers and institutions. The leadership role of the corresponding author is more pronounced.

2   Literature Review

As is known that scientific collaboration is a complex system which is often dominated by the first author and corresponding author. For example, in biological and increasingly in medical science, typically [5], someone is assigned to carry out the research and write a paper as the first author. The other participants with more specialized roles, such as contributing statistical analyses or polishing sentences, sign as co-author in the resulting paper. The corresponding author, however, is responsible for both scientific and non-scientific contributions such as deciding the direction of the research team, designing the roadmap of a project, creating an ideal communication environment for all the co-authors [6], assigning research tasks, checking the logic of the paper, coordinating the completion and submission of the work. And in most cases for Chinese publications, first author and corresponding author belong to the same organization [7]. Therefore, the institution to which the corresponding author belongs to is used in our study to be the research leader.

3   Methods and Data

3.1   Measurement of Scientific Leadership

The prior studies mainly adopt two methods to measure scientific collaboration intensity between two institutions: the "full count" and the "fractional count" [8]. In this paper, I make use of "fractional count", since it relates to the idea of contribution to knowledge production, rather than simply participating in knowledge production. The scientific leadership flow intensity $C_{ab,i}$ from institution a to institution b in paper i is

$$C_{ab,i} = \frac{1}{n_i} \tag{1}$$

where n_i is the number of institutions in paper i. The scientific leadership mass $LM_{a,i}$ that leading institution a in the paper i is

$$LM_{a,i} = \sum_{b=1}^{n_i-1} C_{ab,i} = 1 - \frac{1}{n_i} \tag{2}$$

Here, we don't consider self-leading, so we sum up to $n_i - 1$. The total scientific leadership flows C_{ab} from institution a to institution b is

$$C_{ab} = \sum_{i=1}^{m_b} C_{ab,i} \tag{3}$$

where m_b is the number of papers where a is the leading institution and b is a participating institution. And a's total scientific leadership mass is calculated as

$$LM_a = \sum_{b=1}^{B} C_{ab} \tag{4}$$

where B is the number of institutions that institution a has led (Fig. 1).

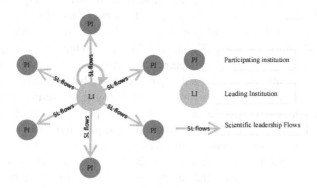

Fig. 1. Scientific leadership from leading institution to participating institution

3.2 Data

We perform a data collection in Thomson Reuters's WoS Core Citation Database, according to this search term "CU = A AND SU = B AND PY = C", where A is *"PEOPLES R CHINA"*, B is research areas in *"Life Sciences & Biomedicine"* field, and C is *2013–2017*. We obtain the complete information of biomedical scientific collaboration between Chinese institutions during 2013–2017. We preliminarily obtain 484903 papers. To avoid noise, we filter the institutions with positive scientific leadership mass in every year and finally obtain 244 institutions.

3.3 Model and Variables

We adopt a gravity model to analyze the determinants of biomedical scientific leadership among different institutions. Specifically, the basic idea of the gravity model stems from Newton's law of universal gravitation, stating that the gravitational force that attracts object i and j are directed related to the mass of i and j and are inversely proportional to the physical distance between i and j. The model has been applied to a broad range of fields. In particular, the model has been extensively applied in a number of studies of scientific collaboration [9]. Given the fractional data and a large number of zeros (many institution pairs have no scientific collaboration), the ordinary least square (OLS) estimates with a censored dependent variable may be biased and inconsistent [3]. Tobit regression, one of the limited dependent variable models, can effectively estimate linear relationship among variables when there was either left- or right-censoring in the dependent variables [10]. We adopt a Tobit regression model where we consider zero scientific leadership value as left censoring of the distribution [4]. To explore the role and its dynamic evolution of proximity in shaping scientific leadership flows, we first conduct a cross-section estimate by the data of 2013–2017, and then we perform cross-section estimates using two sub-period data. The estimation equation is:

$$C_{ij} = \beta_0 + \beta_1 \ln(LM_i) + \beta_2 \ln(LM_j) + \beta_3 \ln(Geoprox_{ij}) + \beta_4 \ln(Cognprox_{ij}) \\ + \beta_5 Instprox_{ij} + \beta_6 Socprox_{ij} + \beta_7 \ln(Econprox_{ij})$$ (5)

The dependent variable C_{ij} is the scientific leadership flow intensity from institution i to institution j during the period 2013–2017. In control variables, LM_i (LM_j) is the institution $i(j)$'s total scientific leadership mass. In addition, time lags are used to avoid endogeneity and reverse causality [3]. LM_i and LM_j refer to the period 2008–2012. The explanatory variables are lagged and capture information for the period 2008-2012 too. Geographical proximity ($Geoprox_{ij}$) is the spatial distance between institution i and j in kilometers. Cognitive proximity ($Cognprox_{ij}$) is the degree of overlap or the closeness of researchers' knowledge [3]. In this paper, we adopt Latent Dirichlet Allocation (LDA) based on keywords of papers to cluster all the papers into 50 topics according to perplexity. And then we embed all the institutions into a 50-dimensional vector according to their publications during 2008–2012. The cognitive proximity in this paper is the cosine similarity of embedding vectors of institution pairs. Institutional proximity ($Instprox_{ij}$) is a dummy variable which takes value 1 when institution i and j are in the same province [3]. Social proximity ($Socprox_{ij}$) is a dummy variable which takes value 1 if i and j has scientific collaborations during 2008–2012 [3]. Economic proximity ($Econprox_{ij}$) indicates the absolute difference in the number of National Natural Science Foundation Project of institution i and j during 2008–2012 [9].

4   Result

Table 1 reports the estimation results of Tobit gravity model. Model 1 is the basic gravity model, which only includes the control variables (LM_i and LM_j) and explanatory variable $Geoprox_{ij}$. Model 2 adds one more explanatory variable to model 1, and model 3 adds one more explanatory variable to model 2 … And finally, model 5 presents the full model, which includes all control variables and explanatory variables.

The positive and significant coefficient of control variables capturing the scientific leadership mass of leading institution LM_i and the scientific leadership mass of participating institution LM_j indicates that scientific leadership flow intensity C_{ij} increases as the value of LM_i and LM_j rise. All coefficients of $ln(LM_i)$ are larger than that of $ln(LM_j)$, revealing that the role played by the leading institution is stronger than that played by participating institution. The negative and significant coefficient of geographical distance suggests that scientific leadership flows decay with physical distance. Cognitive proximity displays a positive and significant coefficient, implying that scientific leadership flows are more likely to occur between institutions with similar research topic background. As for institutional proximity, the regression coefficient is

Table 1. Estimation results of Tobit gravity model

	Model 1	Model 2	Model 3	Model 4	Model 5
$ln(LM_i)$	8.440[***]	5.963[***]	5.999[***]	4.551[***]	4.417[***]
$ln(LM_j)$	7.024[***]	4.433[***]	4.453[***]	3.360[***]	3.232[***]
$ln(Geoprox_{ij})$	−4.246[***]	−4.606[***]	−1.963[***]	−1.600[***]	−1.590[***]
$ln(Cognprox_{ij})$		237.725[***]	241.254[***]	200.344[***]	201.403[***]
$Instprox_{ij}$			15.371[***]	12.547[***]	12.648[***]
$Socprox_{ij}$				13.224[***]	13.210[***]
$ln(Econprox_{ij})$					0.277[***]
_cons	−71.408[***]	−28.875[***]	−47.347[***]	−41.155[***]	−41.178[***]

$^{*}p < 0.10;\ ^{**}p < 0.05;\ ^{***}p < 0.01.$

positive and significant, showing that factors such as similar policies and culture foster scientific leadership flows. The positive and significant coefficient of social proximity suggests that having previous collaborations enhance scientific leadership flows. Previous scientific collaboration may enable mutual trust and confidence. The positive and significant coefficient of economic proximity suggests that scientific leadership flows are more likely to occur between institutions with different economic resources.

Table 2 presents the estimation results for different sub-periods. In order to account for two separate equations in different sub-years, we conduct the Chow test, which is widely used to determine whether the independent variables have significant differences in time series analysis. The result rejects no difference specification (p = 0.000).

Table 2. Estimation results of Tobit gravity model for sub-period

	Model 2013–2014	Model 2016–2017
$ln(LM_i)$	2.181[***]	2.121[***]
$ln(LM_j)$	1.615[***]	1.784[***]
$ln(Geoprox_{ij})$	−0.857[***]	−0.797[***]
$ln(Cognprox_{ij})$	83.603[***]	84.956[***]
$Instprox_{ij}$	4.592[***]	4.970[***]
$Socprox_{ij}$	14.668[***]	12.034[***]
$ln(Econprox_{ij})$	0.069	0.102[***]
_cons	−27.354[***]	−27.994[***]
Chow test	43.91[***]	

$^{*}p < 0.10;\ ^{**}p < 0.05;\ ^{***}p < 0.01.$

It is found that the coefficient for $ln(LM_i)$ and $ln(LM_j)$ is positive and significant in both periods. It's worth noting that the coefficient of scientific leadership mass of leading institution $ln(LM_i)$ is decreasing, while that of participating institution is increasing. Although the role played by the leading institution is still more pronounced than that played by participating institution, their differences are getting smaller. As for geographical proximity, the coefficients in two sub-periods are still negative and significant. However, the coefficient is decreasing too, suggesting that the effect of geographical proximity has declined over time. Besides, the coefficients of cognitive in two sub-periods are still positive and significant. But it is increasing, meaning that scientific leadership flows are more likely to occur between institutions with a similar research background. When it comes to institutional proximity, similar policies and culture significantly foster scientific leadership flows, and the effect is more and more pronounced. The coefficients of social proximity in two sub-periods are positive and significant but decreasing. Previous collaborations do enhance scientific leadership flows. But its influence is also diminishing. It's interesting that the coefficient of economic proximity is positive and statistically insignificant in 2013–2014. But it becomes positive and significant in 2016–2017, indicating that economic proximity is playing an increasing role in scientific leadership flows.

5 Conclusion

In this paper, we originally propose the concept of "scientific leadership" and its measurement in scientific collaboration. Using biomedical papers published by Chinese institutions for the period 2013–2017, we exam the various proximities and their dynamic evolution of scientific leadership flows between institutions from a microscopic perspective. The gravity model (Tobit model) illustrates that both leading institution and participating institution's scientific leadership mass can foster scientific leadership flows, and the leading institution is more pronounced, but their differences are decreasing. The influence of cognitive, institutional and economic proximity are increasing. Scientific flows are more and more likely to occur between institutions with similar scientific background, similar policies and culture and different academic economic resources. But the barrier effect of geographical distance and previous collaboration relationship are fading. Our findings can provide evidence and support for grant allocation policy to facilitate biomedical scientific research and collaborations. Future research could be aimed to apply RL that we proposed to funding data and patent data since only using paper publications is partial and incomplete.

Acknowledgments. This research is supported by the National Natural Science Foundation of China (No. 71573197).

References

1. Navarro, A., Martin, M.: Scientific production and collaboration in Epidemiology and Public Health, 1997–2002. Scientometrics **76**(2), 291–313 (2008)
2. Hoekman, J., Frenken, K., Tijssen, R.J.: Research collaboration at a distance: changing spatial patterns of scientific collaboration within Europe. Res. Policy **39**(5), 662–673 (2010)

3. Fernandez, A., Ferrandiz, E., Leon, M.D.: Proximity dimensions and scientific collaboration among academic institutions in Europe: the closer, the better? Scientometrics **106**(3), 1073–1092 (2016)
4. Boschma, R.A.: Proximity and innovation: a critical assessment. Reg. Stud. **39**(1), 61–74 (2005)
5. Sekara, V.: The chaperone effect in scientific publishing. Proc. Natl. Acad. Sci. U.S.A. **115** (50), 12603–12607 (2018)
6. Wang, L., Wang, X.: Who sets up the bridge? Tracking scientific collaborations between China and the European Union. Res. Eval. **26**(2), 124–131 (2017)
7. Wang, W., Pan, Y.: An investigation of collaborations between top Chinese universities: a new quantitative approach. Scientometrics **98**(2), 1535–1545 (2014)
8. Berge, L.R.: Network proximity in the geography of research collaboration. Pap. Reg. Sci. **96**(4), 785–817 (2017)
9. Acosta, M., et al.: Factors affecting inter-regional academic scientific collaboration within Europe: the role of economic distance. Scientometrics **87**(1), 63–74 (2011)
10. Wooldridge, J.M.: Econometric Analysis of Cross Section and Panel Data (2003)

Author Index

Printed in the United States
By Bookmasters